RENEWALS 458-4574
DATE DUE

Feb 18			
APR 30			
AUG SEP 6			
OCT 2 9			
MAR 2 8			
MAY 0 2			
JLL: 3007799			WHF
MAR 2 2 2004	NO RENEWALS		
NOV 2 1			
GAYLORD			PRINTED IN U.S.A.

Personality and Psychopathology

Personality and Psychopathology

EDITED BY
C. Robert Cloninger, M.D.

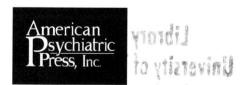

American Psychopathological Association

WASHINGTON, DC
LONDON, ENGLAND

Copyright © 1999 American Psychiatric Press, Inc.
ALL RIGHTS RESERVED
Manufactured in the United States of America on acid-free paper
02 01 00 99   4 3 2 1
First Edition

American Psychiatric Press, Inc.
1400 K Street, N.W., Washington, DC 20005
www.appi.org

Library of Congress Cataloging-in-Publication Data
Personality and psychopathology / edited by C. Robert Cloninger.
    p.   cm. — (American Psychopathological Association series)
    Includes bibliographical references and index.
    ISBN 0-88048-923-5 (alk. paper)
    1. Personality disorders — Complications.   2. Personality.
    3. Psychology, Pathological.   4. Mental illness — Etiology.
    I. Cloninger, C. Robert.   II. Series.
    [DNLM: 1. Mental Disorders — etiology.   2. Personality Disorders —
complications.   3. Personality.   4. Personality Development.
WM 140P467 1999]
RC554.P45 1999
616.89′071—dc21
DNLM/DLC
for Library of Congress   98-30095
                                                                    CIP

Library
University of Texas
at San Antonio

British Library Cataloguing in Publication Data
A CIP record is available from the British Library.

Contents

Part V Treatment and Outcome of Personality Disorders

Contributors

Phillip B. Adams, Ph.D.
Assistant Professor of Clinical Psychology in Psychiatry, College of Physicians and Surgeons of Columbia University, New York, New York

Carmen Bayon, M.D.
Research Fellow in Psychiatry, Washington University School of Medicine, St. Louis, Missouri

Aaron T. Beck, M.D.
Professor of Psychiatry, University of Pennsylvania, Philadelphia, Pennsylvania

Lorna Smith Benjamin, Ph.D.
Professor of Psychology, University of Utah, Salt Lake City, Utah

Devra L. Braun, M.D.
Research Fellow in Psychiatry, Cornell University Medical College, New York Hospital, Westchester Division, White Plains, New York

Magda Campbell, M.D.
Professor Emeritus of Psychiatry, New York University Medical Center, New York, New York

Lee Anna Clark, Ph.D.
Professor of Psychology, University of Iowa, Iowa City, Iowa

C. Robert Cloninger, M.D.
Wallace Renard Professor of Psychiatry, Washington University School of Medicine, St. Louis, Missouri

Patricia Cohen, Ph.D.
Professor of Clinical Public Health, Columbia University Department of Psychiatry, New York, New York

Linda A. Corey, Ph.D.
Professor of Human Genetics, Medical College of Virginia, Richmond, Virginia

Paul T. Costa Jr., Ph.D.
Chief, Laboratory of Personality and Cognition, National Institute on Aging, Johns Hopkins Bayview Campus, Baltimore, Maryland

Jeanette E. Cueva, M.D.
Assistant Professor of Psychiatry, New York Medical College, Valhalla, New York

Wayne C. Drevets, M.D.
Associate Professor of Psychiatry, University of Pittsburgh, Pittsburgh, Pennsylvania

Lindon J. Eaves, Ph.D., D.Sc.
Distinguished Professor of Human Genetics and Psychiatry, Medical College of Virginia, Richmond, Virginia

Albert Ellis, Ph.D.
President, Institute for Rational-Emotive Therapy, New York, New York

John G. Gunderson, M.D.
Chief, Personality and Psychosocial Research Program, McLean Hospital and Harvard Medical School, Belmont, Massachusetts

Katherine A. Halmi, M.D.
Professor of Psychiatry, Cornell University Medical College, New York Hospital, Westchester Division, White Plains, New York

Andrew C. Heath, D.Phil.
Professor of Psychiatry, Washington University School of Medicine, St. Louis, Missouri

Peter R. Joyce, M.D.
Professor of Psychological Medicine, Christchurch School of Medicine, Christchurch, New Zealand

Erin I. Kleifield, Ph.D.
Instructor of Psychology in Psychiatry, Cornell University Medical College, New York Hospital, Westchester Division, White Plains, New York

Armand W. Loranger, Ph.D.
Professor of Psychiatry, Cornell University Medical College, New York Hospital, Westchester Division, White Plains, New York

Pamela A. Madden, Ph.D.
Research Instructor in Psychiatry, Washington University School of Medicine, St. Louis, Missouri

Nicholas G. Martin, Ph.D.
Principal Research Fellow, Queensland Institute of Medical Research, Brisbane, Queensland, Australia

Robert R. McCrae, Ph.D.
Research Psychologist, Personality, Stress, and Coping Section, National Institute on Aging, Johns Hopkins Bayview Campus, Baltimore, Maryland

J. M. Meyer, Ph.D.
Assistant Professor in Human Genetics, Department of Human Genetics, Medical College of Virginia, Richmond, Virginia

Roger T. Mulder, M.D.
Associate Professor of Psychological Medicine, Christchurch School of Medicine, Christchurch, New Zealand

Michael C. Neale, Ph.D.
Associate Professor of Psychiatry and Human Genetics, Department of Psychiatry, Medical College of Virginia, Richmond, Virginia

Bruce Pfohl, M.D.
Professor of Psychiatry, University of Iowa Medical School, Iowa City, Iowa

Katharine A. Phillips, M.D.
Assistant Professor of Psychiatry, Brown University School of Medicine, Butler Hospital, Providence, Rhode Island

Thomas R. Przybeck, Ph.D.
Assistant Professor of Psychiatry, Washington University School of Medicine, St. Louis, Missouri

Ilene C. Siegler, Ph.D., M.P.H.
Professor of Psychology, Department of Psychiatry, Duke University Medical Center, Durham, North Carolina

J. L. Silberg, Ph.D.
Department of Human Genetics, Medical College of Virginia, Richmond, Virginia

Chantal N. Sullivan, B.A.
Assistant, Personality and Psychosocial Research Program, McLean Hospital and Harvard Medical School, Belmont, Massachusetts

Suzanne R. Sunday, Ph.D.
Assistant Professor of Psychology in Psychiatry, Cornell University
Medical College, New York Hospital, Westchester Division, White
Plains, New York

Dragan M. Svrakic, M.D., Ph.D.
Assistant Professor of Psychiatry, Washington University School of
Medicine, St. Louis, Missouri

Joseph Triebwasser, M.D.
Associate, Personality and Psychosocial Research Program, McLean
Hospital and Harvard Medical School, Belmont, Massachusetts

Kimberley Truett, M.S.
Graduate Student, Department of Human Genetics, Medical College
of Virginia, Richmond, Virginia

Niels G. Waller, Ph.D.
Associate Professor of Psychology, University of California, Davis,
California

Ellen Walters, M.S.
Department of Psychiatry, Medical College of Virginia, Richmond,
Virginia

Cynthia Whitehead, B.A.
Research Coordinator, Washington University School of Medicine,
St. Louis, Missouri

Preface

New findings in several fields have converged to clarify the fundamental importance of personality in the development and expression of psychopathology. The frequent occurrence of personality disorders in patients with clinical syndromes like depression became clear with the introduction of multiaxial classification in the APA's DSM-III. Now in DSM-IV specific categories of personality disorder on Axis II have been associated with particular Axis I clinical syndromes. For example, schizophrenia, major depressive disorder, bulimia, and social phobia on Axis I are strongly associated with schizotypal, depressive, borderline, and avoidant personality disorders, respectively, on Axis II. In order to understand the nature of such associations, the American Psychopathological Association invited distinguished experts to examine the relationship between personality and psychopathology. Their task was to examine the relationship of personality traits with psychopathology from several interlocking perspectives—descriptive, developmental, etiological, and therapeutic.

Their reports begin with the description of the frequency and patterns of overlap between personality and psychopathology. The role of depressive personality traits in vulnerability to mood disorders is described by John Gunderson and his colleagues in Chapter 1. The relationship of personality variants to risk of schizophrenia, bipolar disorder, melancholia, and several nonpsychotic syndromes on Axis I and II is described by Robert Cloninger in Chapter 2. Kathy Halmi and colleagues describe associations between personality and eating disorders in Chapter 3. A critical overview of the confusion sometimes introduced by overlap between Axis I and II is provided by Bruce Pfohl in Chapter 4. These initial chapters document the association of personality disorders and other psychiatric syndromes. They also point out both the descriptive utility and the artificiality of the distinction between these axes.

The next set of chapters examines the structure and stability of normal personality traits across the life span, and then relates these traits to the development of psychopathology. Five to seven dimensions of personality have been described in the general population and in samples of psychiatric patients by many investigators, as described in Chapters 2, 6, 7, 9, and 10. Normal personality traits are shown by Patricia Cohen in Chapter 5 to vary along multiple dimensions that develop in stages during childhood and adolescence. However, personality is shown to be moderately stable during adulthood by Paul Costa in Chapter 6. Niels Waller in Chapter 7 shows that the popular five-factor model of personality advocated by Costa neglects two dimensions that are important in both the general population and in psychiatric patients.

The correspondence of personality structure in psychiatric patients to that observed in the general population challenges the assumptions underlying categorical models of personality disorder and clinical syndromes. Accordingly, in the third section, the description of personality disorders is considered from three complementary approaches. Armand Loranger describes a categorical approach based on ratings of item checklists in Chapter 8, which conforms to DSM criteria. Lee Anna Clark describes an alternative method using dimensional ratings of abnormal personality traits in Chapter 9. Dragan Svrakic describes in Chapter 10 a method using dimensional ratings that apply equally well in psychiatric patients and in the general population. Findings with each of these approaches show that people differ quantitatively along several dimensions of personality. Different categories on Axis I and II are associated with different configurations of these quantitative traits.

In the fourth section, the causes of individual differences in personality and psychopathology are examined from genetic, psychosocial, and neurobiological perspectives. Lindon Eaves illustrates in Chapter 11 how twin studies can be used to measure genetic and environmental factors in developmentally complex traits like the social attitude of conservatism. Lorna Benjamin then considers influences from psychosocial factors in childhood (Chapter 12), and Andrew Heath and colleagues examine genetic factors (Chapter 13). Wayne Drevets (Chapter 14) describes how modern neuroimaging methods like positron emission tomography allow specification of the distributed neural networks that support the specific mental operations underlying the development and expression of personality and mental disorders.

In the final section, the role of personality is considered in treatment of psychopathology. Aaron Beck bridges the prior contributions about development and genetics with an evolutionary perspective of the psychotherapy of personality and psychopathology in Chapter 15. Pharmacological approaches to depression and conduct disorders are described based on targeting specific personality traits with particular drugs (Chapters 16 and 17). Albert Ellis (Chapter 18) emphasizes the importance of both rational and emotional components of personality in treating psychopathology.

In summary, these observations show the associations between personality and psychopathology are strong and important whether considered from descriptive, developmental, etiological, or therapeutic perspectives. Together these reports show that recent advances in understanding the genetic, neurobiological, and psychosocial processes that shape the development of personality provide a sound basis for improving the classification and treatment of mental disorders in clinical practice. The interdisciplinary perspective to personality and psychopathology taken here should be informative for everyone interested in the broad field of mental health.

PART I

Role of Personality in Psychopathology

CHAPTER 1

Personality and Vulnerability to Affective Disorders

John G. Gunderson, M.D.
Joseph Triebwasser, M.D.
Katharine A. Phillips, M.D.
Chantal N. Sullivan, B.A.

Significant portions of the psychiatric literature have focused on the interaction between "psychiatric illness" and "personality," and on the possibility of a cause-and-effect relationship between them. For most of this century, the dominant position has been that personality forms the background from which psychiatric illnesses emerge and the context in which they must be understood. Kraepelin (1921), for example, held that "the real, the deeper cause of [manic-depressive illness] is to be sought in a permanent morbid state which must also continue to exist in the intervals between the attacks" (Wetzel et al. 1980, pp. 197–198). In an essay on depression and manic-depressive illness, Abraham (1927) wrote that "in all cycloid illnesses the patient is found to have an abnormal character-formation during his 'free interval'; and . . . this character formation coincides in a quite unmistakable way with that of the obsessional neurotic" (p. 423). Sullivan (1949) stated that "mental disorder must be regarded as the result of the personality relating to the demands of the personal situation" (p. 3). In their famous case studies of patients with manic-depressive illness, Cohen and colleagues

(1954) wrote of "particular patterns of interaction which characterize [the patient's] character and his illness," and of "a manic depressive character in the child" who eventually develops manic-depressive illness (p. 265).

The development of an adult personality can be seen as deriving from the person's genetic or constitutional dispositions, which are often observed in early childhood and referred to as *temperament*. Upon this temperament is superimposed the particular cognitive and interpersonal style, defenses, expectations, and patterns of response that are referred to as *character* and are shaped by environmental learning experiences. One's underlying temperament affects one's environment and is in turn altered by that environment. The ongoing character-shaping experiences continue throughout childhood and adolescence until a relatively stable composite called the adult personality is formed.

In this chapter we review what is known about the types of temperament, character, and personality disorder that make a person particularly vulnerable to the development of depression or other affective disorders. Special attention is given to the depressive personality construct insofar as the controversies that surround it are reflected in DSM-IV (American Psychiatric Association 1994), where it appears in Appendix B—an appendix for categories that need further research.

Temperament

Akiskal, the foremost modern proponent of the application of the temperament construct to affective disorders, divides them into four major subtypes: hyperthymic, cyclothymic, dysthymic (depressive), and irritable (Akiskal and Akiskal 1992) (Figure 1–1). He suggests that all four of these temperaments are largely heritable, and, in addition to predisposing to the subsequent development of certain forms of personality disorder, all four types predispose to both depressive and manic episodes. Indeed he postulates that these temperaments 1) are present in 3%–4% of the population, 2) represent subclinical spectrum variants of the major affective disorders, and 3) are not inherently maladaptive

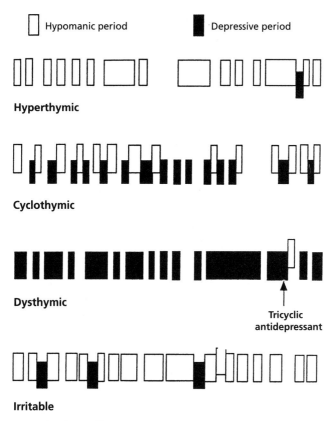

☐ Hypomanic period   ■ Depressive period

Hyperthymic

Cyclothymic

Dysthymic

Tricyclic antidepressant

Irritable

FIGURE 1–1. *The four affective temperaments and their characteristic hypomanic (white blocks) and depressive (black blocks) periods.* [*Adapted from Akiskal and Akiskal 1992.*]

but can become so when they match or "fit" poorly with a particular environment.

A very different perspective on temperament arises from academic psychologists' studies of normal personality. Their goal has been to define largely heritable types—actually *dimensions*—of personality that, like Akiskal's temperaments, are not inherently maladaptive but, unlike Akiskal's temperaments, are derived from factor analytic methods and attempt to identify basic dimensions of personality that pertain to all individuals. The most widely recognized basic system of personality dimensions has been Hans Eysenck's (1953) identification of three factor analytically derived dimensions (neuroticism, extraversion, psychoticism) observed after studying large normal populations. A notable recent development has been the validation given to an expanded set of personality factors, the so-called Big Five, or the five-factor model (Costa and McCrae 1990):

1. Extraversion: outgoing, positive emotionality
2. Agreeableness: warmth, sociability
3. Conscientiousness: responsible, impulsivity
4. Neuroticism: anxious, negative emotionality
5. Openness: inquiring, intellectuality

These five dimensions of personality have been demonstrated to have long temporal stability and sufficient universality to characterize personality types found in multiple cultures (Costa and McCrae 1992; Digman 1990). They also demonstrate variable but substantial levels of heritability (Costa and McCrae 1992). At present only those three dimensions that overlap with Eysenck's system (i.e., neuroticism, extraversion, and psychoticism have been examined prospectively to see whether they relate to the onset of affective disorders.

Table 1–1 summarizes results of the five prospective studies that have looked at temperamental features in persons who developed subsequent major depression. These studies establish that, unlike extraversion or psychoticism, neuroticism (meaning a tendency to be anxiety-prone, emotionally unstable, self-conscious, and easily upset) is a vulnerability marker for major depressive episodes (MDEs). Notably, Hirschfeld et al. (1989) found no overall association between neuroticism or extraversion and the onset of depression until he examined age as a covariate. Then neuroticism surfaced as a personality dimension whose presence in those over age 31 indicated vulnerability to MDEs. In the younger cohort this dimension not only did not predict MDEs but also seemed unstable; indeed, neuroticism seemed to diminish for many youths during the span of years from 17 to 25.

Although there is evidence that high levels of neuroticism characterize people who develop MDEs, there is also evidence that this dimension represents a nonspecific form of vulnerability to a variety of other types of psychopathology—anxiety disorders in particular (Watson et al. 1988). Costa (P.T. Costa Jr., personal communication,

TABLE 1–1.

Premorbid personologic features of patients with depression

	Cognitive	Hostile	Anxious	Emotional	Interpersonally sensitive	Other
Nystrom and Lindegaard 1975	(Ruminative)	(Irritable)	+			Shy, lacks endurance
Angst and Clayton 1986		+	+	(Excitable)		Subordinative
Hirschfeld et al. 1989	(Thoughtful)		(Neuroticism)	+		Dramatic
Boyce et al. 1991			(Neuroticism)		+	
Ernst et al. 1992		+	+		+	

February, 1993) points out that neuroticism is actually a "proxy" title for affective/anxious vulnerability and is also relevant to vulnerability for many personality disorders. Kendler's recent twin study indicates that neuroticism represents the familial form (i.e., is about 70% heritable) by which vulnerability to depressive disorders is transmitted (Kendler 1993).

Relevant to the potential association of the Big Five factors to affective disorders is Tellegen's (1993, in press) recent conceptual critique. He believes the five factors do not provide an adequate representation of personality, and, in particular, he faults them for excluding characteristics of personality that relate to self-esteem or affective-emotional traits. In this regard Tellegen is drawing attention to one of the historically central depictions of temperament: Hippocrates and Galen both used temperament to define emotional, rather than intellectual or interpersonal, styles (Kagan 1989, p. 107). In his own factor analytically derived scheme, Tellegen recognizes both a positive affectivity and a separate negative affectivity factor—factors that are, respectively, complementary to extraversion and neuroticism but involve more mood and social traits (Tellegen and Waller, in press). Tellegen sees both his positive and negative affectivity dimensions as reflecting "built in responsiveness to signals of emotion and emotional-temperamental dispositions." Negative affectivity (also called *negative emotionality*) reflects a constellation of negative traits (nervous, worrying, irritable, overly sensitive, emotionally labile, easily hurt) that might be more specifically expected to represent a form of vulnerability to subsequent depressive disorders. Existing evidence, however, has shown that high negative affectivity is associated with both depressive and anxiety disorders; these conditions are distinguished by the fact that a loss of pleasure (i.e., low positive affectivity) also characterizes depressive states. Still, to our knowledge the predictive (i.e., predisposing) potential of negative affectivity and positive affectivity has not yet been tested (Watson et al. 1988).

Research on temperament in normal children has led to the development and study of a variety of classification schemes (Goldsmith et al. 1987). Buss and Plomin (1984) identify three temperamental types believed to be present in children and in adults, each having significant heritability: emotionality (like neuroticism, meaning easily upset), sociability (similar to extraversion), and activity (vigor, quickness). Buss and Plomin (1984) suggest that the "negative affectivity" components of emotionality, which includes hostility (and which are conceptually linked to Tellegen's modification of the neuroticism construct) are inherited. At present, no longitudinal work has yet established an association between childhood temperament indices and the development of childhood, let alone adult, affective disorders.

Before leaving this area, it should be recognized that "temperaments," as used by Akiskal, or "dimensions," as identified in academic psychology, may themselves represent complex derivatives of heritable dispositions and early childhood experience. Kagan's work indicates that considerable flux in basic "temperamental" characteristics occurs in the first few years of life (Kagan and Moss 1962). Because most indices of childhood temperament fail to show much stability and because the heritability level for these indices can vary over time— often seeming to get stronger with age (Plomin 1986)—it seems as if the obstacles to finding an association between early childhood indices of temperament and adult affective disorder remain formidable. A study by Maziade et al. (1990) is illustrative of the problem. They showed that extreme scores on childhood temperament scales (adopted from Thomas and Chess 1984) have been shown to increase the likelihood of having psychiatric problems. Of relevance is the observation that those children with a type of temperament involving intense emotional reactions, negative moods, and a tendency to withdraw from new stimuli were *not* associated with internalized problems such as childhood depression (as one might expect). This temperament was actually associated with development of externalizing disorders (e.g., oppositional, conduct, attention deficit), but only when the child had parents who themselves had trouble with behavior control.

Character

Characterological attributes usually include the ensemble of cognitive schemas, interpersonal styles, and defensive operations that the growing child accrues as he or she attempts to adapt his or her endogenous dispositions (i.e., temperament) to the vicissitudes of environmental challenges. Even as we deploy this division in this chapter, there is reason to think that defensive style may be significantly genetically determined (Vaillant et al. 1986) and that defenses might thereby be better conceptualized as part of one's temperament. There is no reason to assume that interpersonal and cognitive style are not similarly entwined in their relationship to genes, constitution, and temperament.

Relevant to the characterologic development of vulnerability to depressive disorders are the psychoanalytic observations of children that have suggested that such vulnerability can be traced to the complicated early interactions between children and their primary caregivers. Klein (1932) and later Mahler (1966/1979) both suggested that the vulnerability to adult depression is traceable to an incomplete resolution of the child's normal dilemma of introjecting hostile destructive impulses toward his needed and "loved" caregiver. Incomplete resolution leaves individuals uncomfortable with owning or expressing their hostility, unable to sustain ambivalence, and harshly self-critical (Jacobson 1946, Zetzel 1953). Variations on this developmental failure have been offered as explanations for borderline (Kernberg 1967), passive-aggressive (Whitman et al. 1954), masochistic (Reich 1933), obsessive-compulsive (Freud 1908/1962; Rado 1951), and (as discussed later) depressive types of personality disorder. These observations may offer missing perspectives that can help explain why assessments of temperament prior to age 5 or 7 (when this dynamic "fault" will have been consolidated) are likely to remain limited in their capacity to predict subsequent affective disorder.

Perry (1990) notes that the maturity of a person's usual defensive repertoire correlates with levels of overall functioning and mental health. He prospectively examined the relationship between the defensive styles found in 73 subjects with personality disorders and the recurrence of depressive episodes over a 1-year period (Perry 1990; Perry et al. 1992). The subjects with less mature ("action" and "borderline") defenses did not have more frequent MDEs or other affective episodes, but they were found to have an increased vulnerability to depressive symptoms and to episodes that were more prolonged. He concluded that there is "highly consistent evidence for a hierarchical relationship between the general maladaptiveness of a defense (i.e., their maturity) and . . . the prevalence of . . . affective symptoms, the recurrence rate of depressive symptoms, and overall time spent in symptomatic episodes of . . . affective disorders on follow-up" (p. 560).

Perry's conclusions invite further inquiry. Were the assessments of defense done outside of affective episodes? Can the "borderline" defenses (e.g., splitting or being devaluative) be separated from cognitive styles or trait? Are defensive styles stable over time? If so, at what age does this stability occur, such that the presence of a particular defense mechanism could be a "marker" of vulnerability?

Of relevance may be other findings from the series of prospective studies of premorbid self-reported personality features (Table 1–2). Several studies showed that heightened interpersonal sensitivity characterized those who later became depressed (Boyce et al. 1991; Ernst et al. 1992). Yet, in contrast to expectations (derived from clinicians such as Chodoff [1972]), measures of interpersonal dependency used in Hirschfeld's (1989) study did not differentiate those who became depressed until the subsample that was over 31 was segregated. A more surprising finding is that subjects who develop first-onset depression are premorbidly significantly more ruminative (Nystrom and Lindegaard 1975), analytic, or thoughtful (Hirschfeld et al. 1989). Among women, this extends to greater dreaminess and introspection. Among men, this extends to being relatively uninterested in action and athletics (Hirschfeld 1989) or rating low on masculinity (Clayton et al. 1994).

A fourth perspective on characterological traits that may identify vulnerability to affective disorder comes from six investigators who have dissected the experiences of depressed persons into two qualitatively distinct types, "anaclitic" and "self-critical" (Arieti and Bemporad 1980; Beck 1983; Blatt and Zuroff 1992; Bowlby 1988; Pilkonis 1988; Smith et al. 1988) (see Table 1–2). These studies indicate that traits associated with anaclitic depression involve interpersonal preoccupation, that is, being "socially dependent" (Beck), "anxiously attached" (Bowlby), and having a "dominant other" (Arieti and Bemporad). In contrast, self-critical forms of depression arise in individuals with traits emphasizing "self-reliance" (Bowlby), "dominant goals" (Arieti and Bemporad), or being autonomous (Beck). Depressive patients with the interpersonal/anaclitic type of depression have been shown to be less

TABLE 1–2.

Characterologic characterizations of patients with depression

Contributors (conceptual orientation)	Types and descriptions	
	Interpersonal	Intrapsychic
Bowlby 1969–1988 (Ethological Object Relational)	*"Anxiously Attached"* — Excessively dependent on others. — Seeks interpersonal contact.	*"Self-Reliant"* — Purposely avoids others. — Despises those who pursue intimate relationships.
Blatt 1974–1992 (Psychoanalytic, Cognitive Developmental)	*"Anaclitic/Dependent"* — Feelings of helplessness, weakness, depletion, and being unloved. — Desires being protected, attended to. — Well-being requires love, and assurance. — Difficulty expressing anger.	*"Introjective/Self-Critical"* — Feelings of unworthiness, guilt, and failure to live up to expectations. — Fears loss of approval, recognition, and love. — Highly competitive.
Arieti and Bemporad 1980 (Interpersonal)	*"Dominant Other"* — Needs esteemed other for gratification and self-esteem. — Experiences satisfaction through another. — Clinging, passive, manipulative, and avoids anger.	*"Dominant Goals"* — Seeks love and approval through investment in goals. — Self-worth/esteem requires reassurance. — Seclusive, arrogant, obsessive.

Beck 1983 (Cognitive) personal own	**"Socially Dependent"** – Needs others for safety, help, gratification. – Wishes acceptance, intimacy, understanding, support, guidance, stability, admiration, prestige, and status. – Obtains pleasure from receiving.	**"Autonomous"** – Desire to preserve and increase independence, mobility, rights, freedom of choice, action and expression, and defining boundaries. – Action oriented. – Direct, decisive, positive, dogmatic, and authoritarian.
Pilkonis 1988 (Interpersonal/ Cognitive)	**"Excessive Dependency"** – Feelings of helplessness. – Extreme dependence on others. – Borderline features (affective lability, low frustration threshold, manipulative).	**"Excessive Autonomy"** – Anxiety concerning interpersonal attachment issues. – Lack of interpersonal sensitivity. – Obsessive-compulsive features (rigidity, perfectionism, lack of spontaneity, emphasis on self-control, intellectuality, and productivity).

responsive to pharmacotherapy (Frank et al. 1987) and to respond better to psychotherapy—although less well to psychoanalysis (Blatt 1992). Preliminary evidence of these traits' validity as vulnerability markers is found in work by Mongrain and Zuroff (1989). College students who could be characterized as either dependent ($n = 13$) or self-critical ($n = 15$) were more likely to perceive interpersonal events as stressful compared with 21 students who did not have these traits.

Whereas character traits such as defensive styles, cognitive schemas, or interpersonal style have been persuasively shown to be associated with affective disorders, the more definitive research needed to establish their validity as vulnerability markers will require identification of these traits in samples without current or past mood disorder and the evaluation of their predictive strength. Moreover, it will be of great importance to establish whether and at what age these particular defensive/cognitive/interpersonal styles become stable personality traits.

Depressive (Melancholic) Temperament or Character

A particular type of temperament or character that has relevance to depressive illness is depressive personality disorder (DPD). This disorder may not only predispose to MDEs but also uniquely link the concept of depression and personality. The construct of a depressive personality type can be traced to Hippocrates's "bilious" and Galen's "melancholic" types of temperament; as noted, it is now revived by Akiskal's "dysthymic" temperament. These conceptions are joined by psychoanalytic observations about a depressive, or melancholic, character structure. Both Abraham (1927) and Menninger (1940) attempted to place this into a phase-specific (i.e., oral-sadistic) developmental scheme. Later contributors such as Reich (1933) and Kernberg (1987) were more concerned with the vicissitudes of misdirected, unexpressed, or retroflexed anger in such individuals and, as such, proffer a dynamic formulation for a depressive personality type that has similarities to the formulations that have been made for other personality types (i.e., borderline personality disorder, passive-aggressive personality disorder, obsessive-compulsive personality disorder, masochistic personality disorder).

The historical and clinical significance of this construct prompted renewed interest in the course of DSM-IV's development (Phillips et al. 1990, 1993). Four empirical studies have now shown that adults who meet various criteria for depressive personality represent a substantial population of persons who have significant impairment in functioning. The condition is reliably diagnosed, is associated with a moderate increase in affective disorder in first-degree relatives, and appears stable over time (i.e., more than 1 year). In addition, a significant percentage of persons with DPD have not had prior episodes of major depressive disorder or dysthymia, nor do they meet criteria for other personality disorders (Klein 1990; Klein and Miller 1993; Hirschfeld et al. 1992; Phillips et al. 1992). Only about one-fourth (16%–34%) of those with DPD meet criteria for dysthymic disorder (Figure 1–2), and many dysthymic persons (39%) fail to meet criteria for DPD; moreover, when either the early-onset type of dysthymia or the proposed DSM-IV definition for dysthymia is used, the overlap with DPD actually diminishes (Hirschfeld et al. 1992)! The critical distinction between dysthymia and DPD is that the latter consists of traits

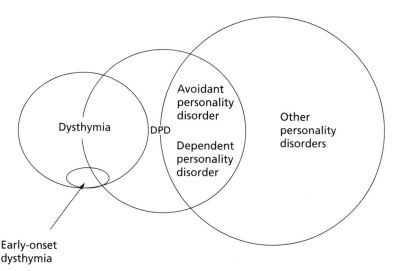

FIGURE 1–2.   *Relation of depressive personality disorders to near-neighbor disorders.*
[*Adapted from Hirschfeld et al. 1992.*]

that need to be *stably* present over a period of many years, whereas the criteria for dysthymic disorder require the presence of depressed *mood* that must be *persistent* only over the preceding 2 years. (Figure 1–2 indicates that avoidant and dependent personality disorders are most apt to overlap; this will be discussed later.)

The thrust of such work impels the diagnostic system to include this construct. But where? "Personologists," impressed with both the conflicts over assertiveness and the masochistic habits that characterize such people (see factors III and IV of Table 1–3), as well as the syndrome's early onset and stability, favor its addition to the group of Axis II disorders. The "affectivists," impressed by the similarity of negativistic descriptive characteristics to the classic symptoms of other depressive disorders (see factor I of Table 1–3), see this as a spectrum variant of depressive disorders that should be added to the Axis I group.

The conflicts about the inclusion of DPD in the DSM classification system are ongoing. But it is clear that there is a need to broaden the system of classification to include personological variants of depressive disorders. With such a change, recognition will be given to people with modest but enduring early-onset depressive traits who can be expected to have a predisposition to the later development of dysthymia and MDEs. It is apparent that within the broader construct of neuroticism is a subgroup of traits (e.g., tense, easily upset, negative emotionality) that are part of the depressive personality construct. Our results (Table 1–4) show that persons with DPD score extremely high on neuroticism (Phillips et al. 1992). It seems likely that DPD represents a more specific form of vulnerability to MDEs. According to Akiskal, persons with MDEs who also have a history of such personality traits will be particularly apt to respond to antidepressants (and they will also have a predisposition to develop other mood disorders). As a footnote to this discussion, it still is not clear whether the depressive personality should be conceptualized as a temperament (i.e., predominately genetic) or characterological (i.e., predominately environmental) problem. Almost certainly the question will stimulate a new generation of research.

Personality Disorders

Fifteen studies have reported the rates of comorbid personality disorders found in samples of patients with affective disorders (Table 1–5).

TABLE 1–3.

Factor analysis

Factors	% of variance
I. Negativistic/depressive Gloomy Pessimistic Negative reactivity Bitter Remorseful Low self-esteem Burdened Worried Critical of others Self-critical	15.4
II. Introverted/tense Introverted Appears quiet Constricted Appears tense Difficulty having fun Appears serious	11.8
III. Unassertive/passive Unassertive Passive Overly dependent Hypersensitive Difficulty being angry	9.8
IV. Masochistic Moralistic Counterdependent Self-denying	7.9

Note. *Four-factor solution with varimax orthogonal transformation. Components listed in order of their loading.*
Source. *Gunderson et al., unpublished.*

Methodological problems confound firm conclusions about the relationships between specific personality disorders and specific mood disorders, but overall impressions probably point toward some basic truths.

TABLE 1–4.

Personality measures for subjects with and without depressive personality

Personality measure	Depressive personality		Significance
	Present (N = 25)	Absent (N = 18)	
NEO-FFI			
Neuroticism	35.2 ± 6.2	29.1 ± 8.3	P = .007
Extraversion	18.3 ± 5.1	21.5 ± 6.1	P = .04
Openness	32.8 ± 5.0	32.1 ± 7.1	NS[a]
Agreeableness	29.8 ± 6.9	32.4 ± 6.0	P = .09
Conscientiousness	25.9 ± 8.0	29.2 ± 8.9	NS

[a]*Not significant.*
Source. *From Phillips KA et al. 1992.*

First, the prevalence of personality disorders is very high in patients with mood disorders (i.e., easily exceeding the rates of 13%–18% found in normal populations) in almost every study that used structured interview or self-report methods of personality disorder assessment. The exceptions derive from those studies that used chart reviews (i.e., Koenigsberg et al. 1985 and Fabrega et al. 1986); in these studies the prevalence rates were close to those expected in normal populations. When rates of personality disorder were assessed in different types of mood disorder by the same investigators (and methods), they were higher in the major depression samples than in bipolar/manic samples.

Second, the types of personality disorder found to be most prevalent in the dysthymic and major depression samples are similar. Specifically, the most common types are avoidant, dependent, and borderline personality disorders, followed by obsessive-compulsive and passive-aggressive personality disorders.

Third, the profile of personality disorders associated with bipolar/manic samples is quite distinct. Although borderline personality disorder is also common in the depressive/dysthymic groups, bipolar disorder is distinct in having higher comorbidity with the other dramatic cluster personality disorders (i.e., the histrionic, antisocial, and narcissistic types).

Because most of the personality disorder types are infrequent in

TABLE 1–5.
Rates of personality disorder in affective disorder samples

| Study | Sample method | | Rates (%) of personality disorder | | | | | | | | | | | |
	N	Type[d]	Any	ST	P	SZ	AS	BP	H	N	AV	DP	OC	PA
Major depression														
Charney et al. 1981	160	IP	CR	34											
Pfohl et al. 1984	78	IP	SI (SIDP)	53	9	1	1	1	23	18	—	15	17	6	4
Koenigsberg et al. 1985	315	MX	CR	23	1	0	0	0.3	4	3	1	0	3	2	1
Fabrega et al. 1986[a]	6,885	MX	CR	9											
Kocsis et al. 1986	26	OP	SCA	40											
Reich et al. 1987	24	OP	SI (SIDP)	50	8	4	4	0	13	21	0	21	29	17	0
			SR (PDQ)	78	35	4	0	4	44	30	0	26	61	48	4
			SR (MCMI)	88	0	0	29	13	21	17	8	38	54	4	42
Shea et al. 1987	249	OP	(PAF)	35	1	5	0	0	2	4	1	13	6	13	1
Alnaes and Torgersen 1988	97	OP	SI (SIDP)	86	6	8	1	0	15	15	2	62	54	21	11
Zimmerman et al. 1988	66	IP	SI (SIDP)	65	5	6	3	15	24	26	8	3	15	11	17
Alnaes and Torgersen 1989	64	OP	SR (MCMI)		3	5	22	6	39	40	5	28	47	9	48
Fogel and Westlake 1990	2,322	IP	CR	16				0.4		23			4	4	
Wetzler et al. 1990	14	MX	SR (MCMI)	86	0	0	21	7	14	0	0	29	21	0	43
Sanderson et al. 1992	197	OP	SI (SCID-II)	50	1	2	0	2	4	4	3	12	15	9	7

(continued)

TABLE 1–5.
Continued

Study	Sample method[e] N	Method	Type[d]	_Rates (%) of personality disorder_ Any	ST	P	SZ	AS	BP	H	N	AV	DP	OC	PA
Dysthymia															
Koeningsberg et al. 1985	68	CR	MX	34	1	0	0	0	6	1	1	0	7	0	0
Fabrega et al. 1986[a]	6,885	CR	MX	32	8										
Kocsis et al. 1986[b]	39	SCA	OP	47							8	10	23	5	17
Alnaes and Torgersen 1988	18	SI (SIDP)	OP	89	15	–	–	0	11	–	11	56	56	33	59
Alnaes and Torgersen 1989[c]	80	SR (MCMI)	OP			10	29	11	51	23	5	40	40	1	
Sanderson et al. 1992	63	SI (SCID-II)	OP	52	2	3	0	2	8	2	6	22	8	13	3
Bipolor or manic															
Koenigsberg et al. 1985	171	CR	MX	9	1	–	0	0	1	0	0	2	2	0	1
Fabrega et al. 1986	6,885	CR	MX	4											
Alnaes and Torgersen 1988	19	SI (SIDP)	OP	84	11	4	5	0	23	26	5	26	47	32	5
Pica et al. 1990	26	SI (SIDP)	IP	62	4	4	4	15	21	50	12	0	0	4	19
Turley et al. 1992	19	SI (SIDP)	IP	58	5	0	5	21		53	11	0	0	5	21
		SR (MCMI-II)		89	5	5	11	47	11	37	47	16	16	5	37

Note. PDQ = Personality Diagnostic Questionnaire, MCMI = Millon Clinical Multiaxial Inventory, PDQ = Personality Disorders Questionnaire, SIDP = Structured Interview for DSM-III Personality Disorders, PAF = Personality Assessment Form, SCID-II = Structured Clinical Interview for DSM-III-R Personality Disorders, ST = Schizotypal, P = Paranoid, SZ = Schizoid, AS = Antisocial, BP = Borderline, H = Histrionic, N = Narcissistic, AV = Avoidant, DP = Dependent, OC = Obsessive-Compulsive, PA = Passive-Aggressive. DSM-III-R-based measurements underlined.

[a] Deferred Axis II diagnoses were included as no personality disorder.
[b] Five others with one personality disorder diagnosis each (3%).
[c] This figure represents the prevalence of personality disorders in the combined groups of pure dysthymic and cyclothymic patients.
[d] IP = inpatient, OP = outpatient, NP = nonpatient, MX = mixed patients.
[e] CR = chart review, SI = structured interview, SR = self-report, SCA = structured clinical assessment.

affective disorder samples, it seems likely that the distinctive patterns of personality types that are unusually prevalent in the depressive and manic forms of affective disorder represent forms of vulnerability. Still, the comorbidity of Axis II disorders found in samples of patients with affective disorders may simply reflect their high prevalence rates, without having a more specific and etiologically significant connection. This possibility is illustrated by extensive research on borderline personality disorder that was prompted by the high rates of comorbid major depression found in borderline personality disorder (40%–60%). The overall conclusion from this extensive research is that borderline personality disorder and depression have a modest and nonspecific etiological association (Table 1–6) (Gunderson and Phillips 1991). Although affect dysregulation is a nonspecific disposition to borderline personality disorder (BPD), there is reason to believe that the characteristic interpersonal style of patients with BPD makes them vulnerable to having the anaclitic type of depression (see Table 1–2; Figure 1–3). Similarly, the other two types of personality disorder most common in samples with major depression (i.e., avoidant and dependent personality disorders) may be personality types that embody (i.e., are "carrier" conditions for) the self-critical and anaclitic personality features, respectively, which are found to characterize the two qualitatively different types of depression (i.e., anaclitic and self-critical). It is not coincidental then that these are the two types of personality disorder most apt to overlap with the newly defined DPD (as shown in Figure 1–2) (Phillips et al. 1992).

Fewer studies have examined the frequency of affective disorders in populations with personality disorders (Table 1–7). Conclusions that can be drawn include first, as might be expected, that Axis II disorders seem to impart a vulnerability to affective illness. The rates of affective disturbance among subjects with Axis II disorders are in the 50% range in many studies and can even approach 100%. Second, as the number of coexisting Axis II disorders increases (probably a measure of greater severity) so does the risk of affective disorders (Torgerson 1984). Third, specific Axis II disorders seem more closely associated with certain affective disorders than with others. Many studies imply, for example, that borderline patients are at greater risk for developing major depression than for developing bipolar disorder. The dissociation be-

TABLE 1–6.

Evaluation of four hypotheses about the interface between borderline personality disorder and depression in 1990

Hypothesis	Comorbidity	Phenomenology	Family prevalence	Drug response	Biological factors	Pathogenesis
Depression is primary (it can produce signs and symptoms of borderline personality disorder)	Refutes[a]	Refutes	Strongly refutes[a]	Strongly refutes	Strongly refutes[a]	Mixed[a]
Borderline personality disorder is primary (it can produce signs and symptoms of depression)	Refutes[a]	Supports	Strongly refutes[a]	Strongly supports[a]	Refutes[a]	Mixed[a]
Depression and borderline personality disorder are unrelated	Supports[a]	Supports[a]	Strongly supports	Supports[a]	Strongly supports[a]	Supports[a]
Both disorders have overlapping, nonspecific sources	Supports	Strongly supports	Supports[a]	Supports[a]	Mixed[a]	Mixed[a]

[a]These evaluations changed from 1985 to 1990.
Source. *Gunderson and Phillips 1991.*

22

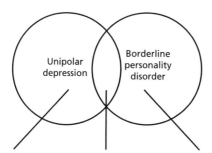

Guilty, remorseful	Depressed affect: early onset,	Empty, lonely
Withdrawn, agitated	sustained	Angry, needy
Suicidality, serious if present	Worthlessness, hopelessness	Repeated suicidal gestures
Stable relationships	Object hunger	Demanding hostile-dependent
Concerned with defeat,	Dependency	relationships
failures	Fragile self-esteem	Concerned with interpersonal
Welcomes caregiving (with		loss, separation
history of independence)		Illusory self-sufficiency
		(with history of dependency)

FIGURE 1–3. *Shared and unshared characteristics of unipolar depression and borderline personality disorder.*
[*Adapted from Gunderson and Phillips 1991.*]

tween certain Axis II disorders and certain Axis I disorders is, in some instances, so clear that certain Axis II disorders seem, if anything, to protect against the development of certain affective illnesses. Two studies have, for example, found the rate of bipolar disorder among subjects with avoidant personality disorder to be lower than in the population at large (Reich 1990; Zimmerman and Coryell 1989).

Discussion

This review indicates the persisting absence of empirically demonstrated connections between childhood indices of temperament and adult mood disorders. On the other hand, this review demonstrates the conclusive evidence for the existence of a nonspecific and probably nonpathological form of vulnerability for the development of MDEs, embodied in the neuroticism construct. The neuroticism construct is linked to "chronic neuroses"—which is a term used to describe people with both anxiety and depressive symptoms who do not meet criteria for existing disorders. At present, neuroticism is probably close to the

TABLE 1–7.
Rates of affective disorder in personality disorder samples

Study	Sample		Instruments	Rates (%)											
	N	Type	Axis I Diagnosis	NoPD	P	SZ	ST	OC	H	DP	AS	AV	BP	PA	Any
Pope et al. 1983	33	IP	DIB (a); CR to assess DSM-III criteria 1, 2, 3									(1) 39 (2) 3 (3) 9			
Torgerson 1984	54	MX	PSE (a); Personality Questionnaire 1, 2, 3				(1) 34 (2) 7 (3) 7								
Modestin and Villyer	26	IP	CI to assess ICD-9 & DSM-III criteria 5									(5) 4			
Zanarini et al. 1989	79	OP	DIB (a); DIPD (a) 1, 2, 3, 4								(1) 59 (4) 3	(1) 78 (2) 45 (3) 0		(2) 100 (3) 0	

24

Study	N		Instrument & Criteria		P	SZ	ST	OC	H	DP	AS	AV	BP	PA	
Zimmermann and Coryell 1989	797	NP	DIS (a) SIDP (a) 1, 2, 3	(1)	9	29	0	65	31	46	29	35	80	62	39	39
				(2)	3	14	0	13	13							
Reich 1990	41	OP	SADS-L (a); PDQ (b) 1, 3													
Reich 1990	170	OP	SADS-L (a); SCID (a) 1, 3													

Note. 1 = Major Depression, 2 = Dysthymia, 3 = Bipolar Disorder, 4 = Cyclothymia, 5 = "Neurotic Depression," 6 = "Reactive Depression," & "Depressive Neurosis," & "Psychotic Depression," & "Neurotic Depression," CR = Chart review, P = Paranoid, SZ = Schizoid, ST = Schizotypal, OC = Obsessive-compulsive, H = Histrionic, DP = Dependent, AS = Antisocial, AV = Avoidant, BP = Borderline, PA = Passive-aggressive.

genetic disposition found to be the backdrop for mixed anxiety/depressive disorders (Boulenger and Lavallee 1993).

Like Tellegen and Waller (in press) we believe that the neuroticism construct needs to include more traits of negative emotionality in combination with an inability to experience positive emotions, to increase its specificity for vulnerability to affective disorder. In this regard, we have highlighted the growing evidence to support a construct of a depressive personality—a construct that shows much in common with neuroticism (e.g., the traits worried, gloomy, tense, guilty). But depressive personality, perhaps because of its distinctions from neuroticism (i.e., critical of self and others, bitter, moralistic, introverted), is a type of psychopathology that is associated with significant impairment, a familial history of depression, and, we expect, a more specific form of disposition to MDEs.

Evaluation of the predisposing nature of character traits, such as defenses, interpersonal style, and cognitive schemas, still requires prospective studies. Nevertheless, the existing work suggests that dependent interpersonal relatedness is a form of vulnerability for some but not all depressions. Other depressions are characterized by more interpersonally distant self-critical traits. The first of these characterizations is present in persons with borderline and dependent personality disorder, whereas the latter characterization better typifies persons with avoidant personality disorder and obsessive-compulsive personality disorder. For the most part these are the types of personality disorder (i.e., borderline, dependent, avoidant) with the highest prevalence in depressive and dysthymic samples. The recurrent theme found in psychoanalytic contributions, an emphasis on retroflexed and inhibited anger, is relevant to these disorders and offers an alternative way of identifying the characterological vulnerability to depressive disorders.

A very different profile of personality disorders is found in association with bipolar disorder; here we observe a higher prevalence of antisocial, narcissistic, and histrionic personality disorder. These personality disorders are not obviously associated with retroflexed aggression or with either the anaclitic or self-critical attitudes found to be associated with depressives. Here the characterological features are expressiveness, impulsivity, lability, and action orientation—features that seem embodied within the hyperthymic and irritable cyclothymic personality constructs and, probably, within the extraversion (or positive emotionality) type of temperament. In general, the fact that distinctive patterns of personality disorder are associated with different forms of mood disorder underscores their role as vulnerability markers and, as Nestadt et al. (1992) recently pointed out, may also indicate that some personality disorders may actually mark invulnerability too.

This chapter indicates that there is already strong evidence for the theory that vulnerability to affective disorders is embedded within personality, whether disordered or not, and that the nature of this diathesis has some specificity for the different types of mood disorder. This conclusion is framed by overriding shifts in the study of the psychopathology of personality and affective disorders. It is increasingly clear that affective disorders are not defined by their time-limited symptomatic episodes. Rather, these episodes fade, and "subclinical" residual symptoms that might better be considered personality traits persist. It is also increasingly clear that personality disorders are not as stable as their definition suggests. Rather, they may change and even remit or relapse in response to developmental issues and in response to their goodness-of-fit with their environment. Both of these shifts call for a reexamination of the distinction between Axis I and Axis II disorders. It seems especially dubious that the Axis I and Axis II groups can be distinguished by their fit with the biological-psychological paradigm. Indeed, it seems most likely that the genetic sources of Axis I disorders will best be understood by a recognition of their phenotypic expression in more enduring personality traits.

References

Abraham K: Selected Papers of Karl Abraham, M.D. New York, Brunner/ Mazel, 1927

Alnaes R, Torgersen S: The relationship between DSM-III symptom disorders (Axis I) and personality disorders (Axis II) in an outpatient population. Acta Psychiatr Scand 78:485–492, 1988

Alnaes R, Torgersen S: Personality and personality disorders among patients with major depression in combination with dysthymic or cyclothymic disorders. Acta Psychiatr Scand 79:363–369, 1989

American Psychiatric Association: Diagnostic and Statistical Manual of Mental Disorders, 4th Edition. Washington, DC, American Psychiatric Association, 1994

Angst J, Clayton P: Premorbid personality of depressive, bipolar, and schizophrenic patients with special reference to suicidal issues. Compr Psychiatry 27:511–532, 1986

Akiskal HS, Akiskal K: Cyclothymic, hyperthymic, and depressive temperaments as subaffective variants of mood disorders, in American Psychiatric Press Review of Psychiatry, Vol 11. Edited by Tasman A, Riba MB. Washington, DC, American Psychiatric Press, 1992, pp 43–62

Arieti S, Bemporad J: Psychological organization of depression. Am J Psychiatry 136:1365–1369, 1980

Beck AT: Cognitive therapy of depression: new perspectives, in Treatment of Depression: Old Controversies and New Approaches. Edited by Clayton PJ, Barrett JE. New York, Raven, 1983, pp 265–290

Blatt SJ: The differential effect of psychotherapy and psychoanalysis with anaclitic and introjective patients: the Menninger Psychotherapy Research Project revisited. J Am Psychoanal Assoc 40:691–724, 1992

Blatt SJ, Zuroff DC: Interpersonal relatedness and self-definition: two prototypes for depression. Clin Psychol Rev 12:527–562, 1992

Boulenger JP, Lavallee YJ: Mixed anxiety and depression: diagnostic issues. J Clin Psychiatry 54 (suppl 1): 3–15, 1993

Bowlby J: Developmental psychiatry comes of age. Am J Psychiatry 145:1–10, 1988

Boyce P, Parker G, Barnett B, et al: Personality as a vulnerability factor to depression. Br J Psychiatry 159:106–114, 1991

Buss AH, Plomin RL: Temperament: Early Developing Personality Traits. Hillsdale, NJ, Lawrence Erlbaum Associates, 1984

Charney D, Nelson J, Quinlan D: Personality traits and disorders in depression. Am J Psychiatry 138:1601–1604, 1981

Chodoff P: The depressive personality: a critical review. Arch Gen Psychiatry 27:666–677, 1972

Clayton PJ, Ernst C, Angst J: Premorbid personality traits of men who develop unipolar or bipolar disorders. Eur Arch Psychiatry Clin Neurosci 243: 340–346, 1994

Cohen M, Baker G, Cohen R, et al: An intensive study of 12 cases of manic-depressive psychosis. Psychiatry 17:103–137, 1954

Costa PT Jr, McCrae RR: Personality disorders and the five-factor model of personality. J Personal Disord 4:362–371, 1990

Costa PT Jr, McCrae RR: The five-factor model of personality and its relevance to personality disorders. J Personal Disord 6:343–359, 1992

Digman JM: Personality structure: emergence of the five-factor model. Annu Rev Psychol 41:417–440, 1990

Ernst C, Schmid G, Angst J: The Zurich study, XVI: early antecedents of depression. A longitudinal prospective study on incidence in young adults. Eur Arch Psychiatry Clin Neurosci 242:142–151, 1992

Eysenck HJ: The Structure of Human Personality. London, Methuen, 1953

Fabrega H, Mezzich J, Mezzich A, et al: Descriptive validity of DSM-III depression. J Nerv Ment Dis 174:573–584, 1986

Fogel BS, Westlake R: Personality disorder diagnoses and age in inpatients with major depressive disorder. J Clin Psychiatry 51:232–235, 1990

Frank E, Kupfer DJ, Jacob M, et al: Personality features and response to acute treatment in recurrent depression. J Personal Disord 1:14–26, 1987

Freud S: Character and anal eroticism (1908), in The Standard Edition of the Complete Psychological Works of Sigmund Freud, Vol 9. Translated and edited by Strachey J. London, Hogarth Press, 1962, pp 169–175

Goldsmith HH, Buss AH, Plomin R, et al: Roundtable: what is temperament? Four approaches. Child Dev 58:505–529, 1987

Gunderson JG, Phillips KA: A current view of the interface between borderline personality disorder and depression. Am J Psychiatry 148:967–975, 1991

Gunderson JG, Phillips KA, Triebwasser J, et al: The Diagnostic Interview for Depressive Personality Disorder. Am J Psychiatry 151:1300–1304, 1994

Hirschfeld RM, Klerman GL, Lavori P, et al: Premorbid personality assessments of first onset of major depression. Arch Gen Psychiatry 46:345–350, 1989

Hirschfeld RM, Shea MT, Phillips KD: Depressive personality disorder in DSM-IV, in 1992 CME Syllabus and Proceedings Summary: American Psychiatric Association 145th Annual Meeting. Washington, DC, American Psychiatric Association, 1992

Jacobson E: The effect of disappointment on ego and superego formation in normal and depressive development. Psychoanal Rev 33:129–147, 1946

Kagan J: Unstable Ideas: Temperament, Cognition, and Self. Cambridge, MA, Harvard University Press, 1989

Kagan J, Moss H: Birth to Maturity. New York, Wiley, 1962

Kendler KS, Neale MC, Kessler RC, et al: A longitudinal twin study of personality and major depression in women. Arch Gen Psychiatry 50:853–826, 1993

Kernberg O: Borderline personality organization. J Am Psychoanal Assoc 15:641–685, 1967

Kernberg O: Clinical dimensions of masochism, in Masochism: Current Psychoanalytic Perspectives. Edited by Glick RA, Meyers DI. Hillsdale, NJ, Analytic Press, 1987, pp 61–79

Klein M: The Psycho-Analysis of Children. New York, WW Norton, 1932

Klein DN: Depressive personality: reliability, validity, and relations to dysthymia. J Abnormal Psychology 99:412–421, 1990

Klein DN, Miller GA: Depressive personality in a nonclinical sample. Am J Psychiatry 150:1718–1724, 1993

Kocsis J, Voss C, Mann J, et al: Chronic depression: demographic and clinical characteristics. Psychopharmacol Bull 22:192–195, 1986

Koenigsberg HW, Kaplan RD, Gilmore MM, et al: The relationship between syndrome and personality disorder in DSM-III: experience with 2462 patients. Am J Psychiatry 142:207–212, 1985

Kraepelin E: Manic-Depressive Insanity and Paranoia. Translated by Barclay RM. Edited by Robertson GM. Edinburgh, E&S Livingstone, 1921

Mahler MS: Notes on the development of basic moods: the depressive affect (1966), in The Selected Papers of Margaret S. Mahler, Vol 2. New York, Jason Aronson, 1979, pp 59–76

Maziade M, Caron C, Cote R, et al: Extreme temperament and diagnosis. Arch Gen Psychiatry 47:477–484, 1990

Menninger K: Character disorders, in The Psychodynamics of Abnormal Behavior. Edited by Brown JF. New York, McGraw-Hill, 1940, pp 384–403

Mongrain M, Zuroff DC: Cognitive vulnerability to depressed affect in dependent and self-critical college women. J Personal Disord 3:240–251, 1989

Nestadt G, Romanoski AJ, Samuels JF, et al: The relationship between personality and DSM-III Axis I disorders in the population: results from an epidemiological survey. Am J Psychiatry 149:1228–1233, 1992

Nystrom S, Lindegaard B: Predisposition for mental syndromes: a study comparing predisposition for depression, neurasthenia and anxiety state. Acta Psychiatr Scand 51:69–76, 1975

Perry CJ: Psychological defense mechanisms and the study of affective and anxiety disorders, in Comorbidity of Mood and Anxiety Disorders. Edited by Maser JD, Cloninger CR. Washington, DC, American Psychiatric Press, 1990, pp 545–562

Perry JC, Lavori PW, Pagano CJ, et al: Life events and recurrent depression in borderlines and antisocial personality disorders. J Personal Disord 4:394–407, 1992

Pfohl B, Stangl D, Zimmerman M: The implications of DSM-III personality disorders for patients with major depression. J Affective Disord 7:309–318, 1984

Phillips KA, Gunderson JG, Hirschfeld RMA, et al: A review of the depressive personality. Am J Psychiatry 147:830, 1990

Phillips KA, Gunderson JG, Kimball CR, et al: An empirical study of depressive personality, in CME Syllabus and Proceedings Summary, American Psychiatric Association 145th Annual Meeting. Washington, DC, American Psychiatric Association, 1992, p 197

Phillips KA, Hirschfeld RMA, Shea T, et al: Depressive personality disorder: perspectives for DSM-IV. J Personal Disord 7(1):30–42, 1993

Pica S, Edwards J, Jackson HJ, et al: Personality disorders in recent-onset bipolar disorder. Compr Psychiatry 31:499–510, 1990

Pilkonis P: Personality prototypes among depressives: themes of dependency and autonomy. J Personal Disord 2:144–152, 1988

Plomin R: Development, Genetics, and Psychology. Hillsdale, NJ, Lawrence Erlbaum Associates. 1986

Pope HG, Jonas JM, Hudson JI, et al: The validity of DSM-III borderline personality disorder. Arch Gen Psychiatry 40:23–30, 1983

Rado S: Psychodynamics of depression from the etiological point of view. Psychosom Med 13: pp 51–55, 1951

Reich W: Charakteranalyse. Leipzig, Sexpol Verlag, 1933

Reich J: Relationship between DSM-III avoidant and dependent personality disorders. Psychiatry Res 34:281–292, 1990

Reich J, Noyes R, Hirschfeld R: A comparison of personality measures in ill and recovered depressed and panic patients. Am J Psychiatry 144:181–187, 1987

Sanderson WC, Wetzler S, Beck AT, et al: Prevalence of personality disorders in patients with major depression and dysthymia. Psychiatry Res 42:93–99, 1992

Shea MT, Glass DR, Pilkonis PA, et al: Frequency and implications of personality disorder in a sample of depressed outpatients. J Personal Disord 1:27–42, 1987

Smith TW, O'Keeffe L, Jenkins M: Dependency and self-criticism: correlates of depression or moderators of the effects of stressful events? J Personal Disord 2:160–169, 1988

Sullivan HS: The theory of anxiety and the nature of psychotherapy. Psychiatry 12:3–12, 1949

Tellegen A: Folk concepts and psychological concept of personality and personality disorder. Psychological Inquiry 4:122–130, 1993

Tellegen A, Waller NG: Exploring personality through test construction: development of the Multi-Dimensional Personality Questionnaire, in Personality Measure: Development and Evaluation, Vol 1. Edited by Briggs SR, Cheek JM. Greenwich, CT, JAI Press (in press)

Thomas A, Chess S: Genesis and evolution of behavioral disorders: from infancy to early adult life. Am J Psychiatry 141:1–9, 1984

Torgerson S: Genetic and nosological aspects of schizotypal and borderline personality disorders. Arch Gen Psychiatry 41:546–554, 1984

Turley B, Bates GW, Edwards J, et al: MCMI-II Personality disorders in recent-onset bipolar disorders. J Clin Psychol 48: 320–329, 1992

Vaillant GE, Bond M, Vaillant CO: An empirically validated hierarchy of defense mechanisms. Arch Gen Psychiatry 43:786–794, 1986

Watson D, Clark LA, Carey G: Positive and negative affectivity and their relation to anxiety and depressive disorders. J Abnorm Psychol 97:346–353, 1988

Wetzel R, Cloninger C, Hong B, Reich T: Personality as a subclinical expression of the affective disorders. Compr Psychiatry 21:197–205, 1980

Wetzler S, Kahn R, Cahn W, et al: Psychological test characteristics of depressed and panic patients. Psychiatry Res 31:179–192, 1990

Whitman RM, Trosman H, Koeing R: Clinical assessment of passive-aggressive personality. Archives of Neurology and Psychiatry 72:540–549, 1954

Zanarini MC, Gunderson JG, Frankenburg, FR: Axis I phenomenology of borderline personality disorder. Compr Psychiatry 30:149–156, 1989

Zetzel ER: The depressive position, in Affective Disorders: Psychoanalytic Contributions to Their Study. Edited by Greenacre P. New York, International Universities Press, 1953, pp 84–116

Zimmerman M, Coryell W: DSM-III in personality disorder diagnoses in a non-patient sample. Arch Gen Psychiatry 46:682–689, 1989

Zimmerman M, Pfohl B, Coryell W, et al: Diagnosing personality disorder in depressed patients: a comparison of patient and informant interviews. Arch Gen Psychiatry 45:733–737, 1988

Measurement of Psychopathology as Variants of Personality

C. Robert Cloninger, M.D.

Dragan M. Svrakic, M.D., Ph.D.

Carmen Bayon, M.D.

Thomas R. Przybeck, Ph.D.

The disorganization of personality was regarded as the fundamental cause of psychoses by Bleuler (1978) and Kraepelin (1919, 1921, 1981) who originated the distinction between schizophrenia and manic-depressive disorder. Kraepelin identified certain personality variants as the basic rudiments or underlying elements that are stable and essential for the development of a psychotic disorder. He noted that the personality variants associated with manic-depressive psychoses, like cyclothymia, were persistent in the intervals between psychotic episodes (Kraepelin 1921).

Likewise, Bleuler and Kraepelin both characterized the fundamental state of schizophrenia as a disorder of voluntary goal-directed

The authors appreciate the helpful comments of Drs. Loren and Jean Chapman, Samuel Guze, and Richard Hudgens, who reviewed an earlier draft.

Supported in part by NIH Grants MH31302, AA07982, and AA08028 to Dr. Cloninger and Spanish Health Ministry Grant FIS 94/5103 to Dr. Bayon.

behavior (Bleuler 1978; Kraepelin 1907/1981). Both regarded hallucinations and delusions as superfluous secondary features of more basic abnormalities in emotional and cognitive processing. Both noted that the "destruction of the will" may precede the onset of more florid secondary symptoms by many years (Bleuler 1978; Kraepelin 1919). Such cases without prominent secondary symptoms are called simple schizophrenia or schizotypal personality.

Unfortunately, the fundamental abnormalities underlying psychoses proved difficult to specify exactly and to rate reliably (Angst and Clayton 1986; Clayton et al. 1994; Hoch and Cattell 1959; Meehl 1962; Svrakic et al. 1993). Consequently, diagnostic criteria were developed that emphasized course of illness and secondary symptoms, while deliberately ignoring character organization (Robins and Guze 1970). Current diagnostic criteria rely on polythetic lists of symptoms, no one of which is essential to the disorder. As a result, diagnosed cases are likely to be etiologically heterogeneous, and some may have neither symptoms nor causes in common.

Fortunately, comprehensive methods for assessment of personality have recently been developed that are highly reliable. Personality can be reliably assessed using self-reports, expert interviews, or collateral informants, thereby producing ratings that show strong agreement across methods (Zimmerman 1994). It is also possible to quantify differences among individuals in etiologically distinct components of personality using tests such as the Temperament and Character Inventory (TCI) (Cloninger et al. 1993). Temperament refers to biases in automatic responses to emotional stimuli and is moderately heritable and stable throughout life regardless of culture or social learning. The TCI distinguishes four independently inherited dimensions of temperament: harm avoidance (HA), novelty seeking (NS), reward dependence (RD), and persistence (P). Character refers to individual differences in self-object relationships, which develop in a stage-like manner as a result of nonlinear interactions among temperament, family environment, and individual life experiences (Svrakic et al. 1996). Three dimensions of character are distinguished by the TCI: self-directedness (SD) (responsible, goal-directed vs. insecure, inept), cooperativeness (CO) (helpful, empathic vs. hostile, aggressive), and self-transcendence (ST) (imaginative, unconventional vs. controlling, materialistic).

In addition, dimensional criteria have recently been proposed as an alternative to symptom checklists for classification of schizophrenia (American Psychiatric Association 1994). These criteria are supported by factor analytic studies showing that schizophrenics differ from one another along three to five dimensions, such as positive symptoms, negative symptoms, and cognitive disorganization, as in DSM-IV (American Psychiatric Association 1994), as well as depression and hostile uncooperativeness (Lindstrom and von Knorring 1993).

Furthermore, beginning with clinical descriptions of schizotypy (Meehl 1962) and early schizophrenia (Hoch et al. 1959), reliable measures of traits have been developed to discriminate individuals prone to psychoses from normal individuals (Chapman et al. 1994b). College students with high scores on one or more of these measures were identified and followed prospectively over a 10-year period (Chapman et al. 1994b). The 182 high scorers on two scales, magical ideation and perceptual aberration, were described as schizotypal and paranoid in follow-up interviews and were more likely to have had a major depressive episode (35% vs. 20%), mania or hypomania (8.2% vs. 1.3%), any psychosis (5.5% vs. 1.3%), and a positive family history of psychosis (15% vs. 7%) than 153 normal controls. In contrast, physical anhedonia, impulsive nonconformity, and Eysenck's psychoticism scale were not predictive of psychosis (Chapman et al. 1994a, 1994b).

Subsyndromal forms of unipolar and bipolar disorder have also been distinguished as variants of personality (Akiskal et al. 1977) or emotionality (Klein et al. 1986; Lovejoy and Steuerwald 1995). In a 12-year prospective study of Swiss army conscripts, the premorbid personalities at age 19 years of men who later developed schizophrenic ($n = 12$), bipolar ($n = 26$), or unipolar depressive ($n = 99$) disorders were compared to the personalities of 2,842 men who remained healthy (Angst and Clayton 1986; Clayton et al. 1994). As measured by the Freiburg Personality Inventory (FPI), the premorbid personalities of those men who later developed depression or schizophrenia were higher than controls in FPI autonomic lability, which measures somatic anxiety and insecurity, such as low TCI SD. Subjects who attempted or completed suicide were also high in FPI aggression, which measures hostile disagreeableness, such as low TCI CO (Clayton et al. 1994). Those who developed bipolar disorders did not differ in premorbid FPI personality traits from those who remained healthy (Angst and Clayton 1986; Clayton et al. 1994), but were lower in FPI aggression than subjects with unipolar depression (Angst and Clayton 1986). This Swiss study has not been independently replicated, but another prospective study of the premorbid temperament of depressive persons showed that they were higher in HA (i.e., anxious, shy, and fatigable) (Nystrom et al. 1975a, 1975b), which often is associated with low TCI SD. Furthermore, depressed persons with personality traits indicative of high TCI CO (e.g., reliance on others) and high TCI ST (e.g., imaginative daydreamers) were more likely than other depressed persons to develop hypomania for the first time during an 11-year prospective study (Akiskal et al. 1995).

These observations suggest the hypothesis that TCI character traits of SD, CO, and ST may be either subsyndromal forms or predictors of susceptibility to psychosis and mood disorders (Bayon et al. 1996). To evaluate this hypothesis, we have studied the pattern of associations between TCI personality traits and symptoms of psychosis and mood disorder in the general population and in psychiatric outpatients. This provided the foundation for a new general model of personality and psychopathology that parsimoniously explains their complex associations. Each possible configuration of TCI character traits has a unique profile of positive and negative emotions, and different risks of psychosis, attempted suicide, and psychiatric hospitalization.

Methods

General Population Survey

Subjects

A stratified random sample of 1,000 noninstititionalized adults, 18 years of age or older, was ascertained in the greater metropolitan area of St. Louis, Missouri. Potential participants were identified at random from standard telephone lists and asked if they were willing to participate in a survey of personality and health sponsored by the National Institutes of Health and approved by the Human Studies Committee of Washington University School of Medicine. In June 1994, 1,740 individuals were solicited for possible participation, and 243 of them declined (14% refusal). From the 1,497 volunteers, a final panel of 1,000 were accepted into demographic strata in numbers representative of the 1990 federal census according to age (18–34, 35–54, 55+), gender, ethnicity (white, black, Hispanic, other), and household location (six counties). The 1,000 selected volunteers were mailed a questionnaire and a $5 prepayment and were paid another $20 upon return of the completed questionnaire. Those who did not return the questionnaire after a few weeks were reminded first with postcards and later with phone calls. Altogether, 866 subjects returned the questionnaire, 804 of which were complete and valid based on checks built into the questionnaire to detect careless or inconsistent responding. The 804 respondents included slightly more women than expected (57% vs. 52%), but were otherwise representative of the general population's demographics, personality, and psychopathology (Cloninger et al. 1991; Robins and Regier 1991).

In June 1995 the 804 who had completed the original questionnaire were mailed a follow-up questionnaire along with a $5 prepayment and an offer of another $20 upon completion; 626 individuals (78%) returned the follow-up questionnaire. Of these, 593 had valid and complete personality inventories. Those completing the follow-up questionnaire did not differ from noncompleters in terms of demographic or psychometric variables except that they were older (mean ages 46 vs. 40 years, $t = 4.97$, $df = 802$, $P < .0001$) and slightly lower in NS (17.5 vs. 18.8, $t = 2.69$, $df = 802$, $P < .01$).

Assessment Procedures

Subjects completed a self-report booklet in 1994 with separate sections for general demographic information, the TCI (Cloninger et al. 1993, 1994), the Inventory of Personal Characteristics (IPC) (Tellegen et al. 1990; Waller and Zavala 1993), the short Michigan Alcoholism Screening Test (Selzer et al. 1975), the NIMH Center for Epidemiological Studies depression scale (CES-D) (Radloff 1977), the Medical Outcome Study short-form General Health Survey (Stewart et al.

1988), which includes the five-item Mental Health Inventory (Berwick et al. 1991), and additional questions described later about psychopathology and mental health treatment. The CES-D asks about 20 depressive symptoms that are rated on a four-point frequency scale for the past week. In a community sample a score of 21 or higher had a sensitivity of 54% and a specificity of 96% for major depression diagnosed by structured interview (Myers and Weissman 1980).

The follow-up questionnaire in 1995 was similar except that the IPC was omitted and a short form of the combined perceptual aberration and magical ideation (PerMag) scale was added to evaluate the prediction of psychosis-proneness (Chapman et al. 1994b). This includes 8 items from the perceptual aberration scale and 7 items from the magical ideation scale. The 15-item scale has a correlation of 0.92 with the 65-item PerMag scale, and its items have an internal consistency reliability (Cronbach's alpha) of 0.80. The test-retest reliability after 1 year for the TCI personality scales was high with correlations between 0.78 and 0.85.

Psychiatric Outpatient Study

Subjects

A consecutive series of 109 outpatients was studied as the patients presented for treatment at the Psychiatry Clinic at Washington University Medical Center in St. Louis. Subjects were not paid but gave informed consent as approved by our Human Studies Committee. Exclusion criteria were age under 18 years, diagnoses of organic brain disorder or mental retardation, and mental status of being too highly agitated or floridly psychotic to complete study questionnaires. Six of 109 subjects were also excluded because of invalid or incomplete tests, leaving 103 with complete and valid data. Their ages ranged from 18 to 78 (mean 44, standard deviation 14 years). There was an excess of women (87 or 80%).

Assessment Procedures

Subjects completed the TCI, the Millon Clinical Multiaxial Inventory (MCMI-II) (Millon 1987), and measures of anxiety and depression described elsewhere (Bayon et al. 1996).

Statistical Analysis

All analyses were carried out with version 6.07 of the SAS statistical software (SAS Institute 1992).

Results

Description of Second-Order Character Interactions

The descriptors of individuals who score high or low on each one of the three TCI character dimensions were known from prior work (Table 2–1) (Cloninger et al. 1993, 1994). Prior to this study, however, no systematic data were available describing individuals with extreme scores on two or more TCI character dimensions. For example, how

TABLE 2–1.
Descriptors of individuals who score high and low on the three character dimensions

Character dimension	Descriptors of extreme variants	
	High	Low
SD	Responsible	Blaming
	Purposeful	Aimless
	Resourceful	Inept
	Self-accepting	Vain
	Disciplined	Undisciplined
CO	Tender-hearted	Intolerant
	Empathic	Insensitive
	Helpful	Hostile
	Compassionate	Revengeful
	Principled	Opportunistic
ST	Self-forgetful	Unimaginative
	Acquiescent	Controlling
	Spiritual	Materialistic
	Enlightened	Possessive
	Idealistic	Conventional

would people high in ST and also low in SD describe themselves? The IPC provided ratings on a four-point scale of 161 words and phrases that people use to describe their attitudes, emotions, and behavior. Descriptors of interactions were identified by correlating each IPC item with the product of two character dimensions. The IPC items that were most strongly correlated with these TCI interactions are shown in Table 2–2.

These descriptions are more fully characterized in Figures 2–1 through 2–3 for clarity. P and SD had parallel influences on the descriptors of character; essentially the same descriptors emerged when the product of SD and P was substituted for SD alone.

In Figure 2–1, high SD and low ST in combination are associated with being logical and well organized; the opposite configuration (low SD and high ST) is associated with being illogical and disorganized. The other diagonal in Figure 2–1 varies from being proactive (inventive, joyful) to being reactive (imitative, cranky). In Figure 2–2, the interactions of ST and CO give rise to variations from suspicious to trusting and from selfish to thoughtful. In Figure 2–3, the interactions of SD and CO give rise to variations from submissive to bullying and from immature to mature.

The descriptors of emotional responses associated with the TCI dimensions are summarized in Table 2–3. The emotions associated with temperament (such as fear, anger, and disgust) are usually called "primary" because they involve automatic preconceptual responses to associative stimuli that occur from infancy onward. In contrast, the emotions associated with character (such as shame vs. hope, scorn vs. empathy, misery vs. joy) are called "secondary" or "complex" because they develop later and are thought to emerge from the interaction of primary emotions with concepts about self-object relationships (Lewis 1992; Svrakic et al. 1996). Both positive and negative emotions are associated with each personality trait, depending on the stimulus conditions.

A Model of Third-Order Interactions: The Character Cube

High and low scorers on the three character dimensions give rise to eight possible configurations shown in Figure 2–4. The labels for these

TABLE 2-2.

Correlations of descriptors from *Inventory of Personal Characteristics (IPC)* of two-way interactions of TCI character dimensions

	Correlation of IPC descriptor with TCI interaction	
TCI interaction	High scores	Low scores
High ST × High SD	+31 exceptional, special	−25 ordinary, indifferent
	+31 imaginative, creative	−22 unimaginative
	+31 cheerful, joyful	−22 easily irritated
High ST × Low SD	+43 often betrayed, misled	−27 don't let things bother
	+41 odd, peculiar	−25 well-organized
	+41 feel sorry for self	−23 put worries out of wind
High ST × High CO	+37 interested in others	−26 sarcastic, scornful
	+32 affectionate, loving	−21 uncommunicative, mean
High ST × Low CO	+44 wicked, evil, vicious	−21 get along with everyone
	+40 do not trust people	−20 respect for authority
High SD × High CO	+38 cheerful, sunny	−47 feel used by others
	+28 peppy, spirited	−39 do not like people
High SD × Low CO	+37 bullying, threatening	−28 willing to accommodate
	+28 vicious, violent	−23 considerate, gentle

Note. IPC descriptors were rated by subjects on four-point scale (definitely true, probably or mostly true, probably or mostly false, and definitely false). TCI dimension scores are sums of about 40 true or false items. Low or reverse TCI scores were computed as the difference of the observed score from the maximal possible score. Pearson correlations were computed between individual IPC item scores and the multiplicative product of the designated TCI dimensions. The highest and lowest correlations are tabulated.

41

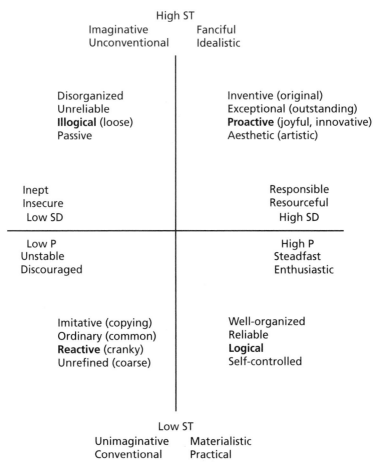

High ST
Imaginative   Fanciful
Unconventional   Idealistic

Disorganized   Inventive (original)
Unreliable   Exceptional (outstanding)
Illogical (loose)   **Proactive** (joyful, innovative)
Passive   Aesthetic (artistic)

Inept   Responsible
Insecure   Resourceful
Low SD   High SD

Low P   High P
Unstable   Steadfast
Discouraged   Enthusiastic

Imitative (copying)   Well-organized
Ordinary (common)   Reliable
Reactive (cranky)   **Logical**
Unrefined (coarse)   Self-controlled

Low ST
Unimaginative   Materialistic
Conventional   Practical

FIGURE 2–1. *Interactions of ST and SD* × *P.*

extreme configurations were based on the descriptive features summarized in Table 2–4 and prior descriptions of personality types in the literature.

For example, individuals who are low in all three character dimensions are described as *melancholic* because they are selfish, immature, and emotionally reactive (see Table 2–4), oscillating between misery and miserliness (i.e., possessive greed) (see Table 2–3). They view life as a difficult competition with hostile adversaries, leading to inevitable suffering. Consequently, those with melancholic characters frequently feel the negative emotions of shame, hate, and misery, but

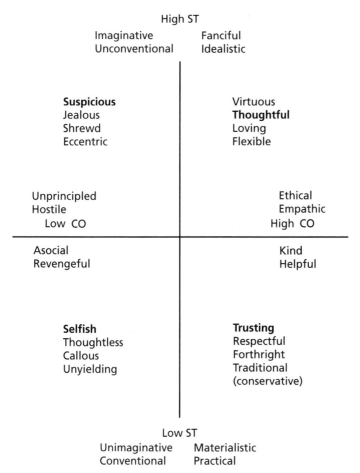

High ST
Imaginative   Fanciful
Unconventional   Idealistic

Suspicious   Virtuous
Jealous   **Thoughtful**
Shrewd   Loving
Eccentric   Flexible

Unprincipled   Ethical
Hostile   Empathic
Low CO   High CO

Asocial   Kind
Revengeful   Helpful

Selfish   **Trusting**
Thoughtless   Respectful
Callous   Forthright
Unyielding   Traditional
    (conservative)

Low ST
Unimaginative   Materialistic
Conventional   Practical

FIGURE 2–2. *Interactions of ST and CO.*

rarely feel positive emotions. Their lack of positive emotional responses, even when something desirable happens, is associated with typical vegetative symptoms of melancholia, such as anorexia and early morning awakening (American Psychiatric Association 1994). The melancholic character constitutes the most common character profile in persons with unipolar depression (Wetzel et al. 1980); this profile is also called the depressive personality (Akiskal et al. 1977; American Psychiatric Association 1994; Kraepelin 1921). Although persons with melancholic characters usually have only recurrent depressions, a substantial minority of persons with bipolar manic-depressive disorder

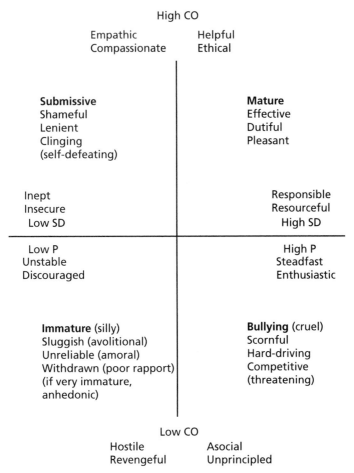

High CO

| Empathic | Helpful |
| Compassionate | Ethical |

Submissive   **Mature**
Shameful   Effective
Lenient   Dutiful
Clinging   Pleasant
(self-defeating)

Inept   Responsible
Insecure   Resourceful
Low SD   High SD

Low P   High P
Unstable   Steadfast
Discouraged   Enthusiastic

Immature (silly)   **Bullying** (cruel)
Sluggish (avolitional) Scornful
Unreliable (amoral)   Hard-driving
Withdrawn (poor rapport) Competitive
(if very immature,   (threatening)
anhedonic)

Low CO

| Hostile | Asocial |
| Revengeful | Unprincipled |

FIGURE 2–3. *Interactions of CO and SD × P.*

have this character type (Kraepelin 1921; Wetzel et al. 1980). The melancholic character has been associated with obsessional or borderline (explosive) temperament profiles (Hirschfeld and Klerman 1979; Svrakic et al. 1996; Wetzel et al. 1980), and this was confirmed in our sample (Table 2–5). The three character configurations that share features in two dimensions with the melancholic are the schizotypal, dependent, and autocratic characters.

Individuals who are low in SD and CO like those with melancholic characters, but high in ST, were designated as disorganized or *schizotypal* because they tend to be illogical, suspicious, and immature

TABLE 2–3.

Effects of reward (+) and punishment (−) on emotional state of four temperaments and three characters

Temperament dimension	High scorers		Low scorers	
	+	−	+	−
HA	Anxious (agitated)	Depressed (retarded)	Cheerful	Fearless
NS	Thrilled	Angry	Placid	Stoic
RD	Affectionate	Disgusted	Aloof	Critical
P	Enthusiastic	Steadfast	Unstable	Discouraged
SD	Secure	Shameful	Vain	Hopeful
CO	Scornful	Compassionate	Empathic	Revengeful
ST	Miserable	Peaceful	Possessive	Joyful

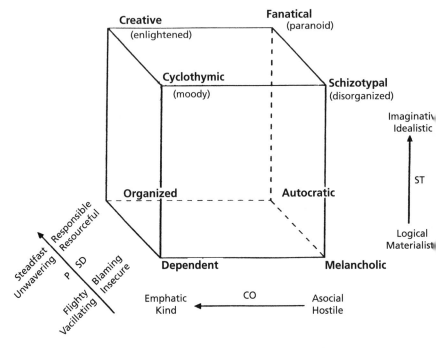

FIGURE 2–4. *The character cube: eight possible configurations of high or low scores on three TCI character dimensions. [Reproduced by permission of the Center for Psychobiology of Personality.]*

(see Table 2–4). This definition corresponds to the original descriptions of schizotypy discussed earlier (Bleuler 1978; Clayton et al. 1994; Kraepelin 1919). Schizotypes are highly suggestible with vivid imaginations and unconventional behavior (i.e., high ST) that is not organized toward realistic goals by analytic reasoning and discipline (i.e., low SD) or toward emotionally rewarding relationships by social values based on trust and ethical principles (i.e., low CO). The schizotypal character was most often associated with borderline (explosive) or sensitive temperaments, found in persons who have frequent approach-avoidance conflicts (i.e., high in both NS and HA) (see Table 2–5).

The *dependent* character is low in SD and ST like the melancholic, but is high in CO. Persons with a dependent character are expected to be submissive, trusting and respectful of others, and emotionally reactive (i.e., touchy, irritable, or hypersensitive to criticism

TABLE 2-4.

Distinguishing second-order features of the eight character types

Character type		Second-order descriptive feature				
	Proactive vs reactive	Logical vs illogical	Suspicious vs trusting	Thoughtful vs selfish	Mature vs immature	Bullying vs submissive
Fanatical	Proactive		Suspicious			Bullying
Creative	Proactive			Thoughtful	Mature	
Organized		Logical	Trusting		Mature	
Autocratic		Logical		Selfish		Bullying
Melancholic	Reactive			Selfish	Immature	
Dependent	Reactive		Trusting		Immature	Submissive
Cyclothymic		Illogical		Thoughtful		Submissive
Schizotypal		Illogical	Suspicious		Immature	

TABLE 2–5.

Distribution of temperament types associated with each character type in the general population

		Observed temperament profiles[a] (row %)[b]								
Character type	#	Obses Hnr	Explo HNr	Avoid HnR	Indep hnr	Aver —	Histr hNR	Relia hnR	Antis hNr	Sensi HNR
Melancholic	124	**30**⁺	**19**⁺	5	8	1	5⁻	0⁻	**19**⁺	14
Schizotypal	101	**20**⁺	**20**⁺	6	2⁻	4	12	4⁻	13	**20**⁺
Dependent	64	**31**⁺	9	8	**3**⁺	2	9	5	3⁻	**30**⁺
Autocratic	77	25	9	0	**25**⁺	4	13	4	18	3⁻
Average	49	27	8	8	10	4	10	8	8	16
Creative	139	4⁻	1⁻	12	15	1	**29**⁺	**20**⁺	7	10
Organized	121	**12**⁻	4⁻	9	15	6	21	**19**⁺	12	2⁻
Fanatical	56	4⁻	5	**18**⁺	**23**⁺	7	18	4	**21**⁺	0⁻
Cyclothymic	73	19	4⁻	12	3⁻	1	**21**⁺	12	4⁻	**23**⁺
Total	804									
Mean		18	9	8	11	3	16	9	12	12

[a]Obsessive (Obses), explosive (Explo), avoidant (Avoid), independent (Indep), average (Aver), histrionic (Histr), reliable (Relia), antisocial (Antis), sensitive (Sensi) based on median splits into high or low harm avoidance (H or h), novelty seeking (N or n), and reward dependence (R or r).

[b]When Mantel-Haenszel estimate of odds ratio is significantly different from 0 (outside of 95% confidence intervals), superscript denotes whether it is positive or negative; row % is also in bold when positive.

and insult) (see Table 2–4), as in other descriptions of dependent or oral traits (Bornstein 1992; Lazare et al. 1970; Walton and Presley 1973). The combination of personal insecurity (i.e., low SD) and their submissive reliance on others (i.e., high CO) makes it disturbing for those with dependent characters to be aware of their faults or to admit them to others, leaving them vulnerable to both vanity and shame (see Table 2–3). This submissive position makes them particularly sensitive to loss of social support, such as rejection or betrayal of their trust, so they are often ambivalent about making friends. Nevertheless, the dependent character is well adapted, like the organized type, under ordinary circumstances. According to this model, rejection or loss of support is expected to evoke irritable denial of personal fault accompanied by self-pity with many sorrowful complaints, insecure vanity with pleasure-seeking hyperactivity, or mixtures of both (see Figure 2–1 and Table 2–3). Their distress can be relieved by desirable events, and so is often associated with atypical depressive symptoms, such as craving for sweets and hypersomnia (American Psychitric Association 1994; Quitkin et al. 1979). Consequently, those with dependent characters are expected to have slightly increased risks of mood disorders, including mostly depression (Bornstein 1992; Hirschfeld and Klerman 1979; Mezzich et al. 1987) and sometimes irritable mania (Kretchmer 1990), particularly when TCI P is low (Osher et al. 1996). The countertype to the dependent person is the fanatical or paranoid type, who is independent and projective of blame.

The *autocratic* character is low in ST and CO like the melancholic, but is high in SD. Those with autocratic characters are logical, selfish, and bullying, which corresponds to prior descriptions of the authoritarian or aggressive personality (Adorno et al. 1950; Heaven 1985; Jabin 1987). They combine hostility with goal-directedness, competitiveness, and preference for hard-driving leadership. Challenges to their control and domination elicit aggressive counterattacks. This is also the "Type A" profile associated with frequent sympathetic hyperarousal (Baker et al. 1984) with increased heart rate, increased blood pressure, and activation of platelets for clotting ("fight or flight response"), which increases risk of coronary heart disease (Byrne et al. 1989; Ray 1990). Those with autocratic characters are expected to have a restricted range of emotions outside of hostility and are rarely joyful

(Adorno et al. 1950). On the other hand, the autocratic countertype, the cyclothymic, is expected to result in persons who are usually cheerful and rarely hostile.

The countertype to the melancholic is the *creative* character. Those with creative characters are high in all three TCI character dimensions (see Figure 2–4). The creative character is proactive, thoughtful, and mature (see Table 2–4), and those with this character type frequently feel the positive emotions of joy, love, and hope (see Table 2–3). This corresponds to the creative leader described by Jung (1939) and Frankl (1978) and to empirical descriptions of creative writers and eminent scientists (Cattell and Drevdahl 1956; Drevdahl and Cattell 1958). Using Cattell's Sixteen Personality Factor Questionnaire, creative writers and scientists were higher in traits related to TCI ST (i.e., imaginative or high in factor M, innovative or high in factor Q_1), TCI CO (i.e., tender or high in factor I, trustful or low in factor L, and empathic or low in factor N), and TCI SD (i.e., self-assured and guilt-free or low in factor O) (Cattell and Drevdahl 1956; Drevdahl and Cattell 1958). Similar profiles of creative individuals have been consistently confirmed (Vernon 1970). The creative character was most likely to occur with histrionic or reliable temperaments, which are low in HA and high in RD (see Table 2–5) (Cloninger et al. 1994; Svrakic et al. 1996).

Persons with the creative configuration are expected to have a low risk of mental disorder. In the rare cases in which all three character dimensions are extremely high, persons with creative characters are motivated largely by meaningful goals and values that extend beyond their private desires. That is, they are motivated by loving generosity with little disturbance from selfish concerns about seeking satisfaction or avoiding suffering. Those with creative characters are sincerely humble and peacefully accepting of whatever happens (see Table 2–3). Without being sought, their joy arises freely from acts of love to the degree that self-interest is forgotten and meaning is invested beyond themselves. Such integrated characters correspond to individuals variously described as enlightened, fulfilled, or self-actualized (Erikson 1963; Frankl 1978; Jung 1939; Kohut 1971; White 1985). In psychoanalytic terms, by means of an all-inclusive identification, they have internalized representations of their self as an integral part of all that is; also, through anticipation, they feel that everything will eventually work out for the best, even if it currently appears frustrating or objectionable.

However, when the character dimensions are all above average, but not extremely high, the individual is creative (generative in Erikson's terms), but not fully integrated (Erikson 1963). Those with such nearly integrated characters tend to be happy and proud overachievers and are at risk for unipolar mania, which occurs rarely (von Zerssen and Possl 1990). However, when unipolar mania occurs, it is consistently associated with slightly above-average adjustment in premorbid personality, similar to that in healthy people without psychiatric disorder (Clayton et al. 1994; von Zerssen and Possl 1990; von Zerssen et al. 1994).

The *organized* character is high in SD and CO like the creative, but low in ST. Persons with organized characters are described as logical, trusting, and mature. This profile is typical of outstanding administrators in empirical studies (Cattell and Drevdahl 1956). Whereas creative leaders are revolutionary and free spirited (Cattell and Drevdahl 1956; Drevdahl and Cattell 1958; Frankl 1978; Jung 1939; Vernon 1970; White 1985), those with an organized character are conservative, taking pride in analytic reasoning, efficiency, consistency, and attention to detail and laws. According to this model, those with an organized character have more interest in power and possessions than those with a creative character.

The *fanatical* character is high in ST and SD like the creative type but is low in CO, which corresponds to the paranoid character described by Kraepelin, who emphasized persistent and coherent goal-directedness combined with suspiciousness, superstitiousness, eccentric fascinations, and other forms of projective thinking in persons with this character type (Kraepelin 1907/1981). The fanatical character configuration emerged in association with contrasting temperament types: antisocial and independent types (unusually defiant, i.e., low in both HA and RD) or the avoidant type (unusually sensitive to social threat, i.e., high in both HA and RD) (see Table 2–5).

The *cyclothymic* character is high in ST and CO like the creative, but is low in SD. Like those with a dependent character, those with cyclothymic character have rejection sensitivity (i.e., low SD and high

CO) associated with atypical depressive symptoms with oscillating vanity and shame (see Table 2–4). However, their higher ST makes them more suggestible, so that they are insecurely joyful and have more frequent mood swings (see Table 2–3). Many patients with bipolar II disorder have the cyclothymic character configuration (Akiskal et al. 1995; von Zerssen and Possl 1990; von Zerssen et al. 1994). It also occurs in many patients with bipolar I psychoses, who most consistently have traits related to high TCI CO, such as sociability and friendliness (Angst et al. 1986; Goodwin and Jamison 1990; Kraepelin 1921; Kretchmer 1990; Millon 1987). In addition, bipolar manic-depressive patients usually have premorbid traits related to high TCI ST (i.e., cheerful, suggestible, vivid imaginations, and broad interests), but a substantial proportion also have traits related to low TCI ST (i.e., irritable, controlling, serious) (Akiskal et al. 1995; Goodwin and Jamison 1990; Kretchmer 1990; von Zerssen et al. 1994).

According to this model, high ST is associated with either joyful creativity or psychosis proneness (schizotypal, cyclothymic, or fanatical), depending on the development of the other two character dimensions. In addition, the risks of both manic and depressive episodes are increased in all character types in which SD is not extremely high. The ratio of elation to irritability, and the ratios of the frequency and duration of manic to depressive episodes, are expected to be highest in creative characters (high ST, CO, and SD), high in cyclothymic characters (high CO and ST only), low in dependent characters (high CO only), and lowest in melancholic characters (low ST, CO, and SD) (Kraepelin 1921; Wetzel et al. 1980). These four types correspond closely to the four fundamental states of manic-depressive disorder distinguished as manic, cyclothymic, irritable, and depressive, respectively, by Kraepelin (Kraepelin 1921; Wetzel et al. 1980) and in recent multidimensional clustering analyses (Angst 1993). In other words, the creative type is the prototype of unipolar manic patients (Clayton et al. 1994; von Zerssen and Possl 1990; von Zerssen et al. 1994), the cyclothymic is the prototype of bipolar manic-depressive patients who are usually cheerful (Akiskal et al. 1995), the reactive dependent is the prototype of atypical depressive patients (American Psychiatric Association 1994; Quitkin et al. 1979) and irritable bipolar patients who are usually depressed (Kretchmer 1990), and the melancholic type is the prototype of unipolar depressive patients with typical vegetative features (Akiskal et al. 1995; von Zerssen and Possl 1990; von Zerssen et al. 1994). Such heterogeneity may explain the variable findings in prior reports about the personality of bipolar patients and their response to lithium (Goodwin and Jamison 1990) and antidepressants (Akiskal 1992; Quitkin et al. 1979).

Tests of the Character Cube Model in the General Population

The hypothesis that the eight character types differ systematically from one another in their experience of positive emotions, negative emotions, and symptoms of psychosis was first tested in the general population. The character cube model makes specific predictions about patterns of similarity and contrast between neighboring character types and countertypes. Consequently, the contrasts predicted by the character cube model were tested by classifying all individuals in a general population into character types and comparing them according to indicators of health (Table 2–6).

Individuals with schizotypal or disorganized character configurations had the highest risks of psychiatric hospitalization, suicide attempts, current depression, and high PerMag scores. Organized people had the lowest risks of any psychopathology, but they were not more cheerful than average. In contrast, creative people were most often cheerful and also had a low risk of any disorders of mood or ideation.

Cyclothymic individuals were both more often cheerful and more often depressed than others, but they were not at increased risk of suicide attempts. On the other hand, autocratic individuals were less likely to be either more cheerful or more depressed than others. Melancholic individuals were depressed and attempted suicide more often than others and were less likely to be cheerful. Dependent individuals were also seldom cheerful, but had nearly average risk of major psychopathology.

Individuals with schizotypal character most frequently had high PerMag scores (43%). High PerMag scores were also more frequent in cyclothymics (22% vs. 7%, Fisher's Exact, 2-tail $P = .002$) and in

TABLE 2–6.

Prevalence of character types in 804 individuals in general population and their differential association with lifetime psychiatric hospitalization, suicide attempts, current depression, cheerfulness, and magical thinking

Character type	#	%	Observed clinical features (%)				
			Mental hospital	Suicide attempt	Currently depressed	Usually cheerful	High PerMag
Organized	121	15.1	2.5	1.7−	0.8−	19.0	0.0−
Autocratic	77	9.6	2.6	2.6	6.5−	6.5−	3.5−
Average	49	6.1	4.1	4.1	12.2	10.2	5.6
Dependent	64	8.0	4.7	4.7	15.6	7.8	4.3
Melancholic	124	15.4	9.7	12.1+	30.7+	4.8−	13.4
Cyclothymic	73	9.1	8.2	6.9	35.6+	26.0+	20.8
Schizotypal	101	12.6	14.9+	15.2+	36.6+	11.9	43.4+
Fanatical	56	7.0	1.8	3.7	12.5	14.3	22.2
Creative	139	17.2	5.1	4.4	2.2	30.9+	6.5−
Mean			6.4	6.5	16.5	15.7	12.8

Note. Mental hospitalization and suicide attempts are ever in lifetime; currently depressed defined as CES Depression score greater than 20; usually cheerful defined as IPC Positive Emotionality score of 60 or more; high PerMag defined by scale score greater than 5.

+ denotes group is significantly increased compared to all others by χ^2, df = 1, P < .05.
− denotes group is significantly decreased compared to all others by χ^2, df = 1, P < .05.

paranoids (21% vs. 7%, Fisher's Exact, two-tail $P = .018$) than all others except schizotypal individuals. All these results confirmed predictions of the character cube model.

Tests of the Character Cube Model in Psychiatric Patients

We next tested the hypotheses derived from the general population sample in a consecutive series of psychiatric outpatients. Axis 1 and Axis 2 psychopathologies were assessed using the MCMI-II scales, which discriminate disorders in the DSM classification system quantitatively. Almost half (43%) of the sample had MCMI scores indicative of a psychotic illness, such as mania, schizophrenia, or delusional disorder. The correlations among the TCI character dimensions and the MCMI scale scores are summarized in Table 2–7.

Scores on the MCMI-II were found to be correlated with the TCI scales as expected from the relations in the general population. High ST was most strongly correlated with features characteristic of psychoses, including schizophrenic, delusional, and manic disorders on Axis I and schizotypal, paranoid, and borderline disorders on Axis II (see Table 2–7). As predicted, ST was also correlated with histrionic personality style.

SD and CO were both low for nearly all disorders, as expected from their general association with personality disorder. In contrast, SD and CO were positively correlated with adaptive personality styles (see Table 2–7).

Discussion

These findings provide a general model of the associations between personality and psychopathology, including psychoses, mood disorders, and personality disorders. All the possible configurations of TCI character dimensions differ systematically from one another in psychotic symptoms and emotional experience. The relationships between

TABLE 2–7.
MCMI-II psychopathology scale scores and TCI profiles (correlations × 100 in 103 psychiatric outpatients)

MCMI psychopathology scales	Character dimensions				Explained variance		
	SD	CO	ST	T	C	T + C
Axis I disorders							
Schizophrenic thought disorder	−49	−46	39	19	44	47
Delusional disorder	−38	−40	40	20	37	42
Bipolar: manic disorder	−15	−12	50	32	28	53
Major depression	−67	−38	16	47	47	58
Dysthymia	−62	−34	20	32	42	46
Anxiety disorder	−54	−27	30	28	36	43
Somatization	−33	−18	42	9	27	30

Axis II disorders						
Schizotypal	**−57**	**−52**	24	30	44	55
Borderline	**−69**	**−50**	**37**	40	63	67
Paranoid	**−34**	**−50**	**38**	10	42	45
Schizoid	**−34**	−29	−9	42	15	43
Antisocial	**−41**	**−53**	30	30	41	49
Avoidant	**−66**	**−43**	10	53	45	65
Adaptive personality styles						
Compulsive	**32**	9	14	19	14	27
Dependent	−7	27	26	23	18	38
Histrionic	1	8	**44**	34	20	47

Note. Correlations of character dimensions greater than 0.30 are in bold (P < .001). T = four temperament dimensions, C = three character dimensions, SD = self-directedness, CO = cooperativeness, ST = self-transcendence.

57

personality and psychopathology found in psychiatric patients were similar in pattern and strength to those observed in the general population. This suggests the hypothesis that the fundamental states underlying severe psychopathology are extreme configurations of character traits that are continuously distributed in the general population.

However, the putative measures of psychosis proneness and mood that we found to be correlated with personality may indicate either antecedents or subsyndromal forms of psychopathology. Consequently, the observed relations of personality to psychopathology may be epiphenomena or early features of progressive psychiatric disorders. Psychopathology has often been described approximately in terms of categorical models of discrete types of disease. However, the frequent occurrence of heterotypic individuals (that is, individuals with intermediate or mixed features) and of transitions in diagnosis over time in the same patient are serious limitations of categorical models that persist despite extensive effort to improve their validity (Angst 1993; Svrakic et al. 1996).

Our current findings document two further limitations of the hypothesis that psychopathology comprises multiple discrete diseases. First, the relations between character and mental health involve a complex pattern of partial similarities and contrasts. Essentially, each character configuration has a unique behavioral profile that can be explained either as eight discrete types or as the nonlinear interaction of three quantitative traits. Not only is the character interaction model more parsimonious, but also it has greater explanatory power by predicting the nonindependent pattern of partial similarities and contrasts observed among the syndromes and allowing for an unlimited variety of intermediate classes. In contrast, the assumption that every distinguishable syndrome represents another discrete disease is statistically degenerate and encourages the proliferation of labels and alternative criteria for unvalidated disorders.

Second, if the correlations between personality and psychopathology were epiphenomena of antecedent cases of psychosis, then the strength of the relationships must depend on the proportion of individuals with psychoses in the sample. Under this hypothesis, the correlation between personality and psychosis should have increased as the proportion of psychotic individuals increased from under 4% in the general population to approximately 40% in the outpatient sample; the possible correlation reaches a maximum in a sample with maximal variance, which occurs with 50% prevalence of a binary trait. Accordingly, the equally strong relationships between psychosis and personality observed in the general population and psychiatric outpatients cast doubt on the hypothesis that these relations are consequences of antecedent psychopathology.

Consequently, the most parsimonious explanation for our results is that interactions among premorbid personality traits are major antecedents of risk for psychopathology. However, much more data is needed to confirm the direction and dynamics of causation definitively. In particular, prospective clinical studies are needed in which personal interviews are conducted with high-risk cases initially and at follow-up. Standard clinical measures of psychopathology should be applied by skilled clinicians. Also, in order to distinguish premorbid personality traits from subsyndromal psychopathology, it is necessary to document the initial health of high-risk cases prior to onset of disorder, which has yet to be done. Furthermore, detailed numerical analysis is needed to confirm that the emergence of psychopathology is a predictable function of the nonlinear dynamics of character development. Such explicit quantitative tests of the development of character and psychopathology as a complex adaptive system are currently being evaluated in our longitudinal data (Svrakic et al. 1996). This includes the possibility of reciprocal interactions between personality and psychopathology, rather than a unidirectional causal chain.

Our findings about schizotypy, perceptual aberration, and magical thinking, as measured by the PerMag scale, confirm earlier findings (Chapman et al. 1994a, 1994b). High PerMag scores were most closely associated with schizotypy but also occurred with other two character types: the cyclothymic (High ST, low SD) or the fanatical (High ST, low CO). The risk of high PerMag scores was nearly average in melancholic types (low SD, low CO, low ST).

The utility of differential diagnosis by character type is also clearly shown in relation to mood disorders. The cyclothymic and the melancholic character were both associated with increased risk for depression, but only the melancholic was associated with suicide attempts and only the cyclothymic was usually cheerful. The differences in character that distinguish the elated cyclothymic, the cranky dependent, and the scornful melancholic may be useful in predicting the greater response of cheerful manic-depressive patients to lithium salts (Goodwin and Jamison 1990).

Like the melancholic individual, the schizotypal personality was also strongly associated with suicide attempts and depression (see Table 2–6); thus, increased risk of suicide attempts was consistently related to the combination of low CO and low SD. Cyclothymic individuals, who are low in SD but high in CO, often experienced depressions but were not more likely than the average person to attempt suicide. In contrast, autocrats, who are high in SD but low in CO, were hostile toward others but unlikely to attempt suicide (see Table 2–6). Therefore, when scornful hostility (i.e., low CO) was combined with vulnerability to shame (i.e., low SD), then the risk of suicide attempts was more than double that in the general population (12%–15% vs. 6.5%). The nonlinear interaction of scorn and shame on the risk of suicide attempts observed here confirms the results of prospective research with attempted and completed suicide (Angst and Clayton 1986; Martin et al. 1985) and psychological autopsies of completed suicides (Clark 1993). In other words, individuals with personality disorders characterized by both low SD and low CO are at increased risk of both attempted and completed suicide. Accordingly, the measurement of TCI character traits may be useful in the clinical evaluation of suicide risk.

The model of emotions elaborated here extends earlier work on primary versus secondary (Lewis 1992) and positive versus negative emotions (Cloninger et al. 1994; Lovejoy and Steuerwald 1995) and integrates it with coincident measurement of stable traits of temperament and character, indicating an underlying continuity between normal emotions and disorders of mood and personality. It also provides an understanding of the emotional conflicts that sustain maladaptive personality configurations and prevent most people from becoming organized or creative.

Here we have largely focused on character dimensions because severe psychopathology appears to be most strongly and consistently related to variation in character structure. Elsewhere, variability in temperament has been shown to differentiate among subtypes of personality disorder (Bayon et al. 1996; Cloninger et al. 1994; Svrakic et al.

1993) and to predict differential response to antidepressants (Joyce et al. 1994; Nelson and Cloninger 1995). Furthermore, the development of character is strongly influenced by nonlinear interactions among the heritable temperament dimensions and social learning in the home and culture (Svrakic et al. 1996). Overall our results suggest the hypothesis that temperament interacts to influence the organization of character, which in turn influences susceptibility to psychopathology.

Lastly, the character types described here represent moderately stable configurations of multiple personality dimensions, rather than permanently fixed or discrete diseases (Angst 1993; Svrakic et al. 1996). The test-retest correlation was 0.78–0.85 for each of the seven TCI dimensions over 12 months, which is highly reliable, but changes in configurations may occur, particularly for individuals with intermediate positions. In the terminology of complex adaptive systems, character configurations are "meta-stable states" whose dynamics are predictable in terms of nonlinear interactions (Svrakic et al. 1996). In other words, the character states most closely associated with psychopathology are moderately stable functions of a complex network of predisposing temperament configurations and environmental stressors. This suggests that it may be productive to focus genetic research on the heritable temperaments dimensions, rather than groupings of genetically heterogeneous character states (Cloninger et al. 1996), and to focus physiological and therapeutic research on the nonlinear dynamics of character organization (Svrakic et al. 1996).

References

Adorno TW, Frenkel-Brunswick E, Levinson DJ, Sanford RN: The Authoritarian Personality. New York, Harper & Brothers, 1950

Akiskal HS: Le déprimé avant la dépression. L'Encéphale 18:485–489, 1992

Akiskal H, Djenderedjian AH, Rosenthal RH, et al: Cyclothymic disorder: validating criteria for inclusion in the bipolar affective disorder group. Am J Psychiatry 134:1227–1233, 1977

Akiskal HS, Maser JD, Zeller PJ, et al: Switching from unipolar to bipolar II.

An 11-year prospective study of clinical and temperamental predictors in 559 patients. Arch Gen Psychiatry 52:114–123, 1995

American Psychiatric Association: Diagnostic and Statistical Manual of Mental Disorders, 4th Edition. Washington, DC, American Psychiatric Association, 1994

Angst J: Today's perspective on Kraepelin's nosology of endogenous psychoses. Eur Arch Psychiatry Clin Neurosci 243:164–170, 1993

Angst J, Clayton P: Premorbid personality of depressive, bipolar, and schizophrenic patients with special reference to suicidal issues. Compr Psychiatry 27:511–532, 1986

Baker LJ, Dearborn M, Hastings JE, et al: Type A behavior in women: a review. Health Psychol 3:477–497, 1984

Bayon C, Hill K, Svrakic DM, et al: Dimensional assessment of personality in an outpatient sample: relations of the systems of Millon and Cloninger. J Psychiatr Res 30:341–352, 1996

Berwick DM, Murphy JM, Goldman PA, et al: Performance of a five-item mental health screening test. Med Care 29:169–176, 1991

Bleuler E: Dementia Praecox or the Group of Schizophrenias. Translated by Zinkin J. New Haven, CT, Yale University Press, 1978

Bornstein RF: The dependent personality: developmental, social, and clinical perspectives. Psychol Bull 112:3–23, 1992

Byrne DG, Reinhart MI, Heaven PC: Type A behavior and the authoritarian personality. Br J Med Psychol 62:163–172, 1989

Cattell RB, Drevdahl JE: A comparison of the personality profile (16 PF) of eminent researchers with that of eminent teachers and administrators, and of the general population. Br J Med Psychol 46:248–261, 1956

Chapman JP, Chapman LJ, Kwapil TR: Does the Eysenck psychoticism scale predict psychosis? A ten year longitudinal study. Pers Individ Diff 17:369–375, 1994a

Chapman LJ, Chapman JP, Kwapil TR, et al: Putatively psychosis-prone subjects 10 years later. J Abnorm Psychol 103:171–183, 1994b

Clark DC: Narcissistic crises of aging and suicidal despair. Suicide Life Threat Behav 23:21–26, 1993

Clayton PJ, Ernst C, Angst J: Premorbid personality traits of men who develop unipolar or bipolar disorders. Eur Arch Psychiatry Clin Neurosci 243:340–346, 1994

Cloninger CR, Przybeck TR, Svrakic DM: The Tridimensional Personality Questionnaire: US normative data. Psychol Rep 69:1047–1057, 1991

Cloninger CR, Svrakic DM, Przybeck TR: A psychobiological model of temperament and character. Arch Gen Psychiatry 50:975–990, 1993

Cloninger CR, Przybeck TR, Svrakic DM, et al: The Temperament and Character Inventory (TCI): A Guide to Its Development and Use. St. Louis, MO, Center for Psychobiology of Personality, Washington University, 1994.

Cloninger CR, Adolfsson R, Svrakic NM: Mapping genes for human personality. Nat Genetics 12:209–210, 1996

Drevdahl JE, Cattell RB: Personality and creativity in artists and writers. J Clin Psychol 14:107–111, 1958

Erikson E: Childhood and Society, 2nd Edition. New York, Norton, 1963

Frankl VE: Man's Search for Meaning: An Introduction to Logotherapy, 3rd Edition. New York, Simon & Schuster, 1978

Goodwin FK, Jamison KR: Manic-Depressive Illness. New York, Oxford University Press, 1990, pp 281–317, 332–367

Heaven PC: Construction and validation of a measure of authoritarian personality. J Pers Assess 49:454–551, 1985

Hirschfeld RMA, Klerman GL: Personality attributes and affective disorders. Am J Psychiatry 136:67–70, 1979

Hoch PH, Cattell JP: The diagnosis of pseudoneurotic schizophrenia. Psychiatr Q 33:17–43, 1959

Jabin N: Attitudes toward disability: Horney's theory applied. Am J Psychoanal 47:143–153, 1987

Joyce P, Mulder R, Cloninger CR: Temperament predicts clomipramine and desipramine response in major depression. J Affective Disord 30:35–46, 1994

Jung CG: The Integration of the Personality. Translated by Dell SM. New York, Farrar & Rinehart, 1939

Klein DN, DePue RA, Slater JF: Inventory identification of cyclothymia. IX. Validation in the offspring of bipolar I patients. Arch Gen Psychiatry 43:441–445, 1986

Kohut H: Analysis of the Self. New York, International Universities Press, 1971

Kraepelin E: Dementia Praecox and Paraphrenia. Translated by Barclay RM and edited by Robertson GM. Edinburgh, Livingstone, 1919, pp 53–54

Kraepelin E: Fundamental states, in Manic-Depressive Insanity and Paranoia. Translated by Barclay RM and edited by Robertson GM. Edinburgh, Livingstone, 1921, pp 117–132

Kraepelin E: Clinical Psychiatry. Original edition, 1907. A facsimile reproduction with an introduction by Carlson ET. Delmar, NY, Scholars' Facsimiles & Reprints, 1981, pp 222–228, 423–433

Kretchmer E: Physique and Character. Translated by Sprott WJH. New York,

Harcourt, Brace & Co, 1926. Reprinted by The Classics of Psychiatry & Behavioral Sciences Library, Birmingham, AL, 1990

Lazare A, Klerman GL, Armor D: Oral, obsessive, and hysterical personality patterns. J Psychiatr Res 7:275–290, 1970

Lewis M: Shame: The Exposed Self. New York, Free Press, 1992

Lindstrom E, von Knorring L: Principal component analysis of the Swedish version of the Positive and Negative Syndrome Scale for schizophrenia. Nord J Psychiatry 47:257–263, 1993

Lovejoy MC, Steuerwald BL: Subsyndromal unipolar and bipolar disorders: comparisons on positive and negative affect. J Abnorm Psychol 104:381–384, 1995

Martin RL, Cloninger CR, Guze SB, et al: Mortality in a follow-up of 500 psychiatric outpatients. II. Cause-specific mortality. Arch Gen Psychiatry 42:58–66, 1985

Meehl PE: Schizotaxia, schizotypy, schizophrenia. Am Psychol 17:827–838, 1962

Mezzich JE, Fabrega H Jr, Coffman GA: Multiaxial classification of depressive patients. J Nerv Ment Dis 175:339–346, 1987

Millon T: Millon Clinical Multiaxial Inventory-II (MCMI-II), 2nd Edition. Minneapolis, MN, National Computer Systems, 1987

Myers JL, Weissman MM: Use of a self-report symptom scale to detect depression in a community sample. Am J Psychiatry 137:1081–1084, 1980

Nelson EC, Cloninger CR: The Tridimensional Personality Questionnaire as a predictor of response to nefazodone treatment of depression. J Affective Disord 35:51–57, 1995

Nystrom S, Lindegard B: Depression: predisposing factors. Acta Psychiatr Scand 51:77–87, 1975a

Nystrom S, Lindegard B: Predisposition for mental syndromes: a study comparing predisposition for depression, neurasthenia and anxiety state. Acta Psychiatr Scand 51:69–76, 1975b

Osher Y, Cloninger CR, Belmaker RH: TPQ in euthymic manic depressive patients. J Psychiatr Res 30:353–357, 1996

Quitkin F, Rifkin A, Klein DF: Monoamine oxidase inhibitors: a review of antidepressant effectiveness. Arch Gen Psychiatry 36:749–760, 1979

Radloff LS: The CES-D Scale: a self-report depression scale for research in the general population. Appl Psychol Meas 1:385–401, 1977

Ray JJ: Authoritarianism as a cause of heart disease: reply to Byrne, Reinhart, & Heaven. Br J Med Psychol 63:287–288, 1990

Robins E, Guze SB: Establishment of diagnostic validity in psychiatric illness: its application to schizophrenia. Am J Psychiatry 126:983–987, 1970

Robins LN, Regier DA (eds): Psychiatric Disorders in America: The Epidemiologic Catchment Area Study. New York, Free Press, 1991

SAS Institute: SAS System for Statistical Analysis. Release 6.07. Cary, NC, SAS Institute, 1992

Selzer ML, Vinokur A, van Rooijen L: A self-administered short Michigan Alcoholism Screening Test (SMAST). J Stud Alcohol 36:117–126, 1975

Stewart AL, Hays RD, Ware JE Jr: The MOS short-form general health survey: reliability and validity in a patient population. Med Care 26:724–735, 1988

Svrakic DM, Whitehead C, Przybeck TR, et al: Differential diagnosis of personality disorders by the seven-factor model of temperament and character. Arch Gen Psychiatry 50:991–999, 1993

Svrakic NM, Svrakic DM, Cloninger CR: A general quantitative theory of personality development: fundamentals of a self-organizing psychobiological complex. Dev Psychopathol 8:247–272, 1996

Tellegen A, Grove W, Waller N: Inventory of Personal Characteristics #7. Minneapolis, MN, Department of Psychology, University of Minnesota, 1990.

Vernon PE (ed): Creativity: Selected Readings. Baltimore, Penguin, 1970

von Zerssen D, Possl J: The premorbid personality of patients with different subtypes of an affective illness. Statistical analysis of blind assignment of case history data to clinical diagnoses. J Affective Disord 18:39–50, 1990

von Zerssen D, Tauscher R, Possl J: The relationship of premorbid personality to subtypes of an affective illness. A replication study by means of an operationalized procedure for diagnosis of personality structures. J Affective Disord 32:61–72, 1994

Waller NG, Zavala J: Evaluating the Big Five. Psychological Inquiry 4:131–140, 1993

Walton HJ, Presley AS: Dimensions of abnormal personality. Br J Psychiatry 122:269–276, 1973

Wetzel RD, Cloninger CR, Hong B, et al: Personality as a subclinical expression of the affective disorders. Compr Psychiatry 21:197–205, 1980

White J (ed): What Is Enlightenment? Boston, Houghton Mifflin, 1985

Zimmerman M: Diagnosing personality disorders: a review. Arch Gen Psychiatry 51:225–245, 1994

Personality Correlates of Eating Disorder Subtypes

Katherine A. Halmi, M.D.

Erin I. Kleifield, Ph.D.

Devra L. Braun, M.D.

Suzanne R. Sunday, Ph.D.

Clinicians have long implicated personality factors in the pathogenesis of eating disorders. Janet (1903) subdivided patients with anorexia into an "obsessional" group and an "hysterical" group. Dally (1969) described patients with anorexia and mixed features of obsessionality and hysteria. By 1980 both Garfinkel et al. (1980) and Casper et al. (1980) were describing impulsive behavior as being associated with the bulimic type of anorexia at a much greater frequency than that present in the restricting type of anorexia.

This chapter presents the changing eating disorder diagnostic criteria and discuss the difficulties in comparing studies of personality and eating disorders in the context of these changing criteria. We present assessments of personality traits and studies of the categorical comorbid diagnoses of personality disorders with eating disorders. The influence of Axis I affective disorders and personality disorders on eating disorder symptoms and general psychopathology is discussed. Finally, a dimensional assessment of personality in eating disorders is presented.

Definition of Eating Disorder Subtypes

Since 1980 studies of the relationship between the personality and eating disorders have yielded widely discrepant results. Some of the difficulties inherent in establishing consistent relationships between personality correlates and eating disorders are due to inconsistencies in terminology and definitions of diagnostic criteria for the disorders between DSM-III (American Psychiatric Association 1980) and DSM-III-R (American Psychiatric Association 1987). Table 3–1 presents the diagnostic criteria of anorexia nervosa and bulimia nervosa in DSM-III, DSM-III-R, and DSM-IV (American Psychiatric Association 1994), respectively. The relationship between bulimia and affective illness may have been artificially inflated by the criteria necessary in DSM-III to meet the diagnoses of bulimia. Specifically, DSM-III required that individuals demonstrate depressed mood and self-deprecating thoughts following eating episodes.

In the DSM-III-R criteria the boundary between anorexia nervosa and bulimia nervosa was blurred. Emaciated patients with anorexia who binged and purged were given two diagnoses, anorexia nervosa and bulimia nervosa. Thus, personality studies of bulimia nervosa using DSM-III-R criteria included both emaciated and normal-weight patients, unless a further refinement of the classification was done independently by the author.

In DSM-IV anorexia nervosa has two subtypes: restricting and bulimic. The two subtypes of bulimia nervosa are purging and nonpurging. Extrapolating from the early studies of Casper et al. (1980) and Garfinkel et al. (1980), one may predict distinct and significant differences in the personality features and diagnoses among these eating disorder subtypes.

Personality Traits and Behaviors

Comprehensive studies investigating personality traits before the onset of anorexia nervosa or bulimia nervosa are cost prohibitive because of

TABLE 3–1.
Diagnostic criteria for anorexia nervosa and bulimia nervosa

A. *DSM-III criteria*

Anorexia nervosa
a. Intense fear of becoming obese, which does not diminish as weight loss progresses
b. Disturbance of body image, e.g., claiming to "feel fat" even when emaciated
c. Weight loss of at least 25% of original body weight or, if under 18 years of age, weight loss from original body weight plus projected weight gain expected from growth charts may be combined to make the 25%
d. Refusal to maintain body weight over a minimal normal weight for age and height
e. No known physical illness that would account for the weight loss

Bulimia nervosa
a. Recurrent episodes of binge eating (rapid consumption of a large amount of food in a discrete period of time, usually less than two hours)
b. At least three of the following:
  1. Consumption of high-calorie, easily ingested food during a binge
  2. Inconsipuous eating during a binge
  3. Termination of such eating episodes by abdominal pain, sleep, social interruption, or self-induced vomiting
  4. Repeated attempts to lose weight by severely restrictive diets, self-induced vomiting, or use of cathartics or diuretics
  5. Frequent weight fluctuations greater than 10 pounds due to alternating binges and fasts
c. Awareness that the eating pattern is abnormal and fear of not being able to stop eating voluntarily
d. Depressed mood and self-deprecating thoughts following eating binges
e. Bulimic episodes not due to anorexia nervosa or any known physical disorder

B. *DSM-III-R criteria*

Anorexia nervosa
a. Refusal to maintain weight over a minimal normal weight for age and height, e.g., weight loss leading to maintenance of body weight 15% below that expected; or failure to make expected weight gain during period of growth, leading to body weight 15% below that expected
b. Intense fear of gaining weight or becoming fat, even though underweight
c. Disturbance in the way one's body weight, size, or shape is experienced; e.g., the person claims to "feel fat" even when emaciated, believes that one area of the body is "too fat" even when obviously underweight

(continued)

69

TABLE 3–1.
Continued

d. In females, absence of at least three consecutive menstrual cycles when otherwise expected to occur (primary or secondary amenorrhea). (A woman is considered to have amenorrhea if her periods occur only following hormone, e.g., estrogen, administration.)

Bulimia nervosa

a. Recurrent episodes of binge eating (rapid consumption of a large amount of food in a discrete period of time)
b. A feeling of lack of control over eating behavior during the eating binges
c. The person regularly engages in either self-induced vomiting, use of laxatives or diuretics, strict dieting or fasting, or vigorous exercise in order to prevent weight gain
d. A minimum average of two binge eating episodes a week for at least three months
e. Persistent overconcern with body shape and weight

C. *DSM-IV criteria*

Anorexia nervosa

a. Refusal to maintain body weight over a minimally normal weight for age and height (e.g., weight loss leading to maintenance of body weight less than 85% of that expected; or failure to make expected weight gain during period of growth, leading to body weight less than 85% of that expected)
b. Intense fear of gaining weight or becoming fat, even though underweight
c. Disturbance in the way in which one's body weight or shape is experienced, undue influence of body shape and weight on self-evaluation, or denial of the seriousness of the current low body weight
d. In postmenarchal females, amenorrhea (i.e., the absence of at least three consecutive menstrual cycles). (A women is considered to have amenorrhea if her periods occur only following hormone, e.g., estrogen, administration.)

Specify type
Restricting type: During the episode of anorexia nervosa, the person does not regularly engage in binge eating or purging behavior (i.e., self-induced vomiting or the misuse of laxatives, diuretics, or enemas).

Binge eating/purging type: During the episode of anorexia nervosa, the person regularly engages in binge eating or purging behavior (i.e., self-induced vomiting or the misuse of laxatives, diuretics, or enemas).

Bulimia nervosa

a. Recurrent episodes of binge eating. An episode of binge eating is characterized by both of the following:

(continued)

TABLE 3–1.
Continued

---

1. Eating, in a discrete period of time (e.g., within any two-hour period), an amount of food that is definitely larger than most people would eat during a similar period of time and under similar circumstances
2. A sense of lack of control over eating during the episode (e.g., a feeling that one cannot stop eating or control what or how much one is eating)

b. Recurrent inappropriate compensatory behavior in order to prevent weight gain, such as self-induced vomiting; misuse of laxatives, diuretics, enemas, or other medication; fasting; or excessive exercise

c. The binge eating and inappropriate compensatory behaviors both occur, on average, at least twice a week for three months

d. Self-evaluation is unduly influenced by body shape and weight.

e. The disturbance does not occur exclusively during episodes of anorexia nervosa.

Specify type

Purging type: The person regularly engages in self-induced vomiting or the misuse of laxatives, diuretics, or enemas.

Nonpurging type: The person uses other inappropriate compensatory behaviors, such as fasting or excessive exercise, but does not regularly engage in self-induced vomiting or the misuse of laxatives, diuretics, or enemas.

---

the large numbers of persons that would need to be examined. Also, the age onset of eating disorders generally precedes the establishment of well-defined personality traits. The next best strategy is to study these patients after recovery from their eating disorder. Strober et al. (1980) showed a decrease in the obsessive-compulsive symptoms of patients with anorexia after treatment but no decrease in trait obsessionality. Patients with anorexia were described as possessing an obsessional character structure marked by heightened industriousness and responsibility, highly regimented behavior and rigid adherence and excessive conformance to rules and standards, social introversion, and limited social spontaneity. The authors postulated that these underlying traits play a facilitative role in the development of obsessive-compulsive symptoms in acute anorexia nervosa.

A study comparing subjects who previously had anorexia with control subjects (Casper 1990) reported greater risk avoidance, greater restraint in emotional expression, and greater conformance to authority in the patients with anorexia. In that same study, subjects who previously had anorexia, compared with their sisters, showed greater self and impulse control, greater industriousness and responsibility, greater interpersonal insecurity and greater minimization of affect, excessive conformance, and more regimentation of behavior.

A study by Wagner et al. (1987) showed patients with anorexia to have a greater sense of personal ineffectiveness, social ineffectiveness, and poor self-esteem compared to a control group. Patients with anorexia often lack childhood experiences that foster personal independence.

Patients with bulimia, on the other hand, were found to possess an impulsive, extroverted style, to show prominent mood lability, to have poor self-control, and to have more interpersonal difficulties compared with patients with anorexia and a control population (Casper et al. 1992).

The demonstration of systematic and pattern differences in personality traits among eating disorder subgroups spurred the investigation of the prevalence of personality disorders (categorical diagnoses) among eating disorders.

Axis II Personality Disorders

Some of the discrepant results in studies of personality disorders and eating disorders could be due to the use of interviews and self-report questionnaires of unproven reliability and specificity and to the use of instruments that may be distorted by Axis I states. As mentioned earlier, differences in the psychiatric terminology between traits and disorders and changes in diagnostic criteria between DSM-III and DSM-III-R may also account for some of the contradictory data.

Personality disorders are often arbitrarily grouped into three clusters. Cluster A includes paranoid, schizoid, and schizotypal personality disorders. Cluster B includes antisocial, borderline, histrionic, and narcissistic personality disorders. Cluster C includes avoidant, dependent, obsessive-compulsive, and passive-aggressive personality disorders. Although many of the studies of personality disorders in eating disorders are contradictory, almost all of the studies have shown a significantly higher preponderance of Cluster B personality disorders associated with patients with bulimia compared with those with anorexia, restricting type.

In one of the earlier studies to report on the full range of personality disorders, Gwirtsman et al. (1983) classified 44% of subjects with bulimia as meeting DSM-III criteria for borderline personality disorder. Similarly Levin and Hyler (1986) found that 63% of subjects with bulimia met criteria for at least one Axis II disorder and that 46% fulfilled criteria for borderline and/or histrionic personality disorders. Finally, Piran et al. (1988) found that the rates of personality disorders among subjects with restricting anorexia nervosa and subjects with bulimia were 86.8% and 97.4%, respectively. The most common diagnosis in the groups with restricting anorexia nervosa was avoidant personality disorder, which occurred in 60% of the patients. The most common diagnosis in the group with bulimia was borderline personality disorder, which occurred in 55.3% of the patients.

Gartner et al. (1989) examined the 12 personality disorders identified by DSM-III-R using the Personality Disorder Examination (PDE) (Loranger et al. 1987) and examining three subtypes of patients with eating disorders. In this study 54% of patients met criteria for at least 1 Axis II diagnosis, 40% met criteria for 2 or more diagnoses, and 17% of the patients had 5–7 Axis II diagnoses.

The most frequent personality disorders, in descending order were borderline (12 diagnoses), self-defeating (11 diagnoses), avoidant (11 diagnoses), obsessive-compulsive (9 diagnoses), dependent (8 diagnoses), narcissistic (4 diagnoses), and histrionic (2 diagnoses). The number of patients in two of the subgroups were too small to make meaningful subgroup comparisons. Subsequent studies using semistructured interviews to assess personality disorders in bulimia patients (as defined in DSM-III-R) showed a range and a prevalence of at least 1 personality disorder from 28% (Herzog et al. 1992) to 77% (Powers et al. 1988). The incidence of personality disorders using semistructured interviews among patients with restricting anorexia ranged from 23% (Herzog et al. 1992) to 80% (Wonderlich et al. 1990).

A number of methodological problems most likely account for

these divergent results. For example, 1) small numbers of subjects were used in some studies, 2) mixed samples of both inpatients and outpatients were used, 3) at times eating disorder patients were not categorized into subtypes but rather lumped together for analyses, 4) different measurement techniques were used in different studies, and 5) many studies did not take into account Axis I state factors of anxiety and depression.

It was clear from these previous studies that the questions they raised could only be answered with an interview-based study of a large enough sample of eating disorder patients to be divided into subtypes. It was also clear that a thorough knowledge of the nature and timing of Axis I comorbidity would be vital in helping to separate Axis I (state) distortions from Axis II personality characteristics. The Structured Clinical Interview for DSM-III-R (SCID) (Spitzer et al. 1989) and Structured Clinical Interview for the DSM-III-R Personality Disorders (SCID II) (Spitzer et al. 1990) were used in a study by Braun et al. (1994), because these interviews were designed to measure disorders, not simply behaviors or symptoms that may be epiphenomena of Axis I states. In this study, subjects were coded as reaching threshold on items only when they could provide particular behavioral examples that occurred at times other than when subjects were in an Axis I state; this would counteract, for example, the tendencies of the patient with dysphoria to overendorse pathology. In this study, 105 female patients with anorexia and/or bulimia nervosa were interviewed. They were divided into four groups: those with restricting anorexia, bulimic anorexia, and bulimia with and without a past history of anorexia. The majority (68.6%) had at least 1 personality disorder, 31.4% had no personality disorders. The patients with bulimia and a history of anorexia were significantly more likely to have 2 or more personality disorders than the sample as a whole.

Of the patients who had personality disorders the vast majority (93.1%) also had Axis I comorbidity. When Axis I and Axis II psychiatric comorbidity were examined together, only 5 of the 71 patients with bulimia (7%) were without other psychiatric comorbidity; in contrast, 23.5% of subjects with restricting anorexia had no psychiatric comorbidity.

Cluster A disorders were diagnosed in only 4.8% of the sample.

Cluster B disorders were diagnosed in 31% of the bulimic subgroups. This contrasts significantly with the restricting anorectic subgroup, none of whom had Cluster B disorders. Borderline personality disorder was by far the most common Cluster B diagnosis and was present in 25.4% of subjects with bulimia. Subjects with restricting anorexia were significantly less likely to have borderline personality disorder than the bulimic subgroups.

Cluster C personality disorders were present in 29.5% of the sample. Avoidant personality disorder was the most commonly prevalent (14.3%), followed by dependent (9.5%), obsessive-compulsive (6.7%), and passive-aggressive (3.8%). The prevalence of Cluster C personality disorders did not vary according to eating disorder subtype. For example, 23.5% of the restricting anorexia subtype, 27.3% of the bulimic anorexia subtype, and 24.5% of the two bulimia subtypes met criteria for avoidant personality disorder. These findings are inconsistent with reports that individuals with anorexia have more Cluster C pathology (Herzog et al. 1992). The differences between these findings may relate to the fact that Herzog and colleagues used outpatient subjects and DSM-III criteria for personality disorders while we used inpatient subjects and DSM-III-R criteria.

Only 6 of the 33 patients with no personality disorder had a history of substance dependence, whereas 36 of 72 patients with at least one personality disorder had such a history. Patients with no personality disorder were significantly more likely to have no affective disorder compared with the sample as a whole.

One issue with the study by Braun and colleagues is whether interviews relying on retrospective patient histories are sufficiently reliable to allow accurate diagnoses of psychiatric disorders and their temporal sequence of development. In addition, state-trait confusion may occur in diagnosing Axis II personality traits in patients currently in a dysphoric or anxious state. Loranger et al. (1991) have presented evidence that a carefully executed interview can yield accurate personality disorder diagnoses in spite of a current Axis I state. The Braun et al. study (1994) tried to prevent state-trait confusion by carefully instructing patients to provide examples of their personality traits from times when they were not depressed, bingeing, or starving and disallowed any examples occurring within those periods.

In another study, Skodol et al. (1993) hypothesized that the inconsistencies in previous studies of personality disorders and eating disorders were attributable largely to 1) the use of different assessment
methods, 2) failure to include meaningful comparison groups, 3) failure to consider base rates of eating disorders and personality disorders,
and 4) restriction to eating disorder clinic patients and/or inpatients.
To remedy these problems, they examined rates of personality disorders
and eating disorders among general samples of inpatient and outpatients using three instruments: the SCID, the PDE, and the Personality
Disorder Questionnaire-R, (PDQ-R) (Wonderlich et al. 1990). Despite
the rather small number of patients with current eating disorders
($n = 21$) (especially for those with anorexia [3 with bulimic anorexia
and 2 with restricting anorexia]), their findings were quite consistent
with earlier described studies in that borderline personality disorder
was associated with bulimia and avoidant personality disorder was associated with anorexia nervosa.

In the Skodol et al. (1993) study, the incidence of personality disorders depended on the diagnostic method employed. The highest
rates were for the PDQ-R, followed by the SCID II, and then the PDE.
The authors suggested the best approach was a more conservative,
consensual method of diagnosis. Using such an approach, the patients
with eating disorders in this study had significantly higher rates of
personality disorders than patients without eating disorders. The authors reported that the odds of a current eating disorder occurring in
conjunction with a personality disorder were about four times more
likely than the odds of an eating disorder occurring alone.

These findings lead to important questions about whether particular patterns of comorbidity exist between personality disorders and
eating disorders. Another key question is whether an individual's personality predisposes or protects her from developing particular Axis I
disorders. Is a woman with a Cluster B personality disorder at risk for
developing bulimia? A prospective study is necessary to demonstrate
whether specific personality disorders actually predispose patients to
develop particular eating disorders. On the other hand, does the development of an eating disorder (especially during adolescent years)
have a formative effect on the personality? Answering these research

questions is vital to the development of more targeted prevention and treatment strategies.

Effects of Depression and Borderline Personality Disorder on Eating Disorder Symptoms and General Psychopathology

Individuals with bulimia who also have a borderline personality disorder have been reported to show elevated eating disorder symptomatology and higher levels of general psychopathology. For example, Johnson et al. (1989) found subjects with borderline bulimia to have elevated Eating Disorder Inventory (EDI; Garner 1983), Symptom Checklist-90 (SCL-90; Derogatis 1977), and Beck Depression Inventory (Beck, 1978) scores as compared with subjects with nonborderline bulimia. Similarly, Cooper et al. (1988) found that the borderline subgroup of eating disorder patients manifested a significantly higher degree of eating disorder and psychiatric symptomatology, especially depression, compared to patients with nonborderline eating disorders. While these studies suggest that borderline personality disorder pathology may affect eating disorder severity, the possible comorbidity of depression further complicates the findings.

Sunday et al. (1993) assessed the relative influence of depression and personality psychopathology in patients with bulimia by examining the incidence of current or lifetime affective disorder and borderline personality characteristics. Core eating disorder symptomatology was measured by the EDI and general psychiatric symptoms were measured by the SCL-90. Assessments of affective disorder and borderline personality disorder were made using the SCID I and II.

Both groups with a current affective disorder diagnosis (those with and without borderline personality characteristics) displayed an elevated overall EDI profile, especially with respect to body dissatisfaction and ineffectiveness. Presence of borderline symptomatology had no effect on eating disorder inventory profiles.

Current affective disorder was associated with an elevation on all of the SCL-90 scales. Borderline personality characteristics influenced only the hostility subscale. These results suggest that the elevated profiles of the EDI and SCL-90 scores for patients with bulimia and borderline personality disorder reported in previous studies may have reflected comorbid affective state.

Assessing Dimensions of Personality

The inconsistencies in identifying personality types using categorical assessment approaches (even with increasingly improved technologies), the overconcern with personality pathology and underemphasis of healthy personality functioning inherent in categorical approaches, and the fact that so many patients with eating disorders met criteria for more than one personality disorder has encouraged conceptualization of personality from a dimensional perspective. The Tridimensional Personality Questionnaire (TPQ) assesses dimensions of personality (Cloninger 1987). The TPQ was developed to operationalize and measure behaviors associated with the following three dimensions of personality: novelty seeking (NS; the tendency towards intense exhilaration and excitement), harm avoidance (HA; the tendency towards intense avoidance of aversive stimuli), and reward dependence (RD; the tendency towards intense response to reward, particularly interpersonal rewards). A fourth dimension, persistence (P), subsequently has been extracted from the original RD scale (see Kleifield et al. 1993). Because of the propensity for patients with eating disorders to demonstrate the extremes of the personality characteristics related to the TPQ, this assessment seemed especially fitting to use for patients with anorexia nervosa and bulimia nervosa. Kleifield et al. (1993) has shown that the TPQ is an internally consistent instrument for use with eating disorder patients. Standardized factor loading following rotation showed that most subscales loaded highly on one of the three factors as predicted by Cloninger (1987).

In another study by Kleifield et al. (1994a), the TPQ was tested in four subgroups of patients with eating disorders and control subjects matched for gender and age. Subjects with restricting anorexia had significantly lower NS scores and higher mean P scores than the bulimic and the control groups. The HA scale and depression scores were positively correlated, whereas the RD scale and depression scores were negatively correlated.

The current level of depression exerted a significant effect on the HA and RD scales but not on the NS scales or the P scale. In this study NS and P presented as robust personality dimensions that not only distinguished among eating disorder subgroups, but distinguished these patients from a normal control group.

A third study by Kleifield et al. (1994b) evaluated the stability of TPQ scores in eating disorder patients by examining the effects of depression on TPQ scores before and after treatment in patients with eating disorders and in control subjects. Subjects with restricting anorexia and bulimic anorexia had low NS scores both before and after treatment and scored significantly lower than the two bulimic groups (bulimia nervosa with and without a past history of anorexia nervosa) and control subjects. On the P scale, subjects with restricting anorexia had scores that were significantly elevated relative to all other groups. Eating disorder diagnostic group differences and treatment effects on the HA scale were due to changes in level of depression. Depression affected RD scores in much the same way with two exceptions; treatment did not affect the adjusted scores of subjects with bulimic anorexia and bulimia with a past history of anorexia after changes in levels of depression were removed. Specifically, the bulimic anorectic group lowered and the bulimic group with a past history of anorexia increased their reward dependence scores across treatment.

These TPQ studies showed the most consistent and stable differences that emerged between the eating disorder diagnostic groups were between the restricting anorectic and the bulimic subgroups. These studies also demonstrated that subjects with restricting anorexia are not only less novelty seeking than the subjects with bulimia, but they were also less novelty seeking than normal subjects. Likewise, the subjects with restricting anorexia showed a tendency toward more rigid and obsessional behavior (elevated P levels) than both bulimic and normal subjects. These findings lend support for viewing the already described personality characteristics as dispositions that not only distinguish eating disorder subgroups, but also distinguish these groups from the normal population. The HA and RD dimensions were significantly influenced by Beck Depression Inventory scores. This again underscores the need to consider the effects of state conditions, most notably depression, when examining personality within a clinical population.

Conclusions

Many investigators have firmly established that personality disorders are highly prevalent among eating disorders. There is a high association of borderline personality disorder in bulimia nervosa and a high association of avoidant personality disorder in anorexia nervosa. These findings parallel the clear differences that emerge between the restricting anorexia group and the two bulimic groups in the personality dimensions in the TPQ, with subjects with bulimia emerging overall as more impulsive and subjects with anorexia as more rigid and obsessive. As such, these character traits may serve as valuable markers to predict the longitudinal course of these disorders. Our original findings have been confirmed in subsequent research by independent groups (Brewerton et al. 1993; Bulik et al. 1995).

The challenge now is to understand why particular personality traits and disorders and eating disorders seem to co-occur and to determine the direction of causality. The evidence revealing the influence of Axis I state factors in mediating the relationship between personality factors and eating disorders demonstrates that the nature of this interaction is more complex than originally thought. It is now time to move beyond descriptive work and into elucidating the causal and mediating mechanisms.

References

American Psychiatric Association: Diagnostic and Statistical Manual of Mental Disorders, 3rd Edition. Washington, DC, American Psychiatric Association, 1980

American Psychiatric Association: Diagnostic and Statistical Manual of Mental Disorders, 3rd Edition, Revised. Washington, DC, American Psychiatric Association, 1987

American Psychiatric Association: Diagnostic and Statistical Manual of Mental Disorders, 4th Edition. Washington, DC, American Psychiatric Association, 1994

Beck AT: Depression Inventory. Philadelphia, PA, Philadelphia Center for Cognitive Therapy, 1978

Braun DL, Sunday SR, Halmi KA: Psychiatric comorbidity in patients with eating disorders. Psychol Med 24:859–867, 1994

Brewerton TD, Hand LD, Bishop ER Jr: The Tridimensional Personality Questionnaire in eating disorder patients. International Journal of Eating Disorders 14:213–218, 1993

Bulik CM, Sullivan PF, Joyce PR, et al: Temperament, character, and personality disorder in bulimia nervosa. J Nerv Ment Dis 183:593–598, 1995

Casper RC: Personality features of women with good outcome from restricting anorexia nervosa. Psychosom Med 52:156–170, 1990

Casper RC, Eckert ED, Halmi KA: Bulimia: its incidence and clinical importance in patients with anorexia nervosa. Arch Gen Psychiatry 37:1030–1035, 1980

Casper RC, Hedeker D, McClough JF: Personality dimensions in eating disorders and the relevance for subtyping. J Am Acad Child Adoles Psychiatry 30:830–840, 1992

Cloninger CR: A systematic method for clinical description and classification of personality variance. Arch Gen Psychiatry 44:573–588, 1987

Cooper JL, Morrison TL, Bigman OL, et al: Bulimia and borderline personality disorder. International Journal of Eating Disorders 7:43–49, 1988

Dally P: Anorexia Nervosa. London, William Heineman Medical Books, 1969

Derogatis LR: SCL-90 Administration, Scoring and Procedures Manuals for the Revised Version. Baltimore, MD, Leonard R. Derogatis, 1977

Garfinkel PE, Moldomsky H, Garner DM: The heterogeneity of anorexia nervosa. Arch Gen Psychiatry 37:1036–1040, 1980

Garner D: The Eating Disorder Inventory, in Anorexia Nervosa: Recent Developments. Edited by Darby PL, Garfinkel P, Garner D. New York, Alan R Liss, 1983, pp 173–184

Gartner AF, Marcus RN, Halmi KA, et al: DSM-III personality disorders in patients with eating disorders. Am J Psychiatry 146:1585–1591, 1989.

Gwirtsman HE, Roy-Byrne P, Yager J, et al: Neuroendocrine abnormalities in bulimia. Am J Psychiatry 140:559–563, 1983

Herzog D, Keller MB, Lavori P, et al: The prevalence of personality disorders in 210 women with eating disorders. J Clin Psychiatry 53:147–152, 1992

Janet P: Les obsessions et la psychastaenie. Paris, Flix Alean, 1903

Johnson C, Tobin D, Enright A: Prevalence and clinical characteristics of borderline patients in an eating-disordered population. J Clin Psychiatry 50:9–15, 1989

Kleifield EI, Sunday SR, Hurt S, et al: Psychometric validation of the Tridimensional Personality Questionnaire: application to subgroups of eating disorders. Compr Psychiatry 34:249–253, 1993

Kleifield EI, Sunday SR, Halmi KA, et al: The effects of depression on the TPQ. Biol Psychiatry 36:68–70, 1994a

Kleifield EI, Sunday SR, Hurt S, et al: The Tridimensional Personality Questionnaire: an exploration of personality traits in eating disorders. J Psychiatr Res 28:413–423, 1994b

Levin AP, Hyler SE: DSM-III personality diagnoses in bulimia. Compr Psychiatry 27:47–53, 1986

Loranger AW, Susman VL, Oldham JM, et al: The personality disorder examination: a preliminary report. J Personal Disord 1:1–13, 1987

Loranger A, Lenzenweger M, Gartner AF, et al: Trait-state artifacts and the diagnoses of personality disorders. Arch Gen Psychiatry 48:720–728, 1991

Piran N, Lerner P, Garfinkel PE, et al: Personality disorders in anorectic patients. International Journal of Eating Disorders 7:589–599, 1988

Powers PS, Coovert DL, Brightwell DR, et al: Other psychiatric disorders among bulimic patients. Compr Psychiatry 29:503–508, 1988

Skodol AE, Oldham JM, Hyler SE, et al: Comorbidity of DSM-III-R, eating disorders and personality disorders. International Journal of Eating Disorders 14:408–413, 1993

Spitzer RL, Williams J, Gibbon M, et al: Structural Clinical Interview for DSM-III-R. New York, New York State Psychiatric Institute, 1989

Spitzer RL, Williams JBW, Gibbon M, et al: Structured Clinical Interview for the DSM-III-R Personality Disorders (SCID-II). Washington, DC, American Psychiatric Press, 1990

Strober M: Personality and symptomological features in young, nonchronic anorexia nervosa patients. J Psychosom Res 24:353–359, 1980

Sunday SR, Levey CM, Halmi KA: Effects of depression and borderline personality traits on psychological state and eating disorder symptomatology. Compr Psychiatry 34:70–74, 1993

Wagner S, Halmi KA, McQuire T: The sense of personal ineffectiveness in patients with anorexia nervosa: one construct or several. International Journal of Eating Disorders 6:495–505, 1987

Wonderlich SA, Swift WJ, Slotnick HB: DSM-III-R personality disorders in eating disorder subtypes. International Journal of Eating Disorders 9:607–616, 1990

CHAPTER 4

Axis I and Axis II: Comorbidity or Confusion?

Bruce Pfohl, M.D.

How Do We Conceptualize Axis I and Axis II?

Since the publication of DSM-III in 1980 (American Psychiatric Association 1980), researchers and clinicians alike have acknowledged the high rate of co-occurrence of Axis I and Axis II disorders. Before addressing the issue of comorbidity between personality disorder diagnoses and Axis I disorders, it is important to consider the implications of placing personality diagnoses on a separate axis from the Axis I disorders. Several decades ago, progress in psychiatry was impeded by a diagnostic manual that categorized psychiatric disorder into organic and functional categories (American Psychiatric Association 1952). Several generations of psychiatrists were encouraged to think that brain anatomy and physiology were important for one class of disorders and irrelevant to another class; that reactions to the psychosocial environment were relevant to one class but not the other. We must be careful not to encourage a similar false dichotomy with the distinction between Axis I and Axis II. It would be a mistake to think of personality disorders as being related to some combination of brain mechanisms and psychosocial factors that have little relevance to Axis I disorders or vice versa.

For purposes of this discussion, the terms *personality disorder* and *Axis II* are used interchangeably even though DSM-IV also includes mental retardation under Axis II. DSM-IV defines *personality disorder* as "an enduring pattern of inner experience and behavior that deviates markedly from the expectations of the individual's culture, is pervasive and inflexible, has an onset in adolescence or early adulthood, is stable over time, and leads to distress or impairment." (American Psychiatric Association 1994, p. 629). Like most definitions, this one is subject to interpretation. Does "stable over time" include the possibility of a marked exacerbation of personality symptoms during periods of Axis I disorder? What if the individual has had a chronic mood or anxiety disorder on Axis I that never remits completely? If starting a new medication results in a remission of both Axis I and Axis II symptoms, can we conclude that there never was a true Axis II disorder to begin with? If an Axis I disorder such as major depressive disorder (MDD) is less responsive to medications when an Axis II disorder is also present, should we think of the latter patient as having an etiologically distinct form of personality disorder?

Table 4–1 presents some hypothetical data that illustrate the problems involved in defining personality disorder and its relationship to Axis I disorders. Let us assume that the resources are available to conduct a longitudinal study of a group of patients from age 15 to age 50 using state-of-the-art structured interviews for Axis I and Axis II. If the diagnostic assessment is repeated yearly by interviewers who are blind to the results of the previous year's assessments, the hypothetical results for one subject might be represented by Table 4–1. Here we see that the subject met criteria for MDD at age 20 and age 27 and had no further diagnosable episodes of affective disorder through age 50.

With respect to Axis II the same subject met criteria for narcissistic personality disorder (NPD) at each yearly assessment. Criteria for borderline personality disorder (BPD) were met during the assessments that took place between age 15 and 20, between age 24 and 27, and at the assessment completed at age 34. The consistency of the diagnosis

TABLE 4–1.

Psychopathology over time: hypothetical data for one subject

Age	Diagnoses			Age	Diagnoses			Age	Diagnoses		
15	—	NPD	BPD	25	—	NPD	BPD	35	—	NPD	BPD
16	—	NPD	BPD	26	—	NPD	BPD	36	—	NPD	BPD
17	—	NPD	BPD	27	MDD	NPD	BPD	37	—	NPD	BPD
18	—	NPD	BPD	28	—	NPD	BPD	38	—	NPD	—
19	—	NPD	BPD	29	—	NPD	BPD	39	—	NPD	—
20	MDD	NPD	BPD	30	—	NPD	BPD	40	—	NPD	—
21	—	NPD	—	31	—	NPD	—	41	—	NPD	—
22	—	NPD	—	32	—	NPD	—	42	—	NPD	—
23	—	NPD	—	33	—	NPD	—	•	•	•	•
24	—	NPD	BPD	34	—	NPD	BPD	50	—	NPD	BPD

of NPD easily fits the "stability over time component of the definition of Axis II. The BPD diagnosis disappears and reappears over time although the overall trend is for the individual not to meet criteria for BPD in later years.

In order to consider the types of observations used to diagnose Axis I and Axis II disorders, let us assume that the yearly assessments for this hypothetical patient allow for the plotting of yearly symptom severity levels as illustrated in Figure 4–1, which represents the same data listed in Table 4–1 plotted as a set of continuous dimensions. The ribbon in the foreground represents the severity of the patient's symptoms on a depression rating scale. Once again, we see that the problems with depression were particularly bad at age 20 and 27. In addition we notice an increase in depressive symptoms at age 34 that was subthreshold for a diagnosis of MDD and we also see that this individual had mild elevations in depressive symptoms throughout much of early adulthood. Though hypothetical, this lack of full remission of depressive symptoms between acute episodes is certainly compatible with published longitudinal studies (Coryell et al. 1990; Matussek and Feil 1983).

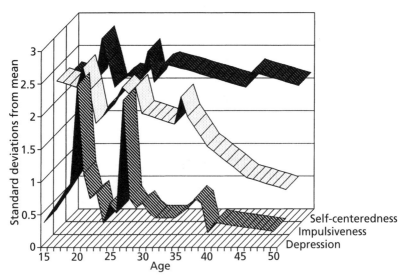

FIGURE 4–1.   *Psychopathology over time: hypothetical data for one subject.*

Let us assume that the variation in the diagnosis of BPD is explained in this patient by variation in the severity of one important component of this disorder, impulsivity. The middle ribbon in Figure 4–1 represents the individual's scores on a hypothetical rating scale for impulsivity. We note that from age 15 through 20, impulsivity scores are two standard deviations above population norms and that this is apparently sufficiently high (in combination with other criteria) to yield a diagnosis of BPD. We also note that this individual appears to experience exacerbations in severity of impulsivity coincident with exacerbations in depressive symptoms. Self-centeredness, an important component of the NPD diagnosis, also shows variation over time.

It clear that even though the severity of self-centeredness and impulsive dimensions decreases with remission in depressive symptoms and with increasing age, these dimensions continue to remain elevated above population norms throughout most of the observation period. The clinical significance of personality symptoms that vary with severity of Axis I disorders is considered later in this chapter.

The three ribbons represent three sets of observations that vary over time. The ribbon representing depressive symptoms shows a greater tendency towards acute exacerbations with a tendency to return to baseline. The ribbons representing the two personality dimensions show lower magnitude variation over time that is at least partially correlated with the depression scores. Differences in pattern of variation is clearly one key component that differentiates how we conceptualize Axis I and Axis II. Are there other differences relevant to how we view these two axes and any associated comorbidity?

Are We Asking the Right Questions?

The questions we ask about the Axis I and Axis II disorders and their relationship are often questions loaded with certain assumptions. The assumptions behind these questions are important to consider because, if the assumptions do not accurately reflect nature, accurate answers become impossible. One particular loaded question is seldom asked openly, yet the answer is built into the structure of how psychopathology is conceptualized and studied by clinicians from different training programs. That question is, "Is real psychiatric disorder Axis I disorder or Axis II disorder?" Clinicians from more biologically oriented training programs are often inclined to answer that psychiatrists should focus their energy into treating well-defined disorders that show a dramatic response to medications or time-limited behavior therapy. Clinicians from more psychoanalytically oriented programs often answer that psychiatrists should focus their energy on treating the underlying personality structure that predisposes patients to various Axis I disorders. Either assumption can interfere with an open-minded exploration of a spectrum of syndromes, some disorders expressing themselves in acute episodes, some expressed over a period of years with less variation, and some falling in between.

I frequently hear another type of loaded question from clinicians consulting those of us with a special interest in personality disorder. The question is often phrased, "Are this patient's symptoms caused by affective disorder or is this really a personality disorder?" I believe that this type of question is prompted by several underlying assumptions that are probably false. The first is that the diagnoses of personality disorder and affective disorder are somehow mutually exclusive. Another is that, if personality disorder is present, the patient is not likely to benefit from medications. This assumption is often supported by another assumption—that chronic psychosocial and occupational problems that respond to antidepressant medications are not really personality disorders, because personality disorders are related to brain mechanisms that have nothing to do with the brain mechanisms that regulate mood.

A third loaded question is, "Is the high comorbidity explained by Axis II disorders predisposing to an Axis I disorder or is it that severe Axis I disorders predispose to Axis II problems?" A more complete set of explanatory options might include the possibility that a diagnosis on Axis I leads to false positive diagnoses on Axis II or perhaps some third factor predisposes to disorders on both axes. Even with these additional possible explanations, it is important not to fall victim to the assumption that the syndromes described in DSM-IV constitute discrete disease entities. With few exceptions, the disorders on Axis I and Axis II represent collections of symptoms organized into syndromes that are defined to provide a useful shorthand for clinicians. At best, these collections of symptoms have some validity with respect to response to treatment, family history, and longitudinal stability. In reality, the boundaries of these syndromes are quite fuzzy. The same medication may be useful for disorders in several different categories, family history studies often find several different syndromes running together, and epidemiologic studies suggest that the presence of almost any psychiatric diagnosis raises the likelihood of a wide variety of comorbid psychiatric diagnoses.

The disorders in the DSM classification system are not diseases with known pathophysiology but clusters of symptoms, some of which may return to a near normal baseline between episodes and some of which are much more chronic. The boundaries between various disorders and between Axis I and Axis II inevitably shift as more is understood about the pathophysiology. Witness the boundary shift between schizophrenia and affective disorder when the response to lithium was recognized as an important clinical variable. In this light, an apparent comorbidity between an Axis I disorder such as MDD and an Axis II disorder such as BPD might indicate that a currently undefined subset of patients with MDD share a common pathophysiology and pathopsychology with a currently undefined subset of patients with BPD.

A safe definition of personality disorder, with as few assumptions made as possible, might read as follows: "Personality disorders represent a class of syndromes defined by the early onset of inflexible and maladaptive traits that are exhibited in a wide range of social and personal contexts and that are relatively stable over a period of years." It is important to realize that this definition does not exclude syndromes that show genetic or familial relationships to Axis I disorders, lessen in severity after several decades, respond to medications, or relate to abnormalities in neurotransmitter systems that may also be relevant to Axis I syndromes. The important point for the present discussion is that Axis I and Axis II are distinguished by syndromal course, not pathophysiologic mechanism.

Axis I and Axis II: Empirical Data

It is now well established that patients with a variety of Axis I disorders often meet criteria for a variety of Axis II disorders. It is not unusual in various clinical series to find one or more comorbid personality diagnoses to be present in approximately half of the patients who meet criteria for MDD (Pfohl et al. 1984), obsessive-compulsive disorder (OCD) (Baer et al. 1992), panic disorder (Noyes et al. 1990), and substance abuse (DeJong et al. 1993, Nace et al. 1991). This contrasts with rates in the range of 10% to 15% in nonclinical populations (Nestadt 1990; Reich et al. 1988; Zimmerman and Coryell 1989).

State Effects on Personality Assessment

The hypothetical data summarized in Figure 4–1 suggest several attributes of the apparent relationship between Axis I and Axis II that can be supported by empirical studies. First, Axis II symptomatology often exacerbates during episodes of Axis I disorders, a finding supported by studies in which the severity of personality symptoms often diminishes when the Axis I condition resolves. Reich and colleagues (1986) found this to be true for a variety of personality dimensions in a group of anxiety disorder patients treated with alprazolam. Other studies suggest that abnormal personality traits show regression toward normality when an Axis I disorder remits (Hirschfeld et al. 1983; Noyes et al. 1990).

Figure 4–1 illustrates that although personality traits may diminish in severity after resolution of the Axis I disorder, baseline personality traits are still elevated relative to population norms. Supportive data are most readily found in studies of patients with MDD. Matussek and Feil (1983) examined 215 subjects who had been in complete remission after an episode of MDD for up to several years. Compared with control subjects, the cases with a prior episode of MDD had higher "autodestructive-neurotic traits." Other personality traits appeared to distinguish particular affective subtypes. Reich and colleagues (1986) examined patients with panic disorder before and after treatment. These patients showed some degree of attenuation of personality trait abnormalities after successful treatment of the Axis I disorder; however, recovered patients with panic disorder continued to score lower than control subjects on trait measures of emotional strength and to score higher than control subjects on interpersonal dependency (Reich et al. 1987).

Hirschfeld and colleagues (1989) measured a variety of personality variables in a series of 400 individuals who had never had an episode of Axis I disorder. They followed the subjects for 6 years. Compared with a never ill control group, the premorbid personality assessments on the 29 who later developed an episode of MDD were remarkable for higher neuroticism, lower emotional stability, and higher dependency. The findings suggest that the comorbidity of personality disorders with Axis I cannot be accounted for by state effects alone.

Implications of Personality Comorbidity for Axis I

Many studies have demonstrated that comorbid personality disorders portend a worse prognosis for patients with a variety of Axis I disorders: major depression (Pfohl et al. 1987; Pilkonis and Frank 1988; Shea et al. 1990), panic disorder (Noyes et al. 1990), eating disorders (Gartner et al. 1989), and OCD (Baer et al. 1992).

The findings of a worse prognosis holds true even when the personality disorder is assessed at the height of the Axis I disorder. A study of panic disorder by Noyes and colleagues (1990) illustrates this point particularly well. Eighty-nine subjects received personality assessment by structured interview at index while fully symptomatic for panic disorder. The severity of personality scores significantly dropped after treatment of the panic disorder; however, personality scores remained higher than those observed in control subjects. Even so, the personality abnormalities measured at index were highly predictive of severity of anxiety symptoms and social adjustment at follow-up three years later.

There is reason to believe that the implications of comorbid personality disorder depends on age, at least among patients with MDD. Two studies have reported that the association of personality disorder with worse outcome with respect to MDD holds only for patients who are at least past their mid-twenties at the time of personality assessment

(Barrash et al. 1993; Hirschfeld et al. 1989). Indeed, certain personality traits may not even be stable in young adults (Finn 1986).

Problems With Categorical Approaches to Axis I and Axis II

Figure 4–1 implies that the severity of certain personality traits may regress toward the mean as the individual gets older. Thus, the categorical system of personality classification may fail to accurately capture differences between individuals as well as changes in the same individual over time. A number of follow-up studies indicate that borderline symptoms do moderate over time such that most of the patients no longer meet criteria for BPD after 10 to 15 years (McGlashan 1986; Paris et al. 1987). Stone (1993) has reviewed longitudinal studies of other personality disorders and found a similar pattern.

Lee Anna Clark (1992) has concisely summarized the problems in using the Axis II categories to account for clinically relevant personality variance. The problems include the relative rarity of patients who meet criteria for just one personality disorder, temporal instability of individual categorical personality disorder diagnoses, marked heterogeneity of symptoms within categories, and lack of statistical evidence for any clear threshold or cutoff for making categorical diagnoses.

Despite population data on personality pathology that appear to fit a continuous distribution, the importance of a continuous dimensional rating of personality pathology might still be dismissed if severity of personality pathology at index evaluation was uncorrelated with severity at follow-up. This does not appear to be the case even for patients with one of the most socially costly personality disorders, antisocial personality disorder. In a 20- to 30-year follow-up of patients previously treated on a psychiatric inpatient unit with a diagnosis of antisocial personality disorder, the amount of antisocial behavior at follow-up was directly correlated with the severity of antisocial symptoms at intake (Black 1993). In other words, a continuous measure of antisocial symptoms is a better predictor of outcome variance than is a categorical diagnosis.

Some authors (Widiger et al. 1989) have suggested that the limitations of Axis II personality categorical diagnoses might be rectified by treating each of the Axis II categories as a dimension. The number of symptoms within each category could be summed up to indicate the severity of borderline or schizotypal traits, for example. The problem with turning the current personality disorder categories into dimensions is that the criteria that make up each disorder are often poorly correlated with other criteria in the same category (Clarkin et al. 1993). Thus, two patients who might both score in the mild to moderate range on BPD might be very different because one might have achieved the moderate score by having problems with impulsivity (criterion 2) and control of anger (criterion 4) whereas another patient could achieve the same score by having problems with marked identity disturbance (criterion 6) and chronic feelings of emptiness and boredom (criterion 7).

To make matters worse, an individual with the personality trait of being easily slighted or hurt by criticism might have this single trait simultaneously scored on three different dimensions: avoidant personality disorder (criterion 1), NPD (criterion 1), and paranoid personality disorder (criteria 4 and 6). This means that a putative link between a given Axis I disorder and the personality trait of being easily slighted or hurt by criticism would be diluted across three different personality disorders.

Spectrum Disorders

The past 10 years have seen increasing use of such terms as the schizophrenia spectrum, the affective spectrum, and the obsessive-compulsive spectrum. These concepts appear to offer another possible explanation for the high rates of comorbidity between certain Axis I and Axis II disorders. For example, a mild loading on a key biologic variable such as dopamine receptor activity could be phenotypically expressed as a subthreshold case of schizotypal personality in which several of the criteria for this disorder are met. A moderate loading on the same variable might result in a personality disorder in which all or most schizotypal personality criteria are met, and a heavy loading might be phenotypically expressed as schizophrenia.

The spectrum concept has been advanced in part because of advances in psychopharmacology. That pharmacologic agents lack specificity has been noted for decades, but this could have been attributed to most agents acting at many different neuroreceptor sites. The development of "cleaner" pharmacologic probes raises the possibility that different categorical disorders may in fact share similar pathologic mechanisms. For example, the actions of fluoxetine are largely limited· to serotonin pathways, yet this agent has been shown to benefit depression, OCD, panic disorder, and body dysmorphic disorder. Abnormalities in serotonin pathways have been linked to certain personality traits such as impulsivity or harm avoidance (Coccaro et al. 1989).

The problem with using the spectrum model to explain comorbidity is that the model implies a quantitative variation in a single dimension. In physics, for example, the electromagnetic radiation spectrum involves a continuous variation in a single physical property—wavelength. In order for a group of psychiatric syndromes to fit the strict spectrum model, differences between syndromes must relate to quantitative variation in a single factor, such as serotonin receptor activity. The truth might be quite different. Perhaps abnormalities in serotonin receptor activity represent a prerequisite for several different psychiatric syndromes, but additional qualitatively different factors contribute to the expression of the apparently related syndromes. In this way, the differences between OCD, body dysmorphic disorder, and obsessive-compulsive personality disorder may not be explained by different positions on the spectrum of serotonin activity but by the presence of other biologic or psychosocial determinants in addition to an abnormality in serotonin activity.

In the case of the Axis I diagnosis of OCD and the Axis II diagnosis of obsessive-compulsive personality disorder, the available data do not support the view that both are part of the same spectrum of disorders. Most investigators have found that other personality disorders are more common than obsessive-compulsive personality disorder among OCD patients (Baer et al. 1992; Pfohl et al. 1987). These findings may relate to the previously noted problem that the current personality disorder categories are composed of individual traits that may cross several personality dimensions. In contrast, the link between schizophrenia and schizotypal personality disorder would appear to fit the spectrum model reasonably well because schizotypal personality disorder is frequently seen in the premorbid history of schizophrenia, and both family history studies (Kendler et al. 1981; Baron et al. 1983) and biologic measures such as smooth pursuit eye movement abnormalities are present in both disorders (Siever et al. 1990).

Conclusions

Any exploration of the high rates of comorbidity between Axis I and Axis II syndromes must begin with the recognition that Axis I and Axis II are distinguished by syndromal course, not pathophysiologic mechanisms. The definition of personality disorder does not exclude syndromes that show genetic or familial relationships to Axis I disorders, lessen in severity after several decades, respond to medications, or relate to abnormalities in neurotransmitter systems that are relevant to Axis I syndromes.

Data collected since the publication of DSM-III in 1980 indicates that there are problems with trying to describe variation in personality pathology using a set of discrete categories. Future studies should also employ personality trait measures because it is possible that Axis I disorders covary not with specific personality categories but with personality traits that cross several different categories.

Although it is true that personality pathology as measured by standard tests and interviews may increase during acute episodes of Axis I disorder, personality pathology measured during acute episodes still has important prognostic implications, and it appears that personality difficulties do not completely resolve even with successful treatment of Axis I disorders. Despite unresolved measurement issues, the negative prognostic implications of comorbid personality disorder on the course of Axis I disorders stand as one of the most reproducible findings in psychiatric research. Indeed, studies of Axis I disorders that fail to measure comorbid personality disorders are as methodologically flawed as studies of personality disorders that fail to assess comorbid Axis I disorders.

References

American Psychiatric Association: Diagnostic and Statistical Manual: Mental Disorders. Washington, DC, American Psychiatric Association, 1952

American Psychiatric Association: Diagnostic and Statistical Manual of Mental Disorders, 3rd Edition. Washington, DC, American Psychiatric Association, 1980

American Psychiatric Association: Diagnostic and Statistical Manual of Mental Disorders, 4th Edition. Washington, DC, American Psychiatric Association, 1994

Baer L, Jenike MA, Black DW, et al: Effect of Axis II diagnoses on treatment outcome with clomipramine in 55 patients with obsessive-compulsive disorder. Arch Gen Psychiatry 49:862–866, 1992

Baron M, Gruen R, Asnis L, et al: Familial relatedness of schizophrenia and schizotypal states. Am J Psychiatry 140:1437–1442, 1983

Barrash J, Pfohl B, Blum NA: "Unstable" personality disorders: prognostic implications for major depression. J Personal Disord 7:155–167, 1993

Black DW: A 30 year follow-up of antisocial personality disorder. Paper presented at annual meeting of American Psychiatric Association, San Francisco, May 1993

Clark LA: Resolution of taxonomic issues in personality. J Personal Disord 6:360–376, 1992

Clarkin JF, Hull JW, Hurt SW: Factor structure of borderline personality disorder criteria. J Personal Disord 7:137–143, 1993

Coccaro EF, Siever LJ, Klar HM, et al: Serotonergic studies in patients with affective and personality disorders: correlates with suicidal and impulsive aggressive behavior. Arch Gen Psychiatry 46:587–599, 1989

Coryell W, Endicott J, Keller M: Outcome of patients with chronic affective disorder: a five-year follow-up. Am J Psychiatry 147:1627–1633, 1990

DeJong AJ, van den Brink W, Harteveld FM, et al: Personality disorders in alcoholics and drug addicts. Compr Psychiatry 34:87–94, 1993

Finn SE: Stability of personality self-ratings over 30 years: evidence for an age/cohort interaction. J Pers Soc Psychol 50:813–818, 1986

Gartner AF, Marcus RN, Halmi K, et al: DSM-III-R personality disorders in patients with eating disorders. Am J Psychiatry 146:1585–1591, 1989

Hamilton M: A rating scale for depression. J Neurol Neurosurg Psychiatry 23:56–62, 1960

Hirschfeld MA, Klerman GL, Clayton PF, et al: Assessing personality: effects of depressive state on trait measurement. Am J Psychiatry 140:695–699, 1983

Hirschfeld RMA, Klerman GL, Lavori P, et al: Premorbid personality assessments of first onset of major depression. Arch Gen Psychiatry 46:345–350, 1989

Kendler KS, Gruenberg AM, Strauss JS: An independent analysis of the Copenhagen sample of the Danish adoption study of schizophrenia. II. Relationship between schizotypal personality disorder and schizophrenia. Arch Gen Psychiatry 38:982–984, 1981

Matussek P, Feil WB: Personality attributes of depressive patients. Arch Gen Psychiatry 40:783–790, 1983

McGlashan TH: The Chestnut Lodge follow-up study. III. Long-term outcome of borderline personalities. Arch Gen Psychiatry 43:20–30, 1986

Nace EP, Davis CW, Gaspari JP: Axis II comorbidity in substance abusers. Am J Psychiatry 148:118–120, 1991

Nestadt, G., Romanoski AJ, Merchant CA, et al: An epidemiological study of histrionic personality disorder. Psychol Med 20:413–422, 1990

Noyes R, Reich J, Christiansen J, et al: Outcome of panic disorder: relationship to diagnostic subtypes and comorbidity. Arch Gen Psychiatry 47:809–818, 1990

Paris J, Brown R, Nowlis D: Long-term follow-up of borderline patients in a general hospital. Compr Psychiatry 28:530–535, 1987

Pfohl B, Stangl D, Zimmerman M: The implications of DSM-III personality disorders for patients with major depression. J Affective Disord 7:309–318, 1984.

Pfohl B, Coryell W, Zimmerman M, et al: Prognostic validity of self-report and interview measures of personality in depressed patients. J Clin Psychiatry 48:468–472, 1987

Pilkonis PA, Frank E: Personality pathology in recurrent depression: Nature, prevalence, and relationship to treatment response. Am J Psychiatry 145:435–441, 1988

Reich J, Noyes R Jr, Coryell W, et al: The effect of state anxiety on personality measurement. Am J Psychiatry 143:760–763, 1986

Reich J, Noyes R Jr, Hirschfeld R, et al: State and personality in depressed and panic patients. Am J Psychiatry 144:181–187, 1987

Reich J, Nduaguba M, Yates W: Age and sex distribution of DSM-III personality cluster traits in a community population. Compr Psychiatry 29:298–303, 1988

Shea MT, Pilkonis PA, Beckham E, Collins JF, Elkin I, Sotsky SM, Docherty JP: Personality disorders and treatment outcome in the NIMH Treatment of Depression Collaborative Research Program. Am J Psychiatry 147:711–718, 1990

Siever LJ, Keefe R, Bernstein DP, et al: Eye tracking impairment in clinically identified patient with schizotypal personality disorder. Am J Psychiatry 147:740–745, 1990

Stone MH: Long-term outcome in personality disorders. Br J Psychiatry 162:229–313, 1993

Widiger TA, Trull TJ, Hurt SW, Clarkin JF, Frances A: A multidimensional scaling of the DSM-III personality disorders. Arch Gen Psychiatry 44:741–746, 1989

Zimmerman M, Coryell W: DSM-III personality disorder diagnoses in a nonpatient sample. Arch Gen Psychiatry 46:682–689, 1989

PART II

What Is Normal Personality Structure and Development?

CHAPTER 5

Personality Development in Childhood: Old and New Findings

Patricia Cohen, Ph.D.

This chapter reviews two aspects of personality development in childhood and adolescence. First, age-related changes characteristic of most children are a starting point for understanding how one stage of development grows out of earlier stages. Clearly the sequence, timing, and endpoints are far from immutable, but this normative sequence provides a point of departure for theoretical and empirical work on nonnormative development. The second focus is on the development of individual differences in personality, where issues of origins and stability of individual differences arise. We present in this chapter some new data relevant to individual differences based on the Children in the Community longitudinal study.

The Development of Personality in Childhood

What is it that changes or develops in childhood, and what are the presumed causes of developmental changes? Biologically, the body matures; strength, extension, and coordination increase and permit exploration of the environment; and energy level, physical capacity, and endurance increase. All of these processes change the cognitive structure of a child. At the same time, the child accumulates knowledge of and experience with the surrounding environment. The environment affects and is affected by ongoing interaction with the child. These interactions are reflected in an increasing degree of differentiation and elaboration of the cognitive function and behavior of the child (Werner 1957) and in the generation of scripts for behavior (Tomkins 1987). In addition to changes associated with physiology and experience, the relevant tasks or developmental challenges and modifications of socially prescribed roles effect changes (Caspi and Bem 1990). A number of theorists, drawing upon the tradition of Piaget (1967) in outlining stages of development, have described critical psychosocial tasks to be accomplished as part of personality development during various age periods (e.g., Erikson 1968; Loevinger 1987).

Among the changes most relevant to personality are the development of the self-concept and the certain aspects of emotional function and expression in childhood. Susan Harter (1992) has summarized some of our knowledge in these two areas.

As Harter (1983) has described it, the self is a cognitive structure around which behavior is organized. This construction is a product of the interaction of biological and social forces and therefore undergoes progressive change throughout life. This structure, in turn, serves to organize behavior by providing a sense of continuity over time and by helping the self to develop scripts for behavior. Table 5–1 presents three aspects of the empirical findings on this development.

One aspect of the development of the cognitive self can be seen in how children describe themselves at different ages. In early childhood children describe themselves by their physical characteristics, typical behaviors, or material possessions. During the years from middle childhood to middle adolescence we see the increasing influence of the social environment on self-description. The ability to describe oneself in terms of motives, goals, and beliefs, with less reference to outside standards, develops gradually in adolescence and adulthood.

The valence of evaluation of the self is another aspect of the development of self in the child. Young children are likely to fuse what they are with what they have learned they ought to be. Negative and

TABLE 5–1.

Aspects of the development of self in childhood

	Early childhood	Middle to late childhood	Early to middle adolescence	Late adolescence
Understanding of self (description)	Physical characteristics, possessions, behaviors	Capabilities compared to others	Characteristics related to approval or disapproval	Personal values and beliefs
Valence of self	All positive, fusion of real and ideal	Positive and negative in different domains	Vacillation from positive to negative; conflict between contradictory abstractions	Self positive and negative in different situations; appropriate
Self-criticism	Cannot criticize self	Observes that others negatively evaluate	Preoccupation with others' evaluations, acceptance	Evaluation according to internalized standards

Source. *Adapted from Harter 1992.*

positive characteristics are polar opposites, and the child can't see that a single person may have both. At older ages a child can admit to negative characteristics in one domain while retaining a positive valence in another. Vacillation between positive and negative self-image in earlier adolescence is gradually replaced with an awareness of the importance of context to behavior.

A third aspect of the development of self is self-criticism. The young child who fuses actual and ideal is not capable of self-criticism. In the elementary school years a growing social awareness leads a child to recognize negative evaluations by others, although acceptance of that criticism is not yet likely. In early and middle adolescence acceptance of the criticism of others may be all too likely until the subsequent development of internalized standards and the ability to evaluate oneself more objectively.

At the same time as these cognitive aspects of the self are developing we also see changes in the role and regulation of emotions (Table 5–2).

Emotions organize behavior and shape personality through signaling the self and others and through regulating perceptions and cognitions (Sroufe 1989). In the first months the emotions control the self, as the infant has little ability to self-regulate. Adaptive functioning and normal personality development are facilitated when the organism stays within certain limits of emotional and physiological arousal. This is facilitated by caretakers, whose earliest function may be understood to involve keeping the infant's level of arousal within optimal limits. Beginning in the first year of life and continuing thereafter, a significant function of development is enhancement of self-control over reactions to stimuli. These control efforts appear to have the goal of improving the predictability of both the inner and external environments and thus avoiding the negative experiences of disorganization and disorientation. In later childhood, emotions are interpreted as caused by others, and others are therefore blamed, threatened, or dominated as the child's resources permit. In this period the child is likely to seek the intervention of an adult. In early and middle adolescence the youth attempts to persuade others about the validity of felt emotions, but continues to attempt to avoid or cover over negative emotions. Full emotional maturity is revealed in self-reflection, shared

TABLE 5–2.
Emotional development in childhood

	Early childhood	Middle to late childhood	Early to middle adolescence	Late adolescence
Causes of negative emotion	Actions of others	Other people (actions, not motives)	Motives, feelings, or intentions of others	Interpersonal, intrapersonal
Emotional regulation	Emotions control self: rage	External solution or avoid: blame, threaten, bully	Persuasion, attempt to disperse affect rather than integrate	Self-reflection negative and shared reflection; emotions as cues and signals
Ego development	Impulsive stage	Opportunistic, self-protective, avoid trouble	Conformist, obey rules, avoid social condemnation	Conscientious, inner rules, moral imperatives

Source. Adapted from Harter 1992.

reflection, and in the use of emotions as cues that intrapersonal or interpersonal psychological work needs to be done.

Ego development as viewed by many theorists may also be seen as an aspect of emotional development. Impulsive behavior tends to characterize early childhood. In middle to late childhood, as described by Erikson (1968), Loevinger (1987), and others, opportunistic and self-protective behaviors dominate as the child seeks to avoid getting in trouble or being dominated by others. Subsequent ages reflect the increased role of social comparison and influence by the opinions of others, as these external standards are gradually internalized. The conscientious stage may characterize later adolescence and adulthood, during which inner rules and moral imperatives take on a major behavioral regulatory role.

The concepts of ego control and ego resiliency (Block and Block 1980) tend to be a partial bridge between the developmental perspective and the individual difference focus. Ego control is both a function that tends to develop over a lifetime and a dimension on which persons of a given age tend to vary importantly. As children develop they tend to learn to delay gratification, anticipate the consequences of their actions, and act cautiously when the situation is ambiguous. Children who have less ego control than their age peers have trouble with these tasks and may be at risk for the "externalizing" behavior disorders. At the other extreme, those who overcontrol may be vulnerable to anxiety and depression, as appropriate external expression of their impulses is suppressed. Ego resiliency refers to the organism's response to change, stress, or challenge. Again, it can be expected that the repertoire of adaptive responses increases as the child ages. However, it is also true that children of a given age differ significantly in the extent to which they show resourceful adaptation to change or act inflexibly with perseverative or disorganized behaviors.

Stage-Specific Risks

Once we have identified certain transitions in the developmental process, it makes sense to examine threats to the successful negotiation of these transitions. The development of attachment to caretakers is a critical issue during the first year. Readiness for this task requires differentiation both of self from nonself and of critical caretakers from others. We do not know as yet the cultural boundaries of this task. It is remarkable to see the difference between 8- or 9-month-old infants reacting to the "strange situation," who tend to be unconcerned, and those infants three or four months later who tend to be greatly upset by their mother's absence. Attachment itself is measured by the child's reaction to the mother at reunion.

A substantial effort of developmentalists has been devoted to understanding the attachment process and its risks (Bretherton and Waters 1985). If theorists are correct, we may see a continuity from this early attachment experience to identification with family and other proximal groups in middle to late childhood, and thereafter to attachment to society at large and the development of an individual identification (Feshbach 1991). By continuity we mean that an adaptive response to each transition facilitates the negotiation of the challenge represented by the next stage. Figure 5–1 presents several of the dimensions along which development proceeds, with a rough indication of the timing and importance of various developmental tasks.

Another important set of experiences in the first year is the interactional reciprocity of mother and infant. As noted earlier, the maternal role can be seen as substantially preoccupied with maintaining an optimal level of infant arousal. One aspect of this task occurs in interactive sequences, where mothers tend to excite or soothe depending on the current state of the infant. Again, it is instructive to note the interaction of individual tendencies and environmental effects. Both premature and postmature infants tend to have difficulty in responding reciprocally to the mother's signals (Field 1982). Nevertheless, patient and persistent caretakers can avoid the potential disruption in the normative establishment of attachment (Bretherton and Waters 1985). Mary Main's (1981) excellent discussion of the potential control function of avoidant responses to the mother at reunion may serve to illustrate the connection between stage of emotional development and risk. According to her analysis, these responses to previously unreciprocating or rejecting mothers have the function of controlling the infant's expression of anger toward the mother and thus the counterintuitive

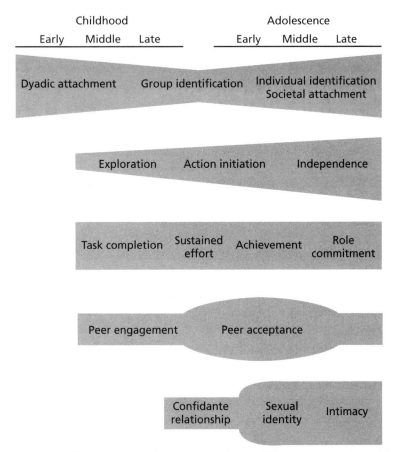

FIGURE 5–1. *Developmental sequences for childhood personality. The thickness of each bar indicates the relative importance of that task compared to other changes occurring during that same period.*

function of maintaining a level of attachment to the needed caretaker. Thus we may see a differentiation even at this age between those infants for whom emotional control has been established, at least in this limited setting and sense, and other poorly attached children whose anger is openly expressed.

Another major dimension begins when infants and toddlers explore objects and the environment . This exploration may evolve into the initiation of action, discussed by Erikson, which begins around ages 3–5. Over time the child learns to explore and initiate activities autonomously. Under optimal socialization experiences the child learns what behaviors are permitted and good and which are bad, thus experiencing shame and conscience and furthering self-control over impulses and emotions. This sequence culminates in the development of independence from caretakers in adolescence.

The development of the skills and habits for task completion are a related trajectory, with school success largely dependent on the ability to apply sustained effort to academic tasks. This effort is expanded in adolescence and adulthood into achievement in domains of special interest and suitability to the individual's capacity, and eventually into commitment to a productive adult role. Erikson (1968) identifies the danger associated with this developmental task of industry to be the emergence of a sense of inferiority. In this light it is interesting to note a connection between the cognitive schemata cultivated in our society and the successful negotiation of this psychosocial task. Our society, stressing individual differences and genetic makeup, has promoted the idea that the major determinant of task success is innate ability. The consequent devaluation of effort may inhibit the development of the habits of industry that have historically characterized our citizens.

Significant peer engagement begins towards the end of early childhood and is moderately important thereafter; however, the strength of ties to the family tend to overwhelm the importance of peers until very late childhood or early adolescence, during which time peer acceptance is of great importance. This importance begins to decline in middle to late adolescence as the youth enters the conscientious stage, with its emphasis on internal standards and moral imperatives (Loevinger 1987).

Another developmental line may be thought of as beginning in late childhood with a close and confiding relationship to selected peers. This line continues with the development of sexual identity in middle adolescence, which is followed by the challenge of intimacy in late adolescence and thereafter (Erikson 1968).

In a sense each of these stage sequences culminates in the development of an individual identity in adolescence and young adulthood in which the self is relatively clearly defined with distinctive traits and capabilities, although it is not seen as static. Identity is most readily established when throughout childhood a comprehensible hierarchy of roles have been presented (Erikson 1968; Harter 1988). The eroding power of clan, ethnicity, and religion in defining a person's proper adult role and broad exposure to a great variety of careers and lifestyles in contemporary Western culture have tended to prolong the establishment of an integrated adult identity, as youth try out a variety of alternatives. It has been shown that early selection of life goals and commitments was predictive of long-term accomplishment and well-being in earlier generations (Clausen 1991). However, it is not clear whether this more extended process will have negative or positive effects on the long-term well-being of the current generation.

In the examination of developmental stage-specific risk it is important to recognize that a developmental transition not well or normatively negotiated does not imply that development is halted at that point. In fact, it never makes sense to think of development as ceasing. Rather, developmentally incompatible environments or events change the trajectory, and development continues along a nonnormative but, in some sense, adaptive pathway.

The Development of Individual Differences in Personality During Childhood

Temperamental Origins of Personality

Personality may be thought of as temperament upon which is overlaid cognitive structures (schemata about the nature of the world and about the nature of oneself), motivational and behavioral patterns that incorporate these basic styles or inclinations in a more or less well-socialized manner, and emotional expression (Buss and Plomin 1975). Temperamental dimensions include relatively stable aspects of individual differences that are thought to be constitutionally based, at least in part. Several researchers have proposed that a genetic basis is an appropriate criterion for the definition of temperamental dimensions (e.g., Buss 1991). Two difficulties have been pointed out with this criterion. First, early childhood is probably the hardest time to identify genetic influences, behavior being so subject to the local influences of internal and external stimuli. Second, at least in later childhood and adulthood it is hard to demonstrate strong differences in trait dimensions with regard to heritabilities (Goldsmith 1983).

As noted elsewhere in this volume, Cloninger (1987) has proposed three primary dimensions, involving behavior initiation, behavior cessation or control, and behavior maintenance. Rothbart (1991) has proposed two dimensions that are somewhat similar to those of Cloninger, reactivity and self-regulation. Other theorists stress the links between emotion and temperament, and Rutter (1987) has focused on the interpersonal aspects of temperament. Aggression, in particular, has been shown to be quite stable from preschool until adolescence (Olweus 1980) and has been proposed for inclusion as a temperament dimension (Rutter 1987). Buss (1991) has tended to emphasize the early traits with the most definite genetic contribution: emotionality, sociability, and activity level. Thus, temperament itself has proved to be somewhat difficult and controversial to define (Strelau and Angleitner 1991). Definitional differences have been accompanied by assessment differences. The investigation of temperament was initiated by Thomas and Chess (1977) and colleagues. They originally proposed nine dimensions (distractibility, persistence, mood, rhythmicity, approach/withdrawal, activity level, adaptability, intensity of reaction, threshold), although they and many other subsequent researchers recognize that these traits can be collapsed into more stable and general factors, and that other individual differences may be as relevant to function. In a literature review Martin et al. (1994) have identified the dimensions common to some of the largest investigations of children at a variety of ages. Factor analyses of individual items from measures covering the Chess and Thomas dimensions have suggested that activity level, task persistence, irritability/manageability, adaptability, and social inhibition/withdrawal are the most common replicable dimensions. These dimensions, in turn, can be collapsed into two more general factors that were originally called *difficult* and *slow to warm up* by Thomas and Chess (1977) and others. These two dimensions are related to those proposed by Cloninger (1987); difficult is probably a combination of behavioral control and behavioral maintenance or reward dependence, while slow to warm up is related to behavioral initiation. Similarly, Rothbart's self-regulation is related to the difficult dimension, while reactivity is related to the slow to warm up conception. Unfortunately it is quite clear that we cannot use factor analysis to determine the "real" number of dimensions, because solutions depend heavily upon the number of factors extracted, as well as the content included in the original items. Thus, it is particularly useful to have theoretically based conceptions to guide us, and these theories should include connections to underlying physiological mechanisms (e.g., Cloninger 1987) or basic functional unities.

Virtually all theorists subscribe to the notion of goodness-of-fit, which suggests that development depends on the fit between the characteristics of the individual and the opportunities and demands presented by the environment. These interactive effects are increasingly complex as the characteristics of the child influence the nature of the environment (Scarr 1992), and environmental characteristics influence the biology of the organism. Thus the tendencies, styles, and expressions that we call temperament gradually acquire cognitive components and become evaluations, attitudes, and habits that are relatively enduring and integrated as personality.

How Stable Is Temperament From the Period of Early Childhood Until Adolescence?

Reviews of the stability of temperament in early childhood (McDevitt 1986) and between early childhood and adolescence and adulthood (Chess and Thomas 1990) have shown that the stability of individual dimensions is not very high and tends to be much less than that of more global dimensions. Significant stability is readily shown over periods of six months to one year in early childhood, but tends to fall off rapidly thereafter. Stability is much increased when temperament measures are pooled over time (Bates et al. 1985), so that, for example, infants who are difficult at both 12 and 18 months are more likely to be difficult at age 36 months than those who were difficult at one but not the other assessment. One of the problems of this research is that the typically small samples of early childhood research may not be sufficiently powerful to detect the small but reliable relationships of these measures over time.

The Relationship Between Temperament and Personality: The Big Five

The field of personality research has been given new energy and direction over the past decade by a near consensus on the main factors that provide the structure within which the myriad of more specific personality traits can be arrayed. Five major, relatively independent dimensions of personality have been identified in studies of adults and in a few studies of children. Reviews of the long history and current status of this work are available (Digman 1989; Goldberg 1993; John 1990). Because these dimensions are presented and discussed elsewhere in this volume (see Chapter 6) we do not review their development here but simply note that a typical set of titles for these factors includes neuroticism/emotionality, extraversion/sociability, agreeableness versus hostility, conscientiousness, and openness to experience/creativity.

Methodological Complications

The literature tends also to be divided between those who focus on dimensions that tend to be approximately normally distributed in the population and those whose concerns are with those most extreme or deviant members of the population (the personality researchers vs. the personality disorder or psychopathology researchers). In the former case the dimensions tend to be measured with items with near-even splits, with a resulting equal focus on both ends of the dimension. In the latter case the measures tend to reflect the presence or absence of a relatively extreme characteristic, and item responses are typically quite skewed.

It is likely that the more symmetrical distributions may be most useful in promoting understanding of normal development. On the other hand, the greater sensitivity to discrimination of the clearly extreme or deviant children may be most useful for identifying the origins and circumstances of problems of psychopathology and resulting service needs. The relatively new field of developmental psychopathology is devoted to determining the accuracy of the presumption that findings based on the population generalize to extreme groups.

New Data on Temperament and Personality in Childhood

Data from the Children in the Community longitudinal study were used to add to our knowledge on the stability and connection between temperament and personality.

Method

The Sample

Families of 976 children ages 1 to 10 were originally randomly sampled based on their residence in two upstate counties of New York in 1975 (Kogan et al. 1977). Leonard Kogan of City University of New York and colleagues designed an interview to measure the problems of children and associated environmental factors with the goal of validating proposed social indicators. A research team led by J. Brook and the author followed up this sample 8, 10, and, most recently, 16 years after the original data collection, interviewing both mothers and youth. About 80% of the original sample is still active in the study; about 75% of those not followed up were among those we were unable to locate because the original interview had not recorded last names. (See Cohen et al. 1993 for a description of sample characteristics and retrieval details.)

Measures of Temperament

The purpose of the original study was to identify the proportion of children in each area who presented clear problems. Eighty-one items reflecting child behavior were factored separately for age and gender groups. The resulting factor structures were sufficiently similar to enable scoring of the same dimensions for these subgroups, although some dimensions are based on slightly different items for different age groups. All scores were standardized by age group. This report is based on eight scales and one item that were scored for children of all ages.

The measures and characteristic items are listed in Table 5–3. They correspond fairly well to the major dimensions found by Martin et al. (1994) in several other published studies. However, because the interview was designed for broad coverage, with relatively few questions for each subject area, the reliabilities are rather poor. We have included aggression to peers for comparison purposes, although it is not usually considered a temperament measure.

As found in other studies, because the temperament measures were correlated with each other, we performed a factor analysis at the scale level. Two factors accounted for the correlations among these scales and corresponded to the dimensions usually labeled difficult and slow to warm up. The first dimension included anger, impulsivity, nonpersistence, and high activity level. The second dimension included fearful, whines/demands, and negative mood, a dimension also related to inhibition/withdrawal as studied by Kagan and colleagues (1988).

Self-Report Personality Measures

At the follow-up interviews we included a number of self-report scales designed to reflect aspects of the child's personality most relevant to mental health problems or substance use or abuse. Because these measures were collected from several sources a certain redundancy was apparent. Therefore we decided to factor the collection of 87 items originally appearing on about 12 scales. The resulting factor structure resembled that found in other studies in large part, but with certain notable differences (see Table 5–3). Given the purposes of the study

TABLE 5–3.

Temperament and personality measures in the Children in the Community study

Scale name	Typical items	Number of items	Reliability
Temperament			
Angry	Cries or complains loudly	6–7	0.30–0.39
Activity level	Moves around a lot when playing	6–7	0.16–0.45
Persistent	Goes back to task when interrupted	3–6	0.52–0.63
Whines/demands	Gets upset at attention to others	6–8	0.46–0.67
Withdrawn	Is timid, fearful	4–5	0.16–0.49
Negative mood	Isn't happy on waking	5–6	NA
Impulsive	Does dangerous things without thinking	1	0.33–0.68
Aggressive	Doesn't get along with peers	4–8	
Personality			
Emotional/neurotic	My feelings are easily hurt.	32	0.87
Sociable/extraverted	Do you usually make friends easily, or do you have trouble making friends?	12	0.66
Conscientious	Preparing for the future is more important for me than enjoying today.	12	0.60
Abrasive/angry	I feel like losing my temper at people.	21	0.79
Slow/dull	Does it take you more time to do things than you or others expect it to?	6	0.56
Confident	I feel that my life is very useful.	17	0.72

and as noted earlier, our measures tend to reflect the problematic end of these dimensions.

Emotional/neurotic, sociability/extraversion, and conscientiousness were readily identified as three of the common factors. The agreeableness factor is represented here negatively by a factor we called abrasive, reflecting hostility, anger, and aggression; the positive end of this bipolar dimension was not included in this study. We did not directly measure the creativity-openness-culture dimension, again reflecting the relative absence of positive descriptors in this domain. However, we found a factor we call slow/dull that may reflect the negative end of the openness factor, at least in part. The factor we called confident, including items of internal locus of control, optimism, and self-esteem, may be similar to the positive affectivity dimension proposed by Tellegen (1985).

Although these common factors are a reasonable match for the presumably nearly orthogonal Big Five personality factors, they were not uncorrelated in these data. We therefore factored the six scales and obtained a clear two-factor solution (see John 1990 for presentation of some other matches between two- and five-factor solutions). The first factor we called ego control as it seems to be a fair match for that construct described by Block and Block (1980). Scales that loaded on this dimension were emotional/neurotic, abrasive, and slow/underachievement (all in the low ego control direction). The second dimension we labeled ego resiliency, again following the Blocks. High loading measures were conscientious, confident, and sociable/extroverted. It is also noteworthy that the scales loading on the first factor were generally composed of negative statements about the self, whereas the scales loading on the second were generally composed of positive statements about the self.

Findings

Temperament Correlations With Age

Because the item sets measuring temperament varied slightly for the 1 year olds, 2–4 year olds, and 5–10 year olds, temperament scores were standardized within each age subgroup, and age changes cannot be examined for the full sample. However, we examined the age correlations within the group of 5–10 year olds and found only one significant age correlation. Aggression toward peers slightly declined with age ($r = -0.09$) according to maternal report. None of the true temperament measures were age related in these early years. Because it is very likely that at least some of these behaviors do change in an absolute sense (for example, impulsive and persistent) we presume that mothers are essentially "correcting for age" when they respond to the questions. When these same questions were asked of the mothers when the children were ages 9–18 several of the measures were negatively correlated with age, including activity level (-0.11), whines/demands (-0.34), anger (-0.14), and aggressive (-0.20).

Stability of Temperament Over an Eight-Year Span

Figure 5–2 provides the correlations with the reassessment eight years later for the total sample and for the younger (originally ages 1–4) and older (ages 5–10) subgroups. All correlation coefficients are statistically significant and have been adjusted for any age effects (but not for unreliability). As can be seen, the highest stabilities were found in the withdrawn, angry, and whines/demands (low adaptability) dimensions. Stabilities tend to be only slightly smaller for the younger children than they are for the older ones. Negative mood tends to be distinctly less stable than most of the other traits. Its instability may have been a consequence of the psychometric weakness of this scale, and it should be replicated with a stronger measure before we conclude that negative mood is less stable than other temperament dimensions. We have included aggression toward peers here for comparison purposes, although it is generally not considered a dimension of temperament. However, several other temperament dimensions were at least as stable as aggression.

We also examined potential gender differences in the stability of temperament, but found none. In addition, we examined the stability of the two more general factors: the correlation over the eight-year span

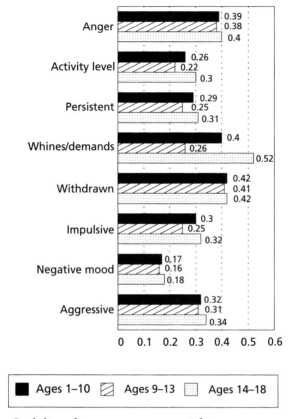

FIGURE 5–2. *Stability of temperament over eight years.*

was 0.42 for both the difficult and the inhibited factors for the total group of children. However, examination of stability in those ages 1–4 and those ages 5–10 showed that whereas the difficult factor was equally stable for younger and older children, the inhibited factor was more stable for older children ($r = 0.47$) than for the younger children ($r = 0.34$), adjustment for age-related changes in means having been made.

In these analyses we have used mothers as the informant regarding the characteristics of the child; therefore, we do not know to what extent the stability in the measures reflects real stability in the child or only stability of the mother's view of the child. This consistency in informant may account for the fact that the stability coefficients are only slightly higher for older children than for younger children.

Early Childhood Temperament as Predictors of Adolescent Personality

There are several reasons why we might expect these relationships to be much smaller. First, there tends to be a change in the level of abstraction, with temperament involving more basic behavioral description. Second, the informant was changed from mother to self-report. Third, the instrument and format are changed, and, as noted earlier, our personality items tend to focus on the pathological extreme rather than on the full distribution of each dimension. Temperament measures were more nearly normally distributed.

We generally found that relationships were higher between the T1 assessments at ages 1–10 and the T3 measures 10 years later than they were between the T1 and T2 measures. This is, of course, contrary to the general rule-of-thumb that more temporally distant measures are less correlated than less temporally distant measures. We take this to reflect the improving validity of the self-reports as the youths mature, as it was particularly true for the younger subsample. However, we should not be surprised that the relationships were all quite modest.

Because of the large number of individual correlations examined here we have used set correlation and replication across age groups and between T2 and T3 as additional criteria for reporting significant relationships, in order to control Type 1 errors. Reported correlations were at least 0.12 and generally less than 0.20.

The set correlation between temperament and personality was significant for the total group (multivariate $R^2 = 0.122$) and for both the younger children ($R^2 = 0.146$) and the older children ($R^2 = 0.179$). Each of the personality dimensions was related significantly to temperament a decade earlier, although the prediction of conscientiousness was marginal.

Those relationships that were present in both older and younger children are shown in Table 5–4.

First, looking at predictions from the higher-order difficult and inhibited measures, the findings are theoretically expectable: children who were more difficult were more neurotic, abrasive, and lower achievers. Children who were more inhibited were more introverted, less conscientious, and had lower levels of self-confidence.

TABLE 5–4.

Significant relationships between early temperament and adolescent personality

Temperament age 1–10		
Factor	Scale	Adolescent personality
Difficult	High activity	Emotional/neurotic
		Abrasive
		Low intellect/achievement
Inhibited	Persists/complies	Introversion
	Whines/demands	Introversion, low confidence
	Fearful	Low intellect/achievement

Note. *Only relationships that were significant (P < .05) in both the older and younger subsamples are reported here.*

Turning to the individual scales, perhaps the biggest surprise was that high activity level in early childhood was a risk for later problems, whereas high anger was not consistently a risk, although it was in the older subsample. Impulsivity similarly was not consistent; it appeared to be a risk for some kinds of problems in the younger sample and for different problems in the older sample.

We examined the relationship between the two general temperament factors, difficult and inhibited, and the two general personality factors, ego control and ego resilience. Difficult children were significantly more likely to have low ego control as adolescents ($r = 0.182$) and inhibited children were significantly more likely to be low on ego resilience as adolescents ($r = -0.190$). These relationships were slightly, but not significantly, smaller for the children who were ages 1–4 at the first assessment than they were for the children who were ages 5–10.

Age Changes and Stability of Personality in Late Childhood and Adolescence

A number of the personality measures showed linear or curvilinear correlations with age, and these were generally consistent at each of the assessments. Older youth tended to report themselves as *less* goal directed than did younger youth at each assessment ($r = -0.12$ and -0.19, respectively). This is, of course, contrary to the expectation that as youth establish an identity they commit themselves to life goals. On the other hand, older adolescents reported themselves as more self-confident ($r = 0.20$ and 0.23, respectively). All other significant age differences were quadratic in shape. Abrasiveness showed a maximum at about age 15 according to both the T2 and T3 assessments. The general ego control factor showed a similar pattern, with lowest levels of self-reported ego control in midadolescence. Emotionality/neuroticism was fairly stable except among late adolescents, among whom it was lower. Underachievement showed a very similar pattern, possibly reflecting the decline in feelings of inadequacy that accompanies the termination of schooling in some youth.

As we would expect from both the older ages and the shorter interval, the personality dimensions in this study were somewhat more stable than the temperament measures had been over the previous period (Figure 5–3). Once again we found higher stabilities for the older children, and the differences tended to be larger than those seen

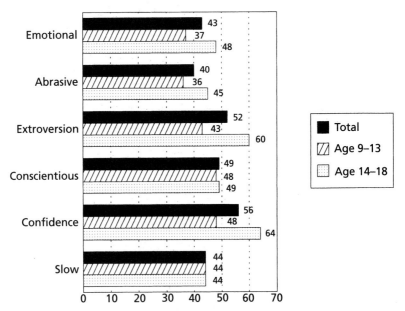

FIGURE 5–3. *Stability of personality over a 2½-year interval.*

on the temperament measures. The higher stabilities in the older children are probably due to a combination of true higher stability in this postpubertal group and higher reliability and validity of the older youths' responses to the personality questions. The measure of self-confidence, which is not one of the Big Five, was the most stable of the dimensions. The relatively lower stability for the slow/underachieving measure suggests that it does measure something other than IQ, which is more stable. This measure may be reactive to changes in school attendance and status. We also examined the stability of the more general ego control and ego resiliency factors and found their stabilities to be 0.50 and 0.63, respectively.

Summary and Discussion of Empirical Findings

In sum, we found modest but significant stability of temperament from early childhood to eight years later for each of the scales examined. These early childhood measures also tended to predict self-reported personality a decade later when it was assessed with a very different instrument, even when children had been as young as age 1–4 at the time of the original assessment. Few other data have shown significant prediction over such a period from such a young age. When teacher ratings of boys' aggressiveness and withdrawal were combined over the first three years of school, they were significantly predicted by avoidant attachment at 18 months (Renken et al. 1989). This was approximately a five-year interval. The findings reported here are not inconsistent with other findings, but reflect the smaller standard errors associated with the unusually large sample size (Lerner and Tubman 1989).

Personality measured by self-report showed moderate to good stability over a 2½-year period, even when the children were as young as ages 9–13 at the time of the first assessment. The previous literature on the stability of personality in childhood has primarily employed teacher or peer ratings or other observational data (Digman 1989; West and Graziano 1989), and stability has tended to be comparable or lower over a period such as the one employed in this study. A number of studies have failed to find significant relationships over a span of four or more years in childhood (e.g., Rubin et al. 1989) but small sample sizes have made such findings ambiguous. The relatively higher stabilities here suggest that a fairly stable self-concept has developed by the late childhood and early adolescent years.

On the whole some pairs of temperament and personality dimensions shared a certain similarity. However, the similarity was even more striking when the two more general factors in each set were examined. The two general factors of temperament and personality are consistent with the ego control and ego resilience described and measured by Block and Block (1980).

Age changes in the personality measures in adolescence were often striking. The decline of self-described conscientiousness over the course of adolescence may reflect the lessening of the strong influence of social conformity that characterized younger adolescents. On the other hand, abrasiveness, and more generally ego control, was most troublesome for those in middle adolescence. This peak may arise from the combination of increasing freedom from adult restraint and supervision and increasingly complex demands for academic and social performance. These problems of heightened emotionality and achievement stress tended to decline in late adolescence as identity is established and new roles become familiar.

References

Bates JE, Maslin CA, Frankel KA: Attachment security, mother-child interaction, and temperament as predictors of behavior-problem ratings at age three years, in Growing Points of Attachment Theory and Research. Edited by Bretherton I, Waters E. Monogr Soc Res Child Dev 50:167–193, 1985

Block JH, Block J: The role of ego-control and ego-resiliency in the organization of behavior, in Minnesota Symposium on Child Psychology, 13. Edited by Collins WA. Hillsdale, NJ, Lawrence Erlbaum Associates, 1980, pp 39–101

Bretherton I, Waters E (eds): Growing points of attachment theory and research. Monogr Soc Res Child Dev 50(1–2, Serial No. 209), 1985

Buss AH: The EAS theory of temperament, in Explorations in Temperament. Edited by Strelau J, Angleitner A. New York, Plenum, 1991

Buss AH, Plomin R: A Temperament Theory of Personality Development. New York, Wiley, 1975

Caspi A, Bem DJ: Personality continuity and change across the life course, in Handbook of Personality Theory and Research. Edited by Pervin LA. New York, Guilford, 1990, pp 549–575

Chess S, Thomas A: Continuities and discontinuities in temperament, in Straight and Devious Pathways from Childhood to Adulthood. Edited by Robins L, Rutter M. Cambridge, England, Cambridge University Press, 1990, pp 205–220

Clausen JS: Adolescent competence and the shaping of the life course. Am J Sociol 96:805–842, 1991

Cloninger CR: A systematic method for clinical description and classification of personality variants. Arch Gen Psychiatry 44:573–588, 1987

Cohen P, Cohen J, Kasen S, et al: An epidemiological study of disorders in late childhood and adolescence. 1. Age and gender specific prevalence. J Child Psychol Psychiatry 34:851–867, 1993

Digman J: Five robust trait dimensions: Development, stability, and utility. J Pers 57: 195–214, 1989

Erikson EH: Identity: Youth and Crisis. New York, WW Norton, 1968

Feshbach S: Attachment processes in adult political ideology: patriotism and nationalism, in Intersections with Attachment. Edited by Gewirtz JL, Kurtines WM. Hillsdale, NJ, Lawrence Erlbaum Associates, 1991, pp 207–226

Field T: Affective displays of high-risk infants during early interactions, in Emotion and Early Interaction. Edited by Field T, Fogel A. Hillsdale, NJ, Lawrence Erlbaum Associates, 1982, pp 101–125

Goldberg L: The structure of phenotypic personality traits. Am Psychol 48:26–34, 1993

Goldsmith H: Genetic influences on personality from infancy to adulthood. Child Dev 54:331–355, 1983

Harter S: Developmental perspectives on the self-system, in Handbook of Child Psychology, Volume IV, Socialization, Personality, and Social Development. Edited by Hetherington EM. New York, Wiley, 1983, pp 275–385

Harter S: Developmental processes in the construction of the self, in Integrative Processes and Socialization: Early to Middle Childhood. Edited by Yawkey TD, Johnson JE. Hillsdale, NJ, Lawrence Erlbaum Associates, 1988, pp 45–78

Harter S: Dimensions of self and emotional development. Presentation at NIMH-sponsored conference, Developmental Approaches to the Assessment of Psychopathology. Bethesda, MD, November 30, 1992

John O: The "Big Five" factor taxonomy: dimensions of personality in the natural language and in questionnaires, in Handbook of Personality Theory and Research. Edited by Pervin LA. New York, Guilford, 1990, pp 66–100

Kagan J, Reznick JS, Snidman N: Biological bases of childhood shyness. Science 240:324–370, 1988

Kogan L, Smith J, Jenkins S: Ecological validity of indicator data as predictors of survey findings. J Soc Serv Res 1:117–132, 1977

Lerner RM, Tubman JG: Conceptual issues in studying continuity and discontinuity in personality development across life. J Pers 57:343–373, 1989

Loevinger J: Paradigms of Personality. New York, WH Freeman, 1987

Main M: Avoidance in the service of attachment: a working paper, in Behavioral Development. Edited by Immelmann K, Barlow GW, Petrinovich L, Main M. Cambridge, England, Cambridge University Press, 1981, pp 651–693

Martin R, Wisenbaker J, Huttunen M: Review of factor analytic studies of temperament measures based on the Thomas-Chess structural model: implications for the Big Five, in The Developing Structure of Temperament and Personality From Infancy to Adulthood. Edited by Halvorsen C, Kohnstamin GA, Martin R. Hillsdale, NJ, Lawrence Erlbaum Associates, 1994

McDevitt S: Continuity and discontinuity of temperament in infancy and early childhood: a psychometric perspective, in The Study of Temperament: Changes, Continuities and Challenges. Edited by Plomin R, Dunn J. Hillsdale, NJ, Lawrence Erlbaum Associates, 1986, pp 27–38

Olweus D: Familial and temperamental determinants of aggressive behavior in adolescent boys: a causal analysis. Dev Psychol 16:644–660, 1980

Piaget J: Six Psychological Studies. New York, Random House, 1967

Renkin B, Egeland B, Marvinney D, et al: Early childhood antecedents of aggression and passive-withdrawal in early elementary school. J Pers 57:257–281, 1989

Rothbart M: Temperament: a developmental framework, in Explorations in Temperament. Edited by Strelau J, Angleitner A. New York, Plenum, 1991, pp 61–74

Rubin KH, Hymel S, Mills RSL: Sociability and social withdrawal in childhood: stability and outcomes. J Pers 57:237–255, 1989

Rutter M: Temperament, personality, and personality disorder. Br J Psychiatry 150:443–458, 1987

Scarr S: Personality and experience, in The Emergence of Personality. Edited by Aronoff J, Rabin AI, Zucker RA. New York, Springer, 1992, pp 49–78

Sroufe LA: Pathways to adaptation and maladaptation: psychopathology as developmental deviation, in The Emergence of a Discipline: Rochester Symposium on Developmental Psychopathology. Edited by Cicchetti D. Hillsdale, NJ, Lawrence Erlbaum Associates, 1989, pp 13–40

Strelau J, Angleitner A: Explorations in Temperament: International Perspectives on Theory and Measurement. New York, Plenum, 1991

Tellegen A: Structures of mood and personality and their relevance in assessing anxiety, with an emphasis on self-report, in Anxiety and the Anxiety Disorders. Edited by Tuma AH, Maser JD. Hillsdale, NJ, Lawrence Erlbaum Associates, 1985, pp 681–716

Thomas A, Chess S: Temperament and Development. New York, Brunner/Mazel, 1977

Tomkins SS: Script theory, in The Emergence of Personality. Edited by Aronoff J, Rabin AI, Zucker RA. New York, Springer, 1987, pp 147–216

Werner H: The concept of development from a comparative and organismic point of view, in The Concept of Development. Edited by Harris DB. Minneapolis, University of Minnesota Press, 1957, pp 125–148

West SG, Graziano WG: Long-term stability and change in personality: an introduction. J Pers 57:175–193, 1989

CHAPTER 6

Continuity and Change Over the Adult Life Cycle: Personality and Personality Disorders

Paul T. Costa Jr., Ph.D.

Robert R. McCrae, Ph.D.

Ilene C. Siegler, Ph.D., M.P.H.*

This chapter is based on three sets of findings that tie together the fields of personality psychology and psychiatry. The first, based on 40 years of factor analytic studies, is that at the highest level individual differences in personality can be described in terms of five broad factors that we call neuroticism, extraversion, openness to experience, agreeableness, and conscientiousness. The five-factor model has been the subject of two *Annual Review* chapters (Digman 1990; Wiggins and Pincus 1992), a special issue of the *Journal of Personality* (McCrae 1992), and dozens of research articles (e.g., Costa and McCrae 1992a). It is a descriptive model derived originally from analyses of natural language trait terms, but it is equally effective in summarizing common themes from questionnaires designed to measure personality from a surprisingly wide variety of different theoretical perspectives (Costa

*Dr. Siegler's work is supported by Grants 1 R01AG12458 from the National Institute on Aging and 1 R01 HL55356 and 1 P01 HL36587 from the National Heart, Lung and Blood Institute.

and McCrae, in press; McCrae 1989), including the needs of Henry Murray (1938), the temperaments of J. P. Guilford (Guilford et al. 1976), the functions and attitudes of C. J. Jung (1923/1971), and the biosocial theory of Robert Cloninger (1988).

The second, much more recent discovery is that these same five factors are strongly linked to the DSM-III-R (American Psychiatric Association 1987) personality disorders (PDs). Since Wiggins and Pincus published the first empirical demonstration in 1989 there have been many confirmations using a variety of measures of the PDs in both normal and clinical samples (e.g., Trull 1992). The extent and interpretation of the links between the five-factor model and disorders of personality is examined at length in a recent book (Costa and Widiger 1994). At a minimum, these findings make it clear that research on normal personality traits is of direct relevance to an understanding of psychopathology.

The third major finding, to which this chapter is largely devoted, is the remarkable stability of personality traits in adulthood. In the 1970s and 1980s, researchers began to publish the results of longitudinal studies that had been initiated in the 1950s and 1960s (Block 1971; Douglas and Arenberg 1978; Finn 1986; Siegler et al. 1979). Despite wide differences in measures, subjects, and periods of the life span studied, all these studies concurred in finding relatively little change in the average level of personality traits and surprisingly high stability of individual differences. Barring interventions or catastrophic events, personality traits appear to be essentially fixed after age 30.

To illustrate the kind of research on which this conclusion is based, we present in some detail new longitudinal data on personality stability from the Baltimore Longitudinal Study of Aging (BLSA) and summarize other research that complements it. We then discuss the issue of continuity and change in the period from adolescence to adulthood and present data from the University of North Carolina (UNC) Alumni Heart Study that speak both to continuity and change in personality between college and the mid-40s, and to the links between the five-factor model and the PDs.

Longitudinal Analyses of the California Q-Set

In 1961 Jack Block published a book called *The Q-Sort Method in Personality Assessment and Psychiatric Research*. The real contribution of the volume was not the Q-sort method—a technique attributable to Stephenson (1953) in which items are ranked in a forced distribution—but the set of items that were to be sorted. Over a period of years, Block and his colleagues had attempted to create a language for personality description that would suffice to communicate all socially or clinically significant aspects of personality. One mark of his success is that each of the five basic factors is well represented in the items. Block tried to avoid statements that were intelligible only within a limited theoretical perspective, hoping that sheer description might help bridge the gap between different schools.

The result was the California Q-Set (CQS; Block 1961). It was originally designed for use by expert raters, but in 1978 Bem and Funder devised a modification of the instrument for self-reports. Essentially, they added clarifying language whenever the original items appeared too technical to be understood by laypersons.

In either version, the instrument uses a Q-sort format. Its 100 items, each printed on a separate card, must be sorted into nine categories, ranging from *extremely uncharacteristic* to *extremely characteristic*; the number of items in each category is specified in advance—five items in the first, eight in the second, and so on. The resulting distribution is approximately normal, and represents the relative salience of various characteristics in the individual's personality. The forced distribution means that the instrument is less susceptible to the influence of certain response sets, such as acquiescence and extreme responding, than are questionnaires that use Likert scales. However, it also can distort the depiction of personality: If 25 items are in fact equally characteristic of an individual, they must arbitrarily be sorted into different categories.

Between August 1981 and January 1985 we administered the self-report version of the CQS to 403 men and women in the BLSA (Shock et al. 1984). Our analyses of these data showed that the five factors could be recovered from CQS data and that the resulting factor scores showed convergent and discriminant validity with alternate measures of the factors (McCrae et al. 1986). They were also significantly correlated with factor scores derived from expert ratings on the CQS based on brief stress and coping interviews conducted on a subset of subjects (McCrae 1991).

Traditionally, a six-year retest interval has been used in the psychological studies of the BLSA (e.g., Douglas and Arenberg 1978), so we instituted repeat Q-sorts in 1987. By the end of 1992, valid retest data had been obtained on 206 men initially aged 20–83, and 67 women initially aged 17–80. The retest intervals ranged from 5.4 to 10.0 years, with a mean interval of 6.6 years.

Stability of the Configuration

In the Q-sort method, items are contrasted with other items to determine which are more salient in the description of the individual. For example, sorters must decide whether the person is better characterized by the statement "Is critical, skeptical, not easily impressed," or by the statement "Is fastidious." Even if one is not very fastidious, one may be more fastidious than skeptical, and if so, the latter item should be sorted higher than the former. The result of all these comparative judgments is a pattern that is intended to capture the unique personality configuration of the individual.

Therefore, a useful way to begin the analysis of these data is to calculate Q-correlations across occasions. That is, for each individual, the item scores at Time 1 and Time 2 are correlated across the 100 items, yielding an index of the consistency of the entire configuration of personality traits.[1] Q-correlations across occasions ranged from 0.12

---

[1]In some respects this procedure may inflate estimates of stability, because the items have different difficulty levels. The item "Is a genuinely dependable and responsible person" is almost always given a high placement, whereas the item "Is guileful and deceitful, manipulative, opportunistic" is almost always considered uncharacteristic; because these item placements are relatively constant, Q-correlations are likely to be positive across any pair of sorts.

to 0.86 with a median of 0.72 for women and 0.71 for men; over three-quarters of the sample had values of 0.60 or higher.[2]

Block's (1971) data provide a useful comparison. He obtained CQS ratings of men and women in junior high school, senior high school, and in the decade of their 30s. When corrected for interrater unreliability, the mean Q-correlations between senior high school and adulthood were 0.56 for men and 0.54 for women. The notably higher levels of Q-correlations seen in the present data may be due to the use of self-reports on both occasions, the shorter retest interval, or the older initial age of our subjects. We can conclude that adults show substantial stability in the configuration of self-reported personality characteristics, at least over a six-year interval.

Of course, there may be exceptions to this generalization. Another way to look at individual Q-sorts is by noting items that change dramatically across occasions. If an item was rated *quite* or *extremely uncharacteristic* at one time and *quite* or *extremely characteristic* at the other, it could be interpreted as evidence of personality change. But this pattern was rare. Of 273 subjects, 239 never showed the pattern, 30 showed it only once, and 3 twice. One subject had four such changes: In 1983 she described herself as hesitant to act, interpersonally distant, self-indulgent, and emotionally bland; whereas in 1989 she considered these among her least characteristic attributes. Are these real changes in personality, or sorting errors? More information—from other observers or additional self–Q-sorts—would be needed to answer that question. In any case, the analysis of item positions makes it clear that the vast majority of adults show little evidence of marked change in any aspect of their personality.

Because most personality measures do not employ Q-sort methods, questions about the stability of trait configurations are rarely asked.

---

[2]In preliminary analyses, five subjects were identified with negative Q-correlations, ranging from −0.06 to −0.77. Unless we are prepared to believe that these individuals had undergone the most profound alterations in every aspect of their personalities over a six-year interval, we must suspect that there is a problem with the data. In our experience, sorting 100 cards into 9 categories is a difficult task, and it is easy to imagine that some of these individuals made the simple mistake of reversing the order of the categories on one of the two occasions. These cases were therefore considered invalid and removed from the analyses. Had they been retained, stability coefficients for the five CQS scales would still have ranged from 0.67 to 0.73 in the total group (cf. Table 6–2).

Instead, longitudinal analyses of personality typically focus on two other questions: Do individuals preserve the same rank ordering over time? and does the group as a whole increase or decrease? The former question is addressed by correlating scores at Time 2 with scores at Time 1; high correlations mean stability of rank order. The latter question can be addressed through cross-sectional comparisons or repeated measures analyses of variance in longitudinal studies; stability of mean levels is indicated by nonsignificant mean differences or changes. Both kinds of analyses are appropriate for the items of the CQS and for scales composed of CQS items.

Stability of Individual Differences

Correlations of test scores on two occasions are interpreted as retest reliability when the two occasions are days or weeks apart—when, that is, it is reasonable to assume that there has been no change in true standing on the measure. Retest reliabilities for personality scales are typically in the range of 0.7 to 0.9 (e.g., McCrae and Costa 1983), which may be regarded as a ceiling on stability coefficients. Single items are inherently less reliable than composite scales, so stability coefficients should also be lower.

When analyses were conducted separately for men and for women, retest correlations were positive and significant for all 100 items in the large sample of men; all of the correlations were positive and 95 of them were significant in the smaller sample of women. The median retest correlation was 0.44 for men and 0.48 for women.

Again, these results can be compared to Block's (1971) findings. Between senior high school and adulthood, the median item retest correlation was 0.26 for men and 0.25 for women. Even when corrected for attenuation the median values, both 0.38, are appreciably smaller than those found in the present study. Adults seem to show more stability than adolescents.

Although our data show general evidence of stability at the item level, there is certainly differentiation among the items—some are more stable than others. The rank-order correlation between stability coefficients in men and in women was 0.48, $P < .001$, suggesting that these differences in stability are replicable. The ten most and least stable items (based on the combined sample) are given in Table 6–1.

The most stable items include such characteristics as talkativeness, compassion, conservatism, and interest in the opposite sex. There are no neuroticism items in this group, but the other four factors are all

TABLE 6–1.

Most and least stable CQS items

CQS item	Six-year retest correlation		
	Men	Women	Total
Most stable			
80. Interested in opposite sex	0.61	0.39	0.59
58. Enjoys sensuous experiences	0.61	0.59	0.61
7. Favors conservative values[a]	0.61	0.59	0.61
26. Is productive	0.61	0.68	0.63
51. Values intellectual matters[a]	0.62	0.69	0.64
35. Has warmth; compassionate	0.59	0.74	0.64
52. Behaves in assertive fashion	0.65	0.68	0.65
18. Initiates humor[a]	0.66	0.72	0.67
4. Is talkative[a]	0.69	0.70	0.69
98. Verbally fluent[a]	0.73	0.74	0.73
Least stable			
76. Tends to project feelings[b]	0.17	0.17[c]	0.17
69. Is sensitive to demands[b]	0.15	0.24	0.17
61. Creates and exploits dependency[b]	0.21	0.06[c]	0.18
36. Is subtly negativistic[b]	0.28	0.24	0.27
12. Self-defensive[b]	0.25	0.38	0.28
50. Unpredictable and changeable	0.23	0.42	0.28
32. Aware of impression on others[b]	0.28	0.26	0.29
22. Feels lack of meaning in life	0.23	0.47	0.29
38. Has hostility toward others	0.26	0.45	0.31
87. Interprets situations in complicated ways	0.39	0.11[c]	0.32

Note. N = 206 *men, 67 women. Except as noted, all correlations are significant,* P < .05.
[a]*One of 15 items showing most interjudge agreement in Funder and Colvin 1988.*
[b]*One of 15 items showing least interjudge agreement in Funder and Colvin 1988.*
[c]*NS.*

represented. Considering that these are individual items, the magnitude of the retest correlations—ranging from 0.59 to 0.73 in the full sample—is remarkable. These data nicely illustrate the basic finding of stability in adult personality.

It is tempting to interpret the least stable items as measuring characteristics that change in adulthood. Tendencies to project feelings onto others, to create and exploit dependency, to be negativistic, self-defensive, and sensitive to anything that can be construed as a demand appear to be undesirable, perhaps pathological traits, and the data in Table 6–1 might suggest that these maladaptive characteristics show little temporal consistency. Could they represent transient psychopathological episodes? Perhaps.

But there is an alternative interpretation: Perhaps these items cannot be easily understood by lay raters and thus show low reliability. Is it reasonable to expect individuals to know whether they project their feelings and motivations? Projection is a defense, and the use of defense mechanisms is supposed to be unconscious. Again, what exactly does it mean to be "sensitive to anything that can be construed as a demand?" Who so construes it, and what does "sensitive" mean? Anxious? Resentful? Vigilant? If individuals cannot interpret an item meaningfully, they are unlikely to respond consistently to it.

There is powerful evidence that this alternative interpretation is correct. In 1988 Funder and Colvin reported a study of interjudge agreement between self-reports and ratings by strangers and friends that might be regarded as a study of item reliability at a single point in time. They listed the 15 CQS items showing the highest average interjudge agreement and the 15 items showing the lowest. As the footnotes to Table 6–1 show, 5 of the 10 items we found to be most stable were among the 15 items Funder and Colvin found to be most reliable across judges; at the same time, 6 of the 10 items we found to be least stable were among the 15 items they found to be least reliable.

The implication is that stability can only be adequately assessed using reliable measures, and scales that aggregate a number of items are likely to be more reliable than individual items. McCrae et al. (1986) provided a way of scoring the five major dimensions of personality from CQS items (see their Table 2, pp. 436–437) using the Time 1 data discussed here. When these scales are created in the present samples for both occasions, the internal consistency coefficients range from 0.59 for openness at Time 2 to 0.86 for neuroticism at Time 1, with a median of 0.73. These are acceptable, though not high, levels of internal consistency, and point to the breadth of content in the scales—a breadth appropriate for measures of the five factors.

Table 6–2 gives the retest correlations for these five scales. Ranging from 0.66 to 0.83, these values are comparable to those found in questionnaire studies using self-reports and observer ratings (Costa and McCrae 1988, 1992c). Further, these values are close to the short-term retest reliability of most personality measures. Given the fallibility of measurement, the stability coefficients in Table 6–2 are about as high as they could possibly be.

Stability of Mean Levels

The analyses in Tables 6–1 and 6–2 concerned the stability of rank ordering of individuals. They do not speak to the question of change in mean level, that is, personality changes that affect the group as a whole in a consistent direction. To take a trivial but revealing example, there was a dramatic change in the age of the sample—mean age at Time 2 being about 6.6 years higher than mean age at Time 1—but the correlation of Time 1 age with Time 2 age is essentially 1.0. Change in mean level is fully compatible with stability in rank ordering.

TABLE 6–2.
Stability coefficients for CQS scales measuring the five-factor model

CQS	Six-year retest correlation		
scale	Men	Women	Total
Neuroticism	0.70	0.81	0.75
Extraversion	0.78	0.78	0.78
Openness to experience	0.74	0.81	0.76
Agreeableness	0.74	0.83	0.77
Conscientiousness	0.75	0.66	0.73

Note. N = 206 men, 67 women. All correlations are significant at P < .001.

Longitudinal studies give direct information on changes in mean levels, but valuable indirect evidence is provided by cross-sectional studies, in which young individuals are compared with old. In the present study, with a continuous age distribution from the 20s to the 80s, correlations of personality scores with age provide a simple summary of age differences that may be due to maturational processes. When the 100 CQS items are correlated with age at Time 1, 24 of them are statistically significant ($P < .05$), but some of these correlations are probably attributable to chance. Corresponding correlations at Time 2 show that 9 of the 24 are replicable. As Table 6–3 shows, these items suggest that older men and women have a certain stodginess: They are moralistic, emotionally bland, and unvarying in their roles. By contrast, younger members of the sample enjoy sensuous experiences, try to push and stretch limits, and eroticize situations. At

TABLE 6–3.

Correlations between age and CQS items and scales

CQS	Correlation with age	
measure	Time 1	Time 2
Items		
41. Is moralistic	0.16*	0.20**
51. Values intellectual matters	0.19**	0.22**
58. Enjoys sensuous experiences	−0.24**	−0.28**
65. Tries to stretch limits	−0.21**	−0.21**
70. Behaves ethically	0.16*	0.19**
73. Eroticizes situations	−0.18**	−0.12*
90. Concerned with philosophical problems	0.19**	0.16**
97. Emotionally bland	0.24**	0.17**
100. Does not vary roles	0.17**	0.15**
Scales		
Neuroticism	−0.11	−0.06
Extraversion	−0.09	−0.12*
Openness to experience	−0.03	−0.05
Agreeableness	0.06	0.11
Conscientiousness	0.21**	0.18**

Note. N = 273. *Only CQS items significantly related to age at both times are reported.*
*$P < .05$. ** $P < .01$.

the level of CQS scales, older individuals appear to be consistently higher in conscientiousness.

All of these correlations are small, however, and like all cross-sectional data, they are subject to alternative interpretations. Older individuals were raised in a more conservative era, and their responses may well reflect generational differences rather than age changes. One way to test that hypothesis is by examining longitudinal changes. If the age differences are due to maturational changes, they should be replicated in longitudinal analyses; if they are due to generational differences (or to other effects such as sample bias) they would generally not be replicated.

Paired *t*-tests provide a statistically powerful way to detect changes over time. Over the 6.6-year interval, only one of the nine CQS items in Table 6–3 showed a significant change: On average, members of the sample scored a bit higher on item 97, replicating the cross-sectional finding that people become slightly less emotional with age. The other age differences are most parsimoniously interpreted as generational or sampling differences. At the level of CQS scales, there was no evidence that individuals became higher in conscientiousness over the interval (despite the suggestion from the cross-sectional findings), nor were there any significant changes in extraversion, openness, or agreeableness. There was a significant decline in neuroticism amounting to about one-fifth of one standard deviation; this effect was not seen in the cross-sectional analyses. Overall, then, it seems fair to conclude that there is very little age-associated change in adult personality as measured by the CQS.

Other Evidence of Stability

If the data just presented were the only information on personality stability we would probably regard them with considerable suspicion. After all, theories like those of Erikson (1950) and Levinson (1977) suggest that there should be continued development in adulthood, and popular stereotypes of aging suggest that rigidity and depression should increase in old age. Adults experience a variety of life events; is it reasonable to think that marriage and divorce, retirement and chronic diseases, social upheavals and personal tragedies leave no mark on an individual's personality? Perhaps some peculiarity of the CQS, or of self-report methods, or of the volunteer BLSA sample leads to an exaggerated estimate of the stability of personality. Perhaps substantially more change would be seen if a longer time interval were examined.

None of these objections seems to be supported by other studies. With regard to instrument, comparable levels of stability are seen using the Sixteen Personality Factor Questionnaire (Siegler et al. 1979), the Guilford-Zimmerman Temperament Survey (GZTS; Costa et al. 1983), the California Psychological Inventory (Block 1977), and the NEO Personality Inventory (NEO-PI; Costa and McCrae 1988).

All these questionnaires, however, depend on self-report, and it has been argued that individuals may have a fixed conception of their personality traits, a crystallized self-concept, that accounts for the apparent stability (Rosenberg 1979). But longitudinal stability has also been demonstrated using spouse and peer ratings on the observer rating form of the NEO-PI (Costa and McCrae 1988, 1992c). It could be countered that friends and spouses also form fixed impressions of the targets' personalities, and perhaps these could explain away the apparent stability. But other studies have used different sets of raters at different times and also found substantial stability (Block 1971; Field and Millsap 1991).

Stability has been documented in a variety of samples, from male veterans (Costa and McCrae 1978) to graduates of a selective women's college (Helson 1993). Perhaps the most impressive documentation of stability in mean levels comes from a cross-sectional study of nearly 10,000 men and women from a national probability sample (Costa et al. 1986). Figure 6–1 shows means for age groups ranging from 35 to 84. Blacks and whites, males and females all show a nearly flat line across this 50-year age span.

Longitudinal studies have rarely covered so long an interval, and it is only longitudinal studies that speak to the stability of individual differences. It has been argued that stability coefficients will decline with time (Conley 1984), and that in fact appears to be the case. For example, we examined stability coefficients in a small group of BLSA men who had completed the 10 GZTS scales on 5 occasions over a

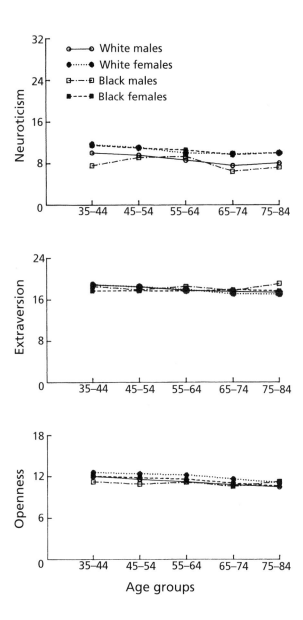

FIGURE 6–1. *Mean levels of neuroticism, extraversion, and openness to experience for 10-year age groups of black and white men and women aged 35 to 84 years. [Adapted from Costa et al. 1986.]*

30-year period. The median stability coefficient for adjacent adminis-
trations (about 6-year intervals) was 0.77; the median coefficient for
the full 30-year interval was reduced to 0.63 (Costa and McCrae
1992c). Stability declines in the long run, but it remains substantial
over the full adult life course.

Of course, some people do change. Although conditions such as
cancer and heart disease do not appear to affect the stability of personality (Costa et al. 1994), dementing disorders clearly do (Siegler et al.
1991). But the most important changes in adulthood occur not near
its end, but at its beginning. The decade between age 20 and 30 sees
a number of changes that are particularly important for an understanding of PDs.

Personality Development
and Personality Disorders

Several studies have provided longitudinal evidence of normative personality change between college age and middle adulthood. Mortimer
et al. (1982) found increased well-being but diminished sociability 10
years after college graduation. Jessor (1983) reported decreased alien-
ation and social criticism and increased achievement motivation over
a similar period. Hann et al. (1986) found that dependability and
warmth increased between high school and mid-30s.

These findings can be translated into the language of the five-factor
model and summarized by saying that as adolescents mature they become lower in neuroticism and extraversion and higher in agreeableness and conscientiousness—less emotional and better socialized. The
same findings can be seen cross-sectionally in Figure 6–2, which compares college age norms and adult norms on the Revised NEO Personality Inventory (NEO-PI-R; Costa and McCrae 1992b). Similar patterns are seen for men and women, and they replicate earlier
cross-sectional findings on the NEO-PI (Costa and McCrae 1989).

These developmental changes are of particular interest to students
of PDs because of the intimate link between personality traits and

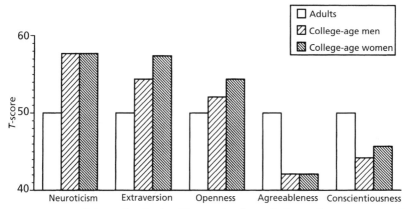

FIGURE **6–2.** *Mean levels (in T-scores) of NEO-PI-R domain scores for adults, college-age men, and college-age women compared with adult norms.*

disorders. Cross-sectional studies in both normal (Costa and McCrae 1990) and clinical (Trull 1992) populations have shown strong and consistent associations between measures of the five major dimensions of personality and a variety of operationalizations of the DSM PDs. For example, as measured by Morey et al.'s (1985) Minnesota Multiphasic Personality Inventory (MMPI; Hathaway and McKinley 1943) PD scales and the Millon Clinical Multiaxial Inventory (Millon 1994), the schizoid PD is negatively related to extraversion, whereas the histrionic PD is positively related. Many PD scales—notably borderline—are related to neuroticism, and several (including narcissistic, antisocial, and paranoid) are related to low agreeableness. Some PDs are characterized by a combination of personality factors: Schizotypal and avoidant PDs combine neuroticism with low extraversion; dependent PD combines neuroticism with agreeableness.

One interpretation of these associations is that PDs are in fact nothing more than maladaptive variants of universal dimensions of personality. If so, we would expect developmental parallels between the two, and the data in Figure 6–2 should suggest hypotheses about age changes in the prevalence of the personality disorders. Neuroticism declines, and neuroticism is a feature common to many PDs. It is therefore not surprising that PDs are less often diagnosed in middle-aged and older patients (Mulder 1991). These findings are not sampling or selection artifacts: The 15-year Chestnut Lodge follow-up study by McGlashan and Heinssen (1989) documented the improvement of patients with borderline PD, noting that many of the characteristics of this disorder "are developmental phenomena common to adolescence that get better with time" (p. 668).

Conscientiousness and agreeableness increase with age, and, as low scores on these dimensions are key features of the antisocial PD (Brooner et al. 1991), we should expect a decline in antisocial PD with age. This is well documented, from Korea (Lee et al. 1990) to New Zealand (Mulder 1991) to the United States. Robins et al. (1991) conducted an epidemiologic study of antisocial PD and found that "this supposedly 'interminable' disorder often remitted in the fourth decade of life" (p. 264), that is, after age 30.

Extraversion declines in the decade of the 20s, and Fogel and Westlake (1990) found that histrionic PD was less common in psychiatric inpatients age 45 and over. Conscientiousness increases, and higher levels of obsessive-compulsive (or anankastic) PD have been reported by Fogel and Westlake (1990) and by Mulder (1991). Schizotypal PD combines high neuroticism with low extraversion or introversion. Because neuroticism decreases while introversion increases, the net maturational effect may be to leave the prevalence of schizotypal PD unchanged. This is consistent with McGlashan's (1986) finding that schizotypal PD patients showed much more modest improvement over time than did borderline PD patients.

Parallels between the developmental course of personality and of the PDs are not perfect. Mulder (1991), for example, found higher rates of paranoid PD in older patients, whereas the normative decline in neuroticism and increase in agreeableness would suggest that paranoid PD should decrease with age. Perhaps this reflects the contribution of age-related cognitive aberrations to the paranoid PD.

In general, however, the parallels between developmental trends in early adulthood in self-reports of personality in normal individuals and in diagnoses of PDs in psychiatric patients is striking and provides another line of evidence for regarding both as manifestations of the same underlying psychological structures.

Stability and Change in Rank Order From Adolescence to Adulthood

Normative developmental trends correspond to changes in the mean levels of variables and do not imply either stability or change in rank ordering. As the CQS data in Table 6–2 illustrate, rank order is very stable in adults over age 30. It is considerably less stable in adolescents; that is, some adolescents increase and some decrease relative to the mean over the decade of the 20s. Retest correlations are correspondingly lowered.

The most direct evidence of lower retest correlations for adolescents is obtained by comparing retest correlations on the same instrument and over the same interval in groups differing in initial age. Finn (1986) examined the 30-year stability of college and middle-aged men on MMPI factor scales and found that the mean stability coefficient was 0.53 for the older cohort, but only 0.38 for the younger. Siegler et al. (1990) gave an indirect demonstration of the same phenomenon by examining correlations between MMPI factor scales and the five NEO-PI factors in two groups. In the first (predictive) group (from the UNC Alumni Heart Study; Siegler et al. 1992a, 1992b) the MMPI was completed when subjects were college students and the NEO-PI was completed when they were adults, about 24 years later. In the second (concurrent) group (from the BLSA) both instruments were completed within a few years of each other by adults. The predictive correlations were roughly half as large as the concurrent correlations, suggesting that about half the variance in personality true scores was stable over the 24-year interval, and about half was not. By contrast, Costa and McCrae (1992c) estimated that about 80% of the true score variance was stable over a comparable interval among older adults.

Is the same true for measures of PDs? We know of no long-term longitudinal study of PD scales, probably because most PDs scales were developed in the past decade. But the indirect method of Siegler et al. (1990) can be applied, because Morey et al.'s (1985) PD scales can be scored from archival MMPI data. Table 6–4 gives 24-year predictive correlations between MMPI PD scales and NEO-PI factors for 1917 men and women, and, for comparison, reproduces the concur-

TABLE 6-4.

Predictive and concurrent correlations between MMPI personality disorder scales and NEO Personality Inventory factors

MMPI personality disorder scale	NEO Personality Inventory factor									
	N		E		O		A		C	
	P[a]	C[b]	P	C	P	C	P	C	P	C
Paranoid	**0.22***	**0.36***	−0.06*	−0.02	0.02	−0.09	**−0.15***	**−0.31***	−0.05	−0.13
Schizoid	0.10*	0.16*	−0.39*	**−0.62***	0.11*	0.06	−0.01	−0.12	0.05	0.14
Schizotypal	0.29*	**0.46***	−0.29*	**−0.48***	0.05	0.00	−0.03	−0.15	0.01	0.04
Antisocial	0.05	0.13	−0.04	0.07	0.09*	0.18*	−0.20*	**−0.35***	−0.18*	**−0.42***
Borderline	0.27*	**0.47***	0.08*	0.19*	0.02	0.09	−0.14*	−0.21*	−0.10*	−0.32*
Histrionic	−0.13*	−0.17*	0.37*	**0.65***	0.03	0.15	−0.06*	0.00	−0.09*	−0.22*
Narcissistic	−0.17*	−0.28*	0.29*	**0.56***	0.05	0.07	−0.17*	−0.18*	−0.02	0.01
Avoidant	0.30*	**0.52***	−0.33*	**−0.54***	0.00	−0.03	0.04	−0.02	0.01	−0.02
Dependent	0.28*	**0.50***	−0.11*	−0.30*	−0.11*	−0.10	0.12*	0.22*	−0.11*	−0.22*
Compulsive	0.25*	**0.50***	−0.02	−0.16*	0.02	−0.07	−0.06*	−0.15	0.01	−0.06
Passive-aggressive	0.21*	**0.39***	−0.09*	−0.17*	0.01	−0.02	−0.12*	−0.16*	−0.16*	**−0.33***

Note. N = 1917 for predictive corrections, 274 for concurrent correlations. Largest correlations are given in boldface.

[a]Predictive correlations.

[b]Concurrent correlations adapted from Costa and McCrae (1990).

*P < .01.

rent correlations for a sample of 274 BLSA adults reported by Costa and McCrae (1990).

Table 6–4 clearly shows that MMPI PD scales are meaningfully and consistently related to NEO-PI factors; data from the predictive sample significantly replicate 30 of the 31 significant correlations previously reported in the concurrent sample. The results are generally consistent with findings using other measures of the PDs: Paranoid PD is related to neuroticism and low agreeableness, antisocial PD to low agreeableness and low conscientiousness, histrionic PD to extraversion. The major discrepancy with other results concerns the compulsive PD, which is unrelated to conscientiousness in these data. In part, this is because the Morey et al. (1985) scales are based on DSM-III criteria (American Psychiatric Association 1980) rather than on DSM-III-R, and in part it is because the MMPI item pool includes few good measures of conscientiousness (Johnson et al. 1984).

A more detailed understanding of the relations between personality traits and PDs can be obtained by examining more specific traits within each of the five broad domains. Most of the UNC alumni who completed the NEO-PI in 1988 were administered a supplemental set of items in 1990; from their responses to both these questionnaires it was possible to score the NEO-PI-R (Costa and McCrae 1992b). The NEO-PI-R divides each domain scale into six facet scales measuring more specific traits. The five largest facet correlates for each of the MMPI PD scales are reported in Table 6–5.

Considering that a quarter century has passed between the administration of PD and personality scales, these data show remarkable specificity. For example, both borderline and dependent PD are characterized at a global level chiefly by high neuroticism, but at the facet level, borderline PD is distinctively associated with angry hostility, impulsiveness, anxiety, and low compliance, whereas dependent PD is associated with self-consciousness, vulnerability, low assertiveness, and low competence. The agreeableness facet of modesty appears only once in Table 6–5, as a negative correlate of the narcissistic PD. Low trust appears to be a distinctive correlate of the paranoid and antisocial PDs. These data provide considerable evidence for the convergent and discriminant validity of many of the MMPI PD scales.

Returning to Table 6–4, one more important conclusion can be

TABLE 6–5.

NEO-PI-R facets related to MMPI personality disorder scales

MMPI personality disorder scale	Revised NEO Personality Inventory facet scales
Paranoid	Angry hostility, anxiety, low trust, self-consciousness, depression
Schizoid	Low gregariousness, low warmth, low assertiveness, low positive emotions, low excitement seeking
Schizotypal	Self-consciousness, depression, low gregariousness, vulnerability, low warmth
Antisocial	Low straightforwardness, low altruism, low compliance, low deliberation, low trust
Borderline	Angry hostility, impulsiveness, depression, anxiety, low compliance
Histrionic	Assertiveness, gregariousness, excitement seeking, warmth, positive emotions
Narcissistic	Assertiveness, low self-consciousness, activity, low modesty, low vulnerability
Avoidant	Self-consciousness, low assertiveness, depression, vulnerability, low gregariousness
Dependent	Self-consciousness, vulnerability, depression, low assertiveness, low competence
Compulsive	Anxiety, angry hostility, depression, vulnerability, self-consciousness
Passive-aggressive	Low self-discipline, angry hostility, depression, impulsiveness, vulnerability

Note. N = 1,687. *The five largest facet correlates of each personality disorder are given,* |r|s = .16 to .37, P < .001.

drawn. The predictive correlations are about half as large as the concurrent correlations, suggesting that only about half the variance in true scores is stable between college and middle adulthood. Theoretically, this means that substantial personality change occurs in the decade of the 20s; practically, it means that personality and PD data collected in college are of somewhat limited utility as predictors of lifelong outcomes.

These data also have implications for the stability of PD diagnoses. The DSM-III-R defines PDs as enduring patterns that "are often recognizable by adolescence or earlier and continue throughout most of adult life" (p. 335). This characterization may be accurate for individuals over age 30, but if the developmental parallels between personality and PDs hold, it may have to be modified for younger patients. Between childhood and middle adulthood, PDs may be relatively fluid, generally decreasing in prevalence but also changing from category to category within the individual. Studies of the reliability of PD diagnoses in adolescents (Edell and McGlashan 1993) support this view. As Korenblum et al. (1990) concluded from a study of 59 adolescents followed from age 13 to 18, "there was a notable lack of consistency with respect to type of personality dysfunction from both a group and individual perspective" (p. 398).

Conclusion

This chapter has reviewed evidence on continuity and change in personality from adolescence through adulthood and has remarked on parallels between normal personality and the PDs. Both can be organized in terms of the broad dimensions of the five-factor model, and both show similar temporal courses. These findings have the profound implication that PDs may be pathological expressions of universal personality dimensions. If so, everything we know about personality traits, from their heritability (e.g., Tellegen et al. 1988) to their cross-observer validity (Funder and Colvin 1997) to their implications for psychotherapy (Miller 1991) may be generalizable to the study and treatment of PDs. The DSM Axis II categorical system has been widely criticized (e.g., Livesley 1991; Widiger 1993); the five-factor model may provide a better basis for understanding personality pathology (Costa and Widiger 1994).

References

American Psychiatric Association: Diagnostic and Statistical Manual of Mental Disorders, 3rd Edition. Washington, DC, American Psychiatric Association, 1980

American Psychiatric Association: Diagnostic and Statistical Manual of Mental Disorders, 3rd Edition, Revised. Washington, DC, American Psychiatric Association, 1987

Bem DJ, Funder DC: Predicting more of the people more of the time: assessing the personality of situations. Psychol Rev 85:485–501, 1978

Block J: The Q-sort Method in Personality Assessment and Psychiatric Research. Springfield, IL, Charles C Thomas, 1961

Block J: Lives Through Time. Berkeley, CA, Bancroft Books, 1971

Block J: Advancing the psychology of personality: Paradigmatic shift or improving the quality of research? in Personality at the Cross-roads: Current Issues in Interactional Psychology. Edited by Magnusson D, Endler NS. Hillsdale, NJ, Lawrence Erlbaum Associates, 1977, pp 37–64

Brooner RK, Costa PT Jr, Felch LJ, et al: The personality dimensions of male and female drug abusers with and without antisocial personality disorder, in Problems of Drug Dependence: Proceedings of the 53rd Annual Scientific Meeting, Committee on Problems of Drug Dependence. Edited by Harris LS. Rockville, MD, National Institute on Drug Abuse, 1991

Cloninger CR: A unified biosocial theory of personality and its role in the development of anxiety states: a reply to commentaries. Psychiatr Dev 2:83–120, 1988

Conley JJ: The hierarchy of consistency: a review and model of longitudinal findings on adult individual differences in intelligence, personality, and self-opinion. Personality and Individual Differences 5:11–26, 1984

Costa PT Jr, McCrae RR: Objective personality assessment, in The Clinical Psychology of Aging. Edited by Storandt M, Siegler IC, Elias MF. New York, Plenum, 1978, pp 119–143

Costa PT Jr, McCrae RR: Personality in adulthood: a six-year longitudinal study of self-reports and spouse ratings on the NEO Personality Inventory. J Pers Soc Psychol 54:853–863, 1988

Costa PT Jr, McCrae RR: NEO-PI/NEO-FFI Manual Supplement. Odessa, FL, Psychological Assessment Resources, 1989

Costa PT Jr, McCrae RR: Personality disorders and the five-factor model of personality. J Personal Disord 4:362–371, 1990

Costa PT Jr, McCrae RR: Four ways five factors are basic. Personality and Individual Differences 13:653–665, 1992a

Costa PT Jr, McCrae RR: Revised NEO Personality Inventory (NEO-PI-R) and NEO Five-Factor Inventory (NEO-FFI) Professional Manual. Odessa, FL, Psychological Assessment Resources, 1992b

Costa PT Jr, McCrae RR: Trait psychology comes of age, in Nebraska Symposium on Motivation: Psychology and Aging. Edited by Sonderegger TB. Lincoln, University of Nebraska Press, 1992c, pp 169–204

Costa PT Jr, McCrae RR: The Revised NEO Personality Inventory (NEO-PI-R), in Handbook of Adult Personality Inventories. Edited by Cheek J, Donahue EM, Briggs SR. New York, Plenum (in press)

Costa PT Jr, Widiger TA (eds): Personality Disorders and the Five-Factor Model of Personality. Washington, DC, American Psychological Association, 1994

Costa PT Jr, McCrae RR, Arenberg D: Recent longitudinal research on personality and aging, in Longitudinal Studies of Adult Psychological Development. Edited by Schaie KW. New York, Guilford, 1983, pp 222–265

Costa PT Jr, McCrae RR, Zonderman AB, et al: Cross-sectional studies of personality in a national sample: 2. Stability in neuroticism, extraversion, and openness. Psychol Aging 1:144–149, 1986

Costa PT Jr, Metter EJ, McCrae RR: Personality stability and its contribution to successful aging. J Geriatr Psychiatry 27:40–59, 1994

Digman JM: Personality structure: Emergence of the five-factor model. Annu Rev Psychol 41:417–440, 1990

Douglas K, Arenberg D: Age changes, cohort differences, and cultural change on the Guilford-Zimmerman Temperament Survey. J Gerontol 33:737–747, 1978

Edell W, McGlashan TH: Instability of personality disorder diagnoses in adolescents. Paper presented at the Conference of the International Society for the Study of Personality Disorders, Cambridge, MA, September 1993

Erikson EH: Childhood and Society. New York, WW Norton, 1950

Field D, Millsap RE: Personality in advanced old age: continuity or change? J Gerontol B Psychol Sci Soc Sci 46:P299–P308, 1991

Finn SE: Stability of personality self-ratings over 30 years: evidence for an age/cohort interaction. J Pers Soc Psychol 50:813–818, 1986

Fogel BS, Westlake R: Personality disorder diagnoses and age in inpatients with major depression. J Clin Psychiatry 51:232–235, 1990

Funder DC, Colvin CR: Friends and strangers: Acquaintanceship, agreement, and the accuracy of personality judgment. J Pers Soc Psychol 55:149–158, 1988

Funder DC, Colvin CR: Congruence of others' and self-judgments of personality, in Handbook of Personality Psychology. Edited by Hogan R, Johnson J, Briggs S. San Diego, CA, Academic Press, 1997, pp 617–648

Guilford JS, Zimmerman WS, Guilford JP: The Guilford-Zimmerman Temperament Survey Handbook: Twenty-five Years of Research and Application. San Diego, CA, EdITS Publishers, 1976

Haan N, Millsap R, Hartka E: As time goes by: change and stability in personality over fifty years. Psychol Aging 1:220–232, 1986

Hathaway SR, McKinley JC: Minnesota Multiphasic Personality Inventory. Minneapolis, University of Minnesota, 1943

Helson R: Comparing longitudinal studies of adult development: toward a paradigm of tension between stability and change, in Studying Lives Through Time. Edited by Funder D, Parke R, Tomlinson-Keasey C, Widaman R. Washington, DC, American Psychological Association, 1993, pp 93–120

Jessor R: The stability of change: psychosocial development from adolescence to young adulthood, in Human Development: An Interactional Perspective. Edited by Magnusson D, Allen VL. New York, Academic Press, 1983, pp 321–341

Johnson JH, Butcher JN, Null C, et al: Replicated item level factor analysis of the full MMPI. J Pers Soc Psychol 47:105–114, 1984

Jung CG: Psychological Types (1923). Translated by Baynes HG and revised by Hull RFC. Princeton, NJ, Princeton University Press, 1971

Korenblum M, Marton P, Golombek H, et al: Personality status: changes through adolescence. Psychiatr Clin North Am 13:389–399, 1990

Lee CK, Kwak YS, Yamamoto J, et al: Psychiatric epidemiology in Korea: part II: urban and rural differences. J Nerv Ment Dis 178:247–252, 1990

Levinson DJ: The mid-life transition: a period in adult psychosocial development. Psychiatry 40:99–112, 1977

Livesley WJ: Classifying personality disorders: Ideal types, prototypes, or dimensions? J Personal Disord 5:52–59, 1991

McCrae RR: Why I advocate the five-factor model: joint analyses of the NEO-PI and other instruments, in Personality Psychology: Recent Trends and Emerging Directions. Edited by Buss DM, Cantor N. New York, Springer-Verlag, 1989, pp 237–245

McCrae RR: The five-factor model and its assessment in clinical settings. J Pers Assess 57:399–414, 1991

McCrae RR (ed): The five-factor model: issues and applications [special issue]. J Pers 60(2):175–525

McCrae RR, Costa PT Jr: Joint factors in self-reports and ratings: neuroticism, extraversion, and openness to experience. Personality and Individual Differences 4:245–255, 1983

McCrae RR, Costa PT Jr, Busch CM: Evaluating comprehensiveness in personality systems: the California Q-Set and the five-factor model. J Pers 54:430–446, 1986

McGlashan TH: The Chestnut Lodge follow-up study: III. Long-term outcome of borderline personalities. Arch Gen Psychiatry 43:20–30, 1986

McGlashan TH, Heinssen RK: Narcissistic, antisocial, and noncomorbid subgroups of borderline disorder: are they distinct entities by long-term clinical profile? Psychiatr Clin North Am 12:653–670, 1989

Miller T: The psychotherapeutic utility of the five-factor model of personality: a clinician's experience. J Pers Assess 57:415–433, 1991

Millon T: Manual for the MCMI-III. Minneapolis, MN, National Computer Systems, 1994

Morey LC, Waugh MH, Blashfield RK: MMPI scales for DSM-III personality disorders: their derivation and correlates. J Pers Assess 49:245–251, 1985

Mortimer JT, Finch MD, Kumka D: Persistence and change in development: the multidimensional self-concept, in Life-Span Development and Behavior, Vol 4. Edited by Baltes PB, Brim OG Jr. New York, Academic Press, 1982, pp 264–315

Mulder RT: Personality disorders in New Zealand hospitals. Acta Psychiatr Scand 84:197–202, 1991

Murray HA: Explorations in Personality. New York, Oxford University Press, 1938

Robins LN, Tipp J, Przybeck T: Antisocial personality, in Psychiatric Disorders in America: The Epidemiologic Catchment Area Study. Edited by Robins LN, Regier DA. New York, Free Press, 1991, pp 258–290

Rosenberg M: Conceiving the Self. New York, Basic Books, 1979

Shock NW, Greulich RC, Andres R, et al: Normal Human Aging: The Baltimore Longitudinal Study of Aging (NIH Publ No 84–2450). Bethesda, MD, National Institutes of Health, 1984

Siegler IC, George LK, Okun MA: Cross-sequential analysis of adult personality. Dev Psychol 15:350–351, 1979

Siegler IC, Peterson BL, Barefoot JC, et al: Hostility during late adolescence predicts coronary risk factors at midlife. Am J Epidemiol 138:146–154, 1992a

Siegler IC, Peterson BL, Barefoot JC, et al: Using college alumni populations in epidemiologic research: The UNC Alumni Heart Study. J Clin Epidemiol 45:1243–1250, 1992b

Siegler IC, Zonderman, AB, Barefoot JC, et al: Predicting personality in adulthood from college MMPI scores: implications for follow-up studies in psychosomatic medicine. Psychosom Med 52:644–652, 1990

Siegler IC, Welsh KA, Dawson DV, et al: Ratings of personality change in patients being evaluated for memory disorders. Alzheimer Dis Assoc Disord 5:240–250, 1991

Stephenson W: The Study of Behavior. Chicago, University of Chicago, 1953

Tellegen A, Lykken DT, Bouchard TJ Jr, et al: Personality similarity in twins reared apart and together. J Pers Soc Psychol 54:1031–1039, 1988

Trull TJ: DSM-III-R personality disorders and the five-factor model of personality: an empirical comparison. J Abnorm Psychol 101:553–560, 1992

Widiger TA: The DSM-III-R categorical personality disorder diagnoses: a critique and an alternative. Psychological Inquiry 4:75–90, 1993

Wiggins JS, Pincus AL: Conceptions of personality disorders and dimensions of personality. Psychological Assessment: J Consult Clin Psychol 1:305–316, 1989

Wiggins JS, Pincus AL: Personality: structure and assessment. Annu Rev Psychol 43:473–504, 1992

CHAPTER 7

Evaluating the Structure of Personality

Niels G. Waller, Ph.D.

American English includes a wealth of personality descriptive words. Comprehensive dictionaries such as *Webster's New International* (1925, 1961), for example, contain nearly 18,000 designators of temperament, mood, social evaluations, and enduring dispositions (Allport and Odbert 1936; Norman 1967). Many of these terms have synonyms or antonyms, and all lexicons are replete with redundancy. Nevertheless, the natural language of personality appears sufficiently rich to capture the most salient nuances of human behavior.

For this reason personality psychologists from many nations (Allport and Odbert 1936; Angleitner et al. 1990; Baumgarten 1933; Brokken 1978; De Raad et al. 1988; Goldberg 1980, 1981; John et al. 1984; Norman 1967; Tellegen and Waller 1987) have meticulously culled trait names from dictionaries hoping to discover the most important and fundamental natural language personality dimensions. There is a

I would like to thank Jack Block, Oliver John, Phil Shaver, Auke Tellegen, and Joe Zavala for helpful comments on earlier drafts of this chapter. Special thanks go to Mr. Zavala for his extraordinary work on the California Twin Study.

growing consensus in the field (Goldberg 1982; Costa and McCrae 1985; Widiger 1993) that five lexically derived factors are "reasonably sufficient for describing at a global level the major features of personality" (McCrae and Costa 1986, p. 1001). Common numbers and names for these factors are I) surgency (or extraversion), II) agreeableness, III) conscientiousness (or dependability), IV) emotional stability (vs. neuroticism) and V) openness to experience (intellect or culture). Collectively they define the so-called Big Five (John 1990) or the five-factor model of personality (FFM; Costa and Widiger 1994; Goldberg 1993; Widiger 1993).

In this chapter I review the history of the FFM and critically examine the evidence behind claims for its comprehensiveness (e.g., McCrae and Costa 1986; Widiger 1993; but see Waller and Ben-Porath 1987; Waller and Zavala 1993). A recurring theme in this review is that the five factors fail to account for important dimensions of self-evaluation. In support of this position, I review work by Tellegen and Waller (1987, in press) demonstrating that at least seven higher-order dimensions, respectfully called the Big Seven, can be captured from the natural language. Five of these dimensions are similar to, although not isomorphic with, the Big Five (McCrae and John 1992). The two remaining dimensions, which tap putatively *evaluative* aspects of self-concept, are labeled positive and negative valence (Tellegen 1993; Tellegen and Waller 1987, in press; Waller and Zavala 1993). Next, using data from more than 1,750 twins and twin-family members, I report the phenotypic factor structure of a newly developed Big Seven questionnaire. I then examine the genetic and environmental architecture of the seven factors of this instrument. Lastly, in line with the focus of this book, I briefly discuss the relevance of the Big Seven for understanding Axis II personality disorders (Waller and Zavala 1993).

Reevaluating the History of Lexical Personality Research

In the early decades of this century, when personology was an inchoate discipline, our field lacked a compelling taxonomy of trait terms. Allport summarized the confused state of the discipline by noting that "each assessor has his own pet units and uses a pet battery of diagnostic devices" (1958, p. 258). Preliminary catalogues of traits, values, motives, and needs were beginning to appear at this time (Murray 1938; Spranger 1928), although the lack of a well-defined and hierarchically structured taxonomy of personality descriptors severely hampered efforts to determine whether these competing systems were comprehensive or merely idiosyncratic. It was a time when a single construct could be called by a dozen different names (McCrae and John 1992). It was also the period when the first multiscaled personality inventories appeared on the scene (Goldberg 1971). Psychologists were interested in mapping the topography of personality. But where were they to go to chart unexplored domains?

A German characterologist named Ludwig Klages provided an early and insightful answer to this question. Klages (1932) asserted that

> whoever, having the right talent, should do nothing but interrogate the words and phrases which deal with the human soul, would know more about [personality] than all the sages who omitted this, and would know perhaps a thousand times more than has ever been discovered by observation, apparatus, and experiment upon man. (p. 74)

This deceptively simple idea has come to be known as the *lexical hypothesis*. It has been elegantly restated by Goldberg (1982), who claims that "Those individual differences that are most salient and socially relevant in people's lives will eventually become encoded into their language; the more important such a difference, the more likely is it to become expressed as a single word" (p. 204).

The lexical hypothesis immediately suggests a source for exploring new domains of personality. Psychologists should study the corpus of natural language personality descriptors; in other words, they should study the dictionary (Figure 7–1).

In the Beginning . . .

Gordon Allport and Henry Odbert conducted one the earliest psycholexical studies of English language trait names. These pioneering

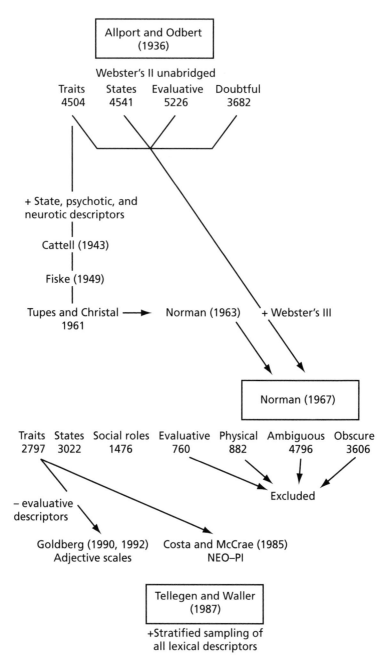

FIGURE 7–1. *Highlights in the history of lexical personality research.*

researchers abstracted and catalogued all "words descriptive of personality or personal behavior (save those that are obsolete) included in Webster's New International Dictionary" (Allport and Odbert 1936, p. 24). Candidate trait names were chosen if they could "distinguish the behavior of one human being from another" (p. 24). Altogether, 17,954 descriptive predicates were culled from the almost 400,000 entries in this lexicon. Next, the pool of candidate trait markers was divided and rationally sorted into four categories. The final categories were published in four columns under the following rubrics: I) personal traits, II) temporary moods or states, III) social evaluations, and IV) metaphorical and doubtful terms.

According to the authors, Column I terms "symbolize most clearly 'real' traits of personality" (Allport and Odbert 1936, p. 26), such as *expansive, friendly, histrionic,* and *industrious.* A total of 4,504 descriptors were deemed authentic trait designators by the authors. Column II terms denote less enduring psychological characteristics such as temporary states, moods, or activities. Example state terms include *happy, anxious,* and *ashamed.* Column III houses the largest number of descriptors in the taxonomy. It also includes many of the so-called evaluative terms that are markers of positive and negative valence. Examples of Column III terms are *evil, worthy, undesirable,* and *seductive.* It is of considerable historical significance that Allport and Odbert believed that social evaluations and other "censorial" predicates—that is, Column III terms—"have absolutely no direct reference to personality" (Allport and Odbert 1936, p. 18). In a later section of this chapter we will consider the implications of this belief. Lastly, Column IV terms denote miscellaneous designations of physique, capacities, and developmental conditions, as well as other residual terms that could not be classified in the first three categories. Examples of Column IV descriptors are *mesmerizable, asexual,* and *Beelzebubian.*

When finished with their Herculean task, Allport and Odbert had classified nearly 18,000 candidate descriptors from a comprehensive register of natural language trait names. Although only 25% of their terms were classified as *genuine* trait referents, the authors realized that their four-fold classification was "at best only approximate and to a certain extent arbitrary" (Allport and Odbert 1936; p. 27; cf. Chaplin et al. 1988). They admitted, for instance, that it was particularly difficult discriminating the Column I terms, which designate enduring dispositions, from the Column II terms, which designate temporary moods, states, and emotions. Commenting on this point they note that whereas "[a]ll people are *anxious* on occasion . . . some individuals . . . are recurrently and characteristically anxious" (p. 28). Therefore, it is "possible to argue that the columns [I and II] should not be kept independent but should be combined for a more ample estimate of the number of *possible* trait-names in the English language" (p. 28). But combining the columns would have resulted in a trait list of mind-boggling size (over 9,000 descriptors!). Perhaps this is why later tax-onomers focused their efforts almost exclusively on the Column I terms of the Allport and Odbert compendium. The first psychologist to seriously organize this reduced list was Raymond Cattell.

Raymond Cattell and the Concept of the Trait Sphere

Soon after the publication of the Allport and Odbert monograph (1936), Raymond Cattell began a series of groundbreaking studies (1943, 1945, 1946) on the factor analytic structure of personality. A votary of multi-variate methods, Cattell (1943) summarized previous work in the area and credited seven defects in the application of factor analysis for the then inconclusive findings on the major personality dimensions. Two entries in his list deserve particular consideration.

Cattell believed that earlier factor analytic work on personality was of limited value because of overreliance on self-report data. Ratings of behavior by judges, he asserted, are superior to "*mere self-ratings* and questionnaire responses" (emphasis added, 1943, p. 478). The reason for this is that a "trait syndrome may 'feel' to the wearer a different garment from the one seen by an outside observer" (1943, p. 478). This idea that consensual validation by judges is a requisite component of personality construct validation was promoted later by McCrae and John (1992). These authors, in a critique of Tellegen and Waller's (1987) positive and negative valence factors, maintain that it is "un-likely that these two factors represent substantive aspects of personality that could be consensually validated" (p. 191). And they ask, "To what specific behaviors could one point that would confirm that an individual [was extreme on positive or negative valence]?" (McCrae and John 1992, p. 191; see also McCrae 1982). My reply to these critics, and my response to Cattell, is that the self-views and other-views of personality need not, and should not, be pitted against one another. Although overt behaviors are frequently used to infer personality traits, private thoughts, feelings, and self-portrayals are also valuable indicators of behavioral coherence. Like other clinically oriented psychologists, I believe that "personality is the *multilevel* pattern of interpersonal responses (*overt, conscious, or private*) expressed by the individual" (emphasis added; Leary 1957, p. 15), and that self- and other-views of personality, even when they differ, should be afforded equal status in the study of lives.

Cattell's other major criticism of personality research concerned the limited sampling of trait terms in previous empirical studies. He noted that "the universe of 'trait elements' for which interrelations have been calculated has been defective in number or in range of personality aspects" (1943, p. 479). Psychologists could correct their myopia by analyzing descriptors from the entire *trait sphere*, which he defined as "the universe of traits, ideally covering all aspects of personality" (p. 482). The elements of the trait sphere were to be sampled from everyday discourse. And in a statement that easily could have been penned by Klages, Goldberg, or other advocates of the lexical hypothesis, Cattell (1943) declared that

> all aspects of human personality which are or have been of importance, interest, or utility have already become recorded in the substance of language. For, throughout history, the most fascinating subject of general discourse, and also that in which it has been most vitally necessary to have adequate, representative symbolism, has been human behavior. (p. 483)

Faced with the problem of obtaining a comprehensive list of natural language trait terms Cattell willingly embraced the earlier taxonomic efforts of Allport and Odbert. Like his predecessors, he believed that the "biophysical trait terms" were the most authentic descriptors of personality. He also agreed with Allport and Odbert that many state terms could function as trait terms and that the evaluative predicates were of no use in a scientific language of personality. He therefore added several hundred state terms and clinical descriptors to the list of purported trait names.

The expanded pool of descriptors contained nearly 5,000 trait designators. In the first of several organizational steps aimed at reducing the size of this unwieldy pool, the trait names were sorted on the basis of semantic similarity into variously sized synonym clusters. Next, antonymous clusters were merged to produce 171 bipolar clusters (Cattell 1945) that were later used in a rating study of 100 male subjects. The relatively large size of the correlation matrix from this study prohibited Cattell in those pre-computer days from using factor analysis or cluster analysis for further semantic distillation. He therefore relied on "intra-cranial" cluster analysis to derive a reduced list of 35 rating scales, which he later dubbed the standard reduced personality sphere. At last, Cattell was in a position to factor analyze a representative sample of personality descriptors.

I have omitted many important and fascinating details from this story, and the reader should consult John et al. (1988; or John 1990) for a scholarly review of Cattell's lexical research. For our purposes it is only necessary that I relate one more aspect of Cattell's work. After conducting numerous studies with his reduced set of rating scales, Cattell concluded that the universe of natural language trait terms could be sufficiently captured by 12 oblique factors (Cattell 1947). In later years Cattell developed his well-known 16-factor model of personality (Cattell et al. 1970).

Subsequent researchers have repeatedly failed to replicate Cattell's findings on the major personality dimensions (Digman and Takemoto-Chock 1981). Three failed replications are particularly noteworthy because of their influence on contemporary views of personality organization. The three studies were conducted by Fiske (1949), Tupes and Christal (1961), and Norman (1963). Since detailed summaries of these studies have been published elsewhere (John et al. 1988; John 1990), I will not review this material in great depth. Instead, I will note that the important and common conclusion of these works is that five, and only five, orthogonal factors are needed to account for the major sources of variance in Cattell's rating scales. The interpretation of these factors was also remarkably consistent across the three investigations. For example, Fiske (1949) labeled his dimensions I) confident self expression, II) social adaptability, III) conformity, IV) emotional control, and V) inquiring intellect. Tupes and Christal (1961) labeled theirs I) surgency, II) agreeableness, III) dependability, IV) emotional stability, and V) culture. Norman (1963) adopted the labels of Tupes and Christal, but renamed Factor III conscientiousness. Today, these factors are collectively called the Big Five (John 1990), and the aforementioned studies are the acknowledged progenitors of the FFM. The following consensually selected adjectives (abstracted from John 1990) are representative Big Five markers: I) talkative, assertive, not quiet, not reserved; II) sympathetic, kind, not fault-finding, not cold; III) organized, thorough, not careless, not disorderly; IV) stable, calm, not tense, not anxious; V) wide interests, imaginative, not commonplace, not simple.

Three classic studies in the history of lexical personality research agreed that Cattell's reduced variable set could be adequately characterized by five higher-order dimensions. Unfortunately, none of these studies addressed the broader issue of whether these same five factors also characterized the universe of trait terms. Cattell obviously made many subjective decisions when reducing his sizable descriptor pool to a mere 35 rating scales. But did he also exclude important trait domains during the process? This question led Norman (1963) to suggest that "it is time to return to the total pool of trait names in the natural language—there to search for additional personality indicators not easily subsumed under one or another of these five recurrent factors" (p. 582).

Norman Returns to the Dictionary

Language systems are evolving systems, and Norman realized that new personality descriptors—and possibly new trait domains—may have been encoded in the language after Allport and Odbert compiled their exhaustive list. He therefore returned to the dictionary and carried out the second major study of American English trait names (Norman 1967). Norman's stated goal was to develop an exhaustive, precise, and well-structured taxonomy of trait names from "all terms in contemporary American English which pertain to aspects of human behavior or personal characteristics" (1967, p. i). To ensure that his taxonomy was exhaustive he began with the 17,954 descriptors from the Allport and Odbert (1936) monograph. He then scanned the latest edition of *Webster's New International Dictionary* (1961) for any additional descriptors that may have entered the natural language during the previous 30 years.

During his search Norman used purposely loose inclusion criteria for deciding when a word was personality descriptive. Nearly 40,000 candidate terms were culled from the dictionary, although most of these were not considered ideal trait indicators. Thousands of terms were semantically redundant, whereas others were simply grammatical, prefixal, or suffixal forms of other terms in the list. It was therefore necessary to develop exclusion criteria to purge this catalogue of the lexical dross.

Norman reasoned that the grammatical cognates (e.g., suffixal variations) could be safely discarded without compromising domain coverage; and by excluding these terms he was able to shorten his list by almost 50%. To Norman's surprise, of the 18,125 surviving terms only 171 descriptors were not included in the original Allport and Odbert classification. Apparently language systems, like other living systems, evolve slowly. In the next phase of the project, four judges sorted the approximately 18,000 terms into 7 (15 lower-order) mutually exclusive categories: stable traits (*cheerful, conscientious, jovial*); temporary states and temporary activities (*hopeful, relaxed, terrified*); social roles and relationships (*dominant, obedient, influential*), evaluative terms and mere quantifiers (*capable, foolish, obnoxious*), physical characteristics and mental health (*suicidal, psychopathic, nymphomaniac*), ambiguous terms (*ding-dong, fiddle-faddle, Germanophobe*), and obscure terms (*emplastic, limpsy, nubigenous*). A goal of this classification was to identify the stable (biophysical) trait terms for further study. Before discussing Norman's classification of the prime terms for stable traits, let us take a closer look at the descriptor categories that were excluded from further study.

Consider, first, the class of evaluative descriptors. Like Allport and Odbert (1936) and Cattell (1943), Norman believed that the natural language "is loaded with terms whose connotations are . . . *purely evaluative*" (1967, p. 5) and that these censorial descriptors should be segregated from the authentic trait names. Norman subsequently barred 760 terms from lexical research because of their supposedly evaluative nature. Some examples from this list include *capable, commonplace, foolish,* and *obnoxious.* Apparently it is difficult to evaluate the *evaluativeness* of a descriptor: Norman's list of censorial predicates is only 14.5% as long as Allport and Odbert's. In addition to evaluative terms, more than 8,000 other trait names were ostracized because they were overly ambiguous, obscure, or metaphorical. Some examples from this second list are *fearful, modest, robust, strong, dreamy, dull, immature, natural, prejudiced, quick, good-looking, simple, slow, thankless,* and *weak.*

If you think that some of these examples are useful trait indicators, take comfort in the fact that you are not alone. All of the italicized descriptors in the preceding paragraph are items in a widely used personality inventory: the Adjective Checklist (Gough and Heilbrun 1983; a total of 64 ACL items are not included in Norman's list of prime terms for stable traits). I draw attention to these examples to illustrate an important point: *When using exclusion rules to organize and pare down trait lists there is always a danger that useful trait indicators will be prematurely excluded from lexical research.* One hopes that meaningful trait dimensions will not also be excluded and that the considerable redundancy in the natural language will guarantee domain coverage. When entire descriptor classes are eliminated, however, such as the evaluative terms or the emotionally toned state indicators, the comprehensiveness of a descriptor pool can no longer be guaranteed. This may account for the finding that 21 Adjective Checklist items (e.g., independent, individualistic, rebellious, suggestible, peculiar, queer, conservative, and prudish) cannot be consensually classified on one of the Big Five factors by a majority of trained judges (John 1989, p. 268).[1]

From a total of approximately 18,000 trait names, Norman selected

---

[1]John's results are somewhat puzzling, however, since Goldberg (1982, p. 210) reintroduced the missing ACL items during the construction of his 1,710-descriptor set.

2,797 descriptors, or nearly 15% of the total, as prime terms for stable traits. He then administered these terms, in sets of 200, to samples of university undergraduates to obtain various itemetric statistics (e.g., item endorsement frequencies for self- ratings and other ratings, social desirability values). On the basis of these statistics 1,200 additional terms were eliminated because they elicited overly extreme self-ratings or were judged too obscure or unclear by a majority of raters. This left Norman with approximately 1,600 predicates for stable traits, and finally he was in a position to tackle the question that motivated his research.

Recall that Norman began this project to determine whether the five robust factors, found in previous lexical research, were by themselves sufficient or merely necessary for describing the global features of personality. To answer this question, he sorted the nearly 1,600 trait terms into 10 categories representing the high and low poles of the five broad factors. The within-category descriptors were sorted into 75 middle-level categories (the labels of which are reported in Goldberg [1990]), and then further sorted into 571 synonym clusters. On the basis of this multilevel classification Norman concluded that the majority of prime terms for stable traits, which included 1,431 adjectives and 175 nouns, could be assigned to one of the poles of the Big Five and that the FFM provided an adequate taxonomy of personality attributes.

Norman's findings were certainly impressive, though by no means conclusive because they were based on the subjective judgments of a single investigator. In other words, Norman's rational classification could not speak to the *empirical* structure of his descriptor pool. The first investigator to classify these descriptors using empirical methods was Lewis Goldberg (1981, 1982, 1990, 1992, 1993).

More than any other researcher, Goldberg has systematically studied the empirical structure of natural language personality predicates. Because the details of this work have been summarized elsewhere (Briggs 1992; Goldberg 1990, 1992, 1993), for our purposes a brief review of his primary findings will suffice. In a nutshell, Goldberg factor analyzed numerous subsets of Norman's reduced descriptor pool, using a variety of different methods of factor extraction and rotation, and he concluded that "analyses of any reasonably large sample of English trait adjectives in either self- or peer descriptions will elicit a variant of the Big-Five factor structure, and therefore that virtually all such terms can be represented within this model" (1990, p. 1223). Moreover, based on his factor analytic results, Goldberg developed several Big Five adjective scales (Goldberg 1990, 1992) that can be used to quickly assess an individual's standing on the five pervasive factors. Costa and McCrae (1989) have also developed a popular questionnaire measure of the five-factor structure. Because these instruments, and other Big Five measures (Hogan 1986), are increasingly being used in personality research, it is appropriate at this time to ask whether the FFM truly offers a comprehensive paradigm for personality description.

Tellegen and Waller Go Back to the Dictionary: Round Three

There are reasons to suspect that the FFM fails to account for important personality dimensions and that it offers a slanted view of the five natural language personality factors (Waller and Ben-Porath 1987; Waller and Zavala 1993). Consider the following: Allport and Odbert (1936), Cattell (1943), Norman (1967), and Goldberg (1990) endorsed a definition of traits that excludes the majority of emotion and mood descriptors and the vast number of evaluative terms that are encoded in the natural language. Yet we now know that mood descriptors and other emotion-laden terms are meaningfully related to well-validated personality traits (Tellegen and Waller, in press; Watson and Clark 1992, and references cited therein). We also know that *Self-evaluations are a psychological reality for most people*" (Bedner et al. 1989, p. 103). And prominent psychiatrists (Peck 1983) and social psychologists (Darley 1992) have asserted that even the extremely evaluative predicate *evil* has a legitimate place in a comprehensive taxonomy of personality attributes. Isn't it at least possible, therefore, if not highly probable, that the nature of the Big Five has been systematically skewed by the exclusion of potentially important descriptor classes?

To answer this question, Auke Tellegen and I (Tellegen 1993; Tellegen and Waller 1987, in press; Waller and Zavala 1993) revisited the lexicon and conducted the third major study of English language trait names. Like our predecessors, we culled a large number of descriptors from a contemporary and authoritative dictionary (*The American Heritage Dictionary of the English Language*), though we used a unique set of rules for discerning personality descriptive words. On the one hand, we wanted to avoid using overly restrictive inclusion criteria that might prevent us from discovering important and unexplored trait domains. On the other hand, we realized that overinclusive rules, if they were indiscriminately applied to the more than 400,000 entries in the dictionary, would leave us with a descriptor set that was prohibitively large.

Faced with this dilemma, we decided that it was critically important not to blacklist any class of trait indicators from our list. We also reasoned that the most general dimensions in the natural language would be represented by many, rather than few trait names. (Recall that Norman sorted nearly 1,600 descriptors into five semantic categories.) We therefore concluded that we needed only to abstract a representative, rather than an exhaustive, set of descriptors from the lexicon and that we could accomplish this task most efficiently by using a stratified sampling scheme. Our procedure was first to partition the dictionary into 25-page segments. Next, the first trait designator on a page that satisfied our purposely liberal inclusion criteria was chosen from up to eight target pages in each partition. Terms were considered personality descriptive if they could be meaningfully inserted into one or both of the following generative phrases: *Tends to be X* or *Is often X*. Notice that our grammatical hurdles do not exclude state descriptors or evaluative terms.

Four hundred personality descriptors were selected and assembled in two questionnaire booklets. Our questionnaire was not simply an adjective rating scale, however. Rather, our items were designed to conform as closely as possible to the original dictionary definitions. By using this format we could be relatively confident that our subjects would understand the meanings of our items. Recall that Norman and Goldberg eliminated thousands of terms from their lists because they were judged either ambiguous or obscure. For example, the adjective *gesticulative* is a relatively ambiguous and obscure trait descriptor (cf. Goldberg and Kilkowski 1985). The personality characteristic that is tapped by the item: *Makes gestures, especially to add force or emphasis during speech, gesticulative,* (number 149 in our questionnaire booklet) is easily grasped by most individuals. The dictionary defines *gesticulative* as follows: [tending to] make gesture, especially to do so to add force or emphasis during speech.

Tellegen and Waller (1987) collected self-descriptions on 400 lexically derived items from 585 University of Minnesota undergraduates. These students were also given the 35 Cattell variables that have played such an important part in the history of the FFM. The subjects were instructed not to rate how they felt at this moment but how they usually or generally or typically felt, thought, or acted, and to mark their answer sheet accordingly, using a four-point scale. The ratings were correlated, and factor solutions of between 5 and 20 factors were extracted and rotated to the varimax position. A seven-factor solution provided the most compelling and psychologically meaningful description of the data. The seven Tellegen and Waller factors, with a sample of abbreviated markers, are as follows: I) positive valence (*important, outstanding, special, first-rate*); II) negative valence (*evil, vicious, wicked, worthless*); III) positive emotionality (*cheerful, social, convivial, spirited*); IV) negative emotionality (*nervous, anxious, prone to have mood swings, cycloid*); V) conventionality (*conservative, mossbacked; not eccentric, not odd*); VI) agreeableness (*agreeing, not stubborn, not bad-tempered, not sarcastic*); and VII) dependability (*deliberate, careful, resolute, consistent*).

Notice that five of these factors closely resemble, although differ in important respects from, the five dimensions of the FFM. Positive emotionality resembles extraversion or factor I of the Big Five , but emphasizes the positive emotional core of this dimension (see Watson and Clark 1992, for a similar interpretation). Likewise, negative emotionality accents the negative emotional core of neuroticism. The two agreeableness factors are similar, as our choice of the same name implies, and Tellegen and Waller's dependability factor was clearly recognizable as Big Five conscientiousness. Interestingly, Tellegen and Waller's conventionality factor more closely resembled the obverse of openness to experience (McCrae and Costa 1986) than intellect (Goldberg 1993), suggesting that McCrae and Costa's interpretation of factor V may be more aligned with the natural language.

The most striking difference between the Tellegen and Waller findings and other lexical results was the emergence of two broadly defined evaluative factors. Previous investigators (Osgood et al. 1957; Peabody 1967, 1970, 1978) have assumed that evaluation is best conceived as a single bipolar dimension anchored by the terms *good* and *bad*. Tellegen and Waller discovered that in the domain of self portrayals two orthogonal evaluative factors can be extracted from lexical descriptors that have not been purged of their evaluative indicators. Positive valence measures a sense of self-worth and personal value at moderate levels and a grandiose sense of self-importance and specialness at the upper extreme. Negative valence taps self-perceptions of evilness or awfulness. These authors also demonstrated the authenticity of positive and negative valence by showing that they were not artifacts of item difficulty (Tellegen 1993; Tellegen and Waller, in press; Waller and Zavala 1993). Later I will discuss the psychological meaning of these dimensions in greater detail after describing a conceptual validation study of the Big Seven.

The Robustness of the Big Seven

Tellegen et al. (1991) developed an experimental Big Seven research questionnaire to examine the structural robustness of the seven-factor model. The questionnaire was called *The Inventory of Personal Characteristics* (IPC-7). As part of an ongoing study of the genetic and environmental influences on personality development, I administered the IPC-7 to approximately 1,800 twins and twin-family members of the California Twin Study. This sample of genetically informative subjects has allowed me to investigate the factor structure of the IPC-7 and to conduct a biometric analysis of the seven-factor model. The results of these analyses follow.

Data from 1,754 community-dwelling volunteers were used in the factor analysis of the IPC-7. At the time of testing the 600 male and

1,154 female subjects in this sample had mean ages of 44.22 (SD = 17.15, range = 15–87) and 39.41 (SD = 16.73, range = 15–90) years, respectively. The item responses were ipsatized (i.e., person centered) to minimize the effects of extreme response style (Goldberg 1992; Hamilton 1968) and then correlated to produce a 161 × 161 inter-item correlation matrix. The linear and quadratic effects of gender and age were partialled from the matrix to attenuate the influence of these variables on the resulting factor structure. Several factor solutions were extracted (using principal axes with iterated communalities) and rotated to the varimax position.

The eigenvalue plot from the ipsatized correlation matrix suggested that a seven-factor solution best accounted for the major sources of variance in the IPC-7. (The first 15 ranked eigenvalues were 13.62, 9.17, 6.80, 5.41, 5.13, 3.97, 2.95, 2.49, 2.19, 2.11, 1.84, 1.71, 1.64, 1.62, 1.60.) Factor solutions from five to nine factors were therefore extracted and examined for psychological meaningfulness. The seven-factor solution provided the most compelling psychological structure.[2] The varimax-rotated factor loadings from this solution are reported in Table 7–1.

When viewing this table one is immediately impressed by the almost perfect simple structure in the pattern of factor loadings. The majority of items load on a single factor and relatively few items exhibit factorial complexity. The seven factors are also easily recognized as the seven dimensions of the Big Seven. This is not altogether surprising. The IPC-7 was partly constructed to tap Tellegen and Waller's (1987, in press) seven-factor model. Nonetheless, it is comforting that in an independent sample, which is considerably more heterogeneous then Tellegen and Waller's (1987) student sample, the most unique features of the Big Seven are unequivocally replicated. There are two large and psychologically meaningful evaluative factors that are essentially uncorrelated. The correlation between positive and negative valence in

---

[2]A five-factor solution made no psychological sense. Factor I in the five-factor solution was a mixture of positive valence, (reversed) agreeableness and (reversed) negative emotionality. Factor II combined conscientiousness and conventionality markers. Factor III was an emotionality factor defined by reversed negative emotionality and positive emotionality markers. Factor IV contained negative emotionality and (reversed) agreeableness items and factor V contained all of the negative valence markers.

TABLE 7–1.
Seven primary factors of the natural language

Abbreviated items	PVAL	NVAL	PEM	NEM	C	A	CNV
Outstanding, superior	69	-03	05	-11	-00	-05	-11
Impressive, remarkable	67	-05	10	-10	-03	-02	-06
Excellent, first rate	61	-03	07	-15	07	00	-02
Exceptional, special	60	-00	07	-10	-09	00	-15
Deserve to be admired	54	-08	11	-07	-01	00	-01
Important, significant	53	-06	12	-17	01	01	00
High-ranking, powerful	51	02	15	-13	03	-15	01
Of high quality	51	-05	05	-14	03	-01	-03
Influential, have status	50	-05	15	-14	09	-07	-01
Elegant, refined	47	-10	08	-02	03	09	08
Skilled, highly qualified	46	-14	08	-18	11	-04	-17
Talented, gifted	45	-05	03	-10	10	-04	-26
Sophisticated	40	-11	13	-10	-04	-01	-07
Without equal, matchless	37	07	-08	-12	14	-02	-02
Noble	36	-08	06	-05	-09	05	11
Imaginative, creative	**33**	-07	12	-09	-11	01	-31
Do not use imagination much	**-31**	00	-16	03	08	03	22
An ordinary, everyday person	**-51**	-08	-03	00	09	12	**33**
Average, unremarkable	**-58**	-04	-12	07	05	10	25
Not exceptional, not that special	**-66**	-05	-14	-05	05	03	11
Wicked, evil	03	**70**	-00	-06	00	01	-00

Cruel, mean	00	63	−00	−09	05	−09	−02
Awful	−03	59	−00	−01	02	00	05
Deserve to be hated	−08	53	−00	−01	03	00	−00
Dangerous to others	02	52	01	−04	−03	−09	−07
Mentally disturbed, sick	02	50	06	00	−00	12	−11
Treacherous, disloyal	−04	49	06	−08	04	12	−06
Disgusting, sickening	−07	47	00	−04	03	00	−04
Vicious, nasty	−02	47	00	05	−07	−25	02
Depraved, perverted	01	46	07	00	−06	03	−07
Insane, crazy	−00	44	04	−01	−22	00	−20
Rough, violent	02	41	02	−06	−08	−23	−02
Deceitful, two-faced	−08	39	00	04	−07	02	−06
Immoral	−06	39	03	−00	−11	01	−07
Deserve to be disliked	−12	36	−08	06	00	−17	−02
Bullying, threatening	−00	33	04	−03	−05	−25	00
Gregarious	09	07	69	−11	−10	−05	01
Like to be with people, sociable	−00	02	63	−06	−09	07	−00
Talkative	03	10	61	03	−10	−20	01
Lively, animated	15	01	56	−08	−12	−08	−14
Peppy, spirited	19	−07	55	−13	−08	−01	01
Playful	07	−02	45	−14	−18	02	−12
Warm, friendly	05	−00	43	−10	−04	29	06
Vigorous, energetic	19	−06	40	−16	01	−04	−10
Cheerful, sunny disposition	00	−04	40	−32	−05	25	05
Liked, popular	17	−03	38	−19	−00	11	06

(continued)

TABLE 7–1.
Continued

Abbreviated items	PVAL	NVAL	PEM	NEM	C	A	CNV
Laugh easily	−06	−00	38	−18	−12	03	−07
Affectionate, loving	05	01	36	−02	−03	14	−01
Carefree	−00	−05	32	−29	−24	22	02
Interested in others	−09	03	31	−06	−01	11	−18
Do not trust a lot of people	−12	06	−35	22	−03	−26	06
Uninterested in others	−06	−01	−36	−01	−01	−13	12
Don't show feelings	−14	−06	−44	−11	−00	04	01
Do not like a lot of people	−04	04	−44	11	−02	−18	00
Don't talk much, uncommunicative	−13	−11	−57	−04	03	−19	01
Prefer to be alone, a loner	−07	−04	−57	03	05	00	−10
Reserved, distant	−06	−13	−61	06	07	01	04
Quiet	−14	−18	−61	−00	11	26	−01
Feelings are easily hurt	−19	−06	−08	58	00	07	−00
Often feel sorry for myself	−19	−04	−11	54	−05	03	01
Often feel guilty for no reason	−20	−02	−09	53	−06	07	−00
Nervous, high-strung	−07	−00	−09	52	01	−11	00
Often jumpy and jittery	−11	−03	−05	52	−10	−08	03
Irritated by minor setbacks	−19	−01	−09	51	−00	−20	04
Prone to feel threatened, helpless	−19	−02	−17	49	−07	14	05
Bothered by painful memories	−10	01	−07	49	−05	−06	−04
Lose sleep over worries	−05	−06	04	47	04	−02	04

	A	B	C	D	E	F	G
Often feel betrayed by others	−12	03	−17	47	−13	−07	03
Quick to feel embarrassed	−27	−14	−21	45	05	12	04
Feel used by others	−12	03	−14	44	−12	02	07
Quick to blame myself	−28	−11	−07	44	−02	09	−09
Easily startled	−10	−09	−02	39	−06	06	12
Easily manipulated by others	−21	−06	−07	37	−15	27	08
Prone to have bad dreams	−01	07	−01	34	−06	−02	−04
Easily deceived, misled	−22	−05	−02	30	−19	16	03
Stay calm in an emergency	00	−04	00	−35	03	−01	−12
Quickly get over embarrassment	06	04	19	−43	−07	−03	04
Relaxed, low key	−05	−05	−10	−44	−07	38	−03
Do not worry about little things	02	04	−00	−61	−14	06	−03
Can put worries out of mind	01	−01	01	−63	−10	09	−00
Not easily upset	00	−05	02	−63	00	22	−04
Don't let things frustrate me	00	−01	01	−67	−04	14	−02
Do things in an orderly manner	07	−03	−09	04	65	−03	08
Well-organized	09	−05	04	−04	65	−04	05
Keep belongings neat and tidy	05	−01	03	05	55	−00	10
Careful in making decisions	02	−07	−15	−08	51	07	02
Like to have a place for everything	00	−00	−03	07	50	01	18
Punctual, get thing done on time	−00	−05	01	−05	45	−04	04
Consistent, predictable	−09	−10	−10	−05	44	13	18
Logical and reasonable	01	−07	−15	−08	40	07	−01
Disciplined, self-controlled	09	−06	−08	−17	39	05	09
Like to do things by the rules	−09	−11	−09	04	35	16	33

(continued)

175

TABLE 7–1.
Continued

Abbreviated items	PVAL	NVAL	PEM	NEM	C	A	CNV
Dutiful, carry out obligations	–14	00	–05	–01	34	02	08
Conscientious, scrupulous	01	–09	–05	–08	34	03	–01
Deliver what I promise	–01	–01	03	–11	32	–01	–02
Have some wild ideas	06	–01	12	01	–36	–15	–31
Do things that surprise and puzzle	05	01	05	05	–37	–12	–12
Fast and careless	–02	–04	09	–03	–38	–09	–15
Do not like to have detailed plans	–07	–05	–05	–15	–40	03	–12
Stop activity before completing it	–10	–05	–01	08	–41	02	–04
Do things spur of the moment	03	01	21	–07	–41	–05	–12
Spontaneous, impulsive	07	–04	32	–12	–43	–10	–16
Like to "play things by ear"	–02	–07	15	–16	–43	–03	–16
Like to be a bit disorganized	–10	–00	01	–13	–51	00	–26
Get into arguments, argumentative	–11	06	02	13	–14	–52	–05
Stubborn, obstinate	–10	01	–08	13	–04	–48	03
Others think I am quarrelsome	–14	13	–02	12	–07	–47	–01
Headstrong, willful	12	–02	10	–00	–07	–45	00
Rather fight than make a concession	01	–07	01	–01	–02	–44	01
Tough, uncompromising	03	–05	–08	–01	05	–44	–01
Strong, forceful	24	–04	17	–15	06	–43	–10
Unyielding, unbending	–03	–05	–12	15	01	–41	07
Do not hide views	04	06	30	–10	–00	–39	–16

Unpleasant if necessary	−08	05	−10	00	−02	**−38**	−06
Sarcastic, scornful	−14	08	−14	08	−06	**−34**	−15
Like to please others	−16	−05	13	17	04	**31**	06
Polite, tactful	01	−02	02	−04	17	**32**	13
Get along with almost everyone	−09	00	28	−20	01	**34**	11
Don't complain about poor service	−19	−07	−17	−04	−02	**32**	−02
Try to avoid difficulties with people	−12	−02	−11	11	05	**35**	08
Agreeable, willing to accommodate	−14	−02	10	−08	01	**41**	−01
Considerate, gentle	03	−01	08	−05	09	**41**	−03
Dislike arguments and conflict	−12	−04	−10	10	06	**43**	15
Easy on others, lenient	−12	−05	06	−12	−11	**47**	−00
Apt to give in to avoid disagreement	−14	01	−12	14	−01	**51**	11
Hold traditional values and beliefs	−06	−09	03	−01	15	05	**57**
Conservative	−13	−07	−16	−03	14	01	**56**
Home discipline would stop crime	−02	−03	−03	00	−00	−07	**46**
Conventional	−18	−09	−05	−01	20	07	**45**
Most parents are too permissive	−08	−04	−09	01	−01	−09	**42**
Thought of as old fashioned	−13	−11	−17	02	08	00	**39**
Have a natural respect for authority	−08	−08	04	06	13	23	**38**
Want my family well behaved	−06	−10	−06	06	19	05	**33**
Dislike foul language	−02	−10	−05	01	14	18	**31**
Different, unlike others	21	06	−17	−00	−17	−07	**−30**
Have wide-ranging interests	12	−07	14	−17	−12	−00	**−32**
Curious, inquisitive	03	−04	09	−11	−06	−05	**−33**
Weird	−12	27	−07	00	−26	−04	**−38**

(continued)

TABLE 7–1.
Continued

Abbreviated items	PVAL	NVAL	PEM	NEM	C	A	CNV
Odd, peculiar	−10	17	−21	11	−21	−02	−40
Strange	−13	16	−18	03	−24	−03	−42
Progressive, favor social reform	00	−08	10	−05	02	−01	−46
Unusual, unconventional	14	−04	−05	−03	−27	−12	−49
Politically radical	00	05	−00	−01	−06	−05	−52
Deserve respect and recognition	29	−00	00	00	03	00	−00
Flawless	27	00	00	−18	06	09	13
Stupid	−21	26	09	−01	05	17	−00
Deserve disapproval	−16	19	−01	09	−10	−05	05
Can experience real joy	00	−05	21	−19	−04	00	−09

Skeptical	−11	−03	−25	01	07	−20	−07
Humorless	−07	03	−28	03	06	04	14
Dependable, reliable	−15	−24	−05	−11	28	01	01
Cautious, circumspect	−10	−11	−22	09	26	05	15
Thrify	−10	−13	−15	−08	18	00	07
Decent	−07	−07	00	−08	08	04	−03
Naively enthusiastic	−07	−03	14	07	−24	−16	05
Often find myself in an argument	−15	−03	−06	10	−17	−29	−16
Steadfast	10	−04	−01	−20	21	−25	−00
Straightforward, forthright	07	−02	04	−20	17	−22	−10
Fairminded	−00	−01	−02	−17	16	17	−15
Unselfish	07	−03	20	−06	−01	26	−00
Want to have a good reputation	−00	−06	12	02	10	09	21

Note. PVAL, Positive Valence; NVAL, Negative Valence; PEM, Positive Emotionality; NEM, Negative Emotionality; C, Conscientiousness; A, Agreeableness; CNV, Conventionality. Factor loadings ≥ 0.30 in boldface. N = 1,754 community-dwelling volunteers.

the obliquely (promax) rotated solution for these data was 0.03. The highest correlation between any pair of factors in this solution was only 0.37 (between conscientiousness and conventionality).

Widiger (1993) and McCrae and John (1992) question the authenticity of positive and negative valence and suggest that these dimensions represent maladaptive variants of the existing Big Five. Widiger believes that "Negative valence . . . could suggest extreme antagonism [i.e., low Agreeableness]. Positive valence . . . may suggest excessively low Neuroticism" (1993, pp. 85–86). McCrae and John (1992) characterized agreeableness as the classic dimension of character "describing good versus evil" (p. 197). Our findings indicate that neither of these views is correct. Prototypical negative valence markers, such as *evil, wicked, awful,* and *deserve to be hated* are virtually uncorrelated with the agreeableness factor in Table 7–1. Representative positive valence markers, such as *outstanding, superior,* and *excellent,* share less than 2% of their variance with negative emotionality (corresponding to Big Five neuroticism). In other words, positive and negative valence are authentic dimensions of personality and self-appraisal that fall outside of the FFM.

It should be emphasized, however, that these factors do not account for all of the evaluative descriptors in the natural language. Indeed, numerous censorial predicates show meaningful relations to the other factors in the five-factor structure. Consider how the evaluative terms broaden the interpretation(s) of factor V.

Goldberg (1993, p. 27) has noted that it is "somewhat of a scientific embarrassment" that there is still no consensus concerning the exact nature of factor V, which is variously labeled intellect (Digman and Takemoto-Chock 1981; Peabody and Goldberg 1989), intellectance (Hogan 1986), openness to experience (McCrae and Costa 1985, 1987), or culture (Norman 1963; Tupes and Christal 1961). Notice that in Table 7–1 the openness to experience markers *wide ranging interests, curious, inquisitive,* and (secondarily) *creative* load most strongly on the factor that we have called conventionality. Tellegen and Waller (1987, in press) labeled this dimension conventionality in their earlier work because of the overwhelming number of terms dealing with conventional versus progressive attitudes, values, and beliefs that were present in their stratified sample of natural language personality descriptors. John (1990, p. 76) has also noted that in previous work by Goldberg (1990) "Nonconformity (nonconforming, unconventional, rebellious) loaded positively, and Conventionality (traditional, conventional, unprogressive) loaded negatively, on Factor V in all four samples" of Goldberg's analysis of the Norman descriptors. McCrae and Costa (1985) have also stressed the relation between conventionality and factor V, although these authors favor a broader interpretation of this dimension which they call openness to experience. Our results suggest that conventionality may be the more appropriate label if one is referring to the natural language dimension, and that openness to experience is a better title if one is referring to the broader psychological dimension (i.e., the dimension that relates to traits like absorption, which have few common-language predicates; cf. McCrae 1990). Notice also that the evaluative descriptors: *odd, peculiar,* and *strange* are salient markers of low conventionality, demonstrating that the evaluative terms, beside defining positive and negative valence, also broaden and clarify the boundaries of other major personality dimensions.

People who are relatively "closed" to new experiences describe themselves in conventional terms; they espouse traditional values and beliefs and have a natural respect for authority and rules. Individuals who are "open" to their environment willingly embrace new experiences, thoughts, and values and describe themselves as being progressive and radical. Being excessively open in a rule-bound society has its dangers, however. If you have memories of past lives, believe that you were abducted by aliens, or experience an occasional hallucination, other *less open* individuals may describe you as being *odd, strange,* and *peculiar.* Eventually you may begin to believe them.

A Twin-Family Study of the Big Seven

In this section I report the results of an ongoing twin-family study of the genetic and environmental architecture of the Big Seven. The data in the following analyses were obtained from 313 monozygotic (MZ) pairs, 91 dizygotic (DZ) pairs, and 149 married couples from the California Twin Study. For purposes of this study I constructed seven-factor scales from the highest-loading markers in Table 7–1. These scales were used to generate the twin and spouse correlations and the covariance matrices for the biometric analyses. The familial correlations and internal consistency reliability estimates (α, Cronbach 1951) for the seven scales are reported in Table 7–2.

At least three aspects of this table warrant comment. First, notice that the seven dimensions of the IPC-7 can be reliably measured with scales of moderate length. The alpha reliability coefficients, which estimate the proportion of reliable variance in the scale scores, range from 0.79 to 0.88, with a mean value of 0.85. These values are impressively high for broad-band factor scales. Secondly, note that the MZ correlations are uniformly higher than the corresponding DZ correlations for all seven dimensions. This suggests that genetic factors are an important source of variance on these scales. Thirdly, note that the spouse correlations for three scales are essentially 0.0 (negative valence, negative emotionality, and conscientiousness) whereas for the remaining scales they are smallish (positive valence, positive emotionality) to moderate (conventionality). Considered together, these findings suggest that genes play an important role in determining trait variation on the seven natural language personality dimensions.

TABLE 7–2.

Familial correlations and internal consistency reliabilities for seven natural language personality dimensions

Scale names	# items	r_{MZ}	r_{DZ}	$r_{spouses}$	α reliability
Positive valence	19	0.48	0.32	0.15	0.88
Negative valence	15	0.34	−0.03	0.05	0.82
Positive emotionality	15	0.50	0.09	0.11	0.87
Negative emotionality	21	0.55	0.32	−0.01	0.88
Agreeableness	16	0.33	0.17	0.03	0.79
Conscientiousness	21	0.48	−0.06	−0.04	0.86
Conventionality	17	0.60	0.36	0.41	0.83

Note. N = 313 MZ and 91 same sex DZ twin pairs, and 149 spouse pairs. Standardized reliabilities computed on ipsative scores after partialling the linear and quadratic effects of age and gender from the data. N = 1,754 community-dwelling volunteers.

To test this hypothesis more rigorously, several biometric models were fit to the twin-family covariances using a method known as multiple-group covariance structure analysis (Heath et al. 1989; Neale and Cardon 1992). An advantage of this method over less formal biometric procedures (e.g., Falconer 1961) is that when the assumptions of the model are valid or at least approximately so (e.g., all genetic and environmental effects are additive, the absence of a special twin environment) the method provides maximum likelihood (or generalized least squares) estimates of the genetic and environmental parameters and a χ^2 measure of model fit. The χ^2 index can be used to compare the relative performance of competing models of the same data.

I will not discuss here the mathematical rationale of the biometric models in any detail. Readers who are interested in learning more about these procedures can consult Neale and Cardon (1992), Eaves et al. (1989), or Loehlin (1992) for lucid tutorials. For our purposes it is necessary only to know that the procedure estimates the genetic and environmental variance components (or path coefficients) for a specific model by minimizing the discrepancy between the observed and model-implied family covariances. The expectations for the model-implied covariances were derived by Fisher (1918) and are reported in Table 7–3. Notice that this approach accommodates additive and nonadditive quantitative genetic models both with and without assortative mating. All models in this section were tested with a program written by this author for multiple-group covariance structure analysis (written in GAUSS [APTECH 1993]).

The genetic and environmental variance components for the seven natural-language personality scales are reported in Table 7–4. We will first consider the results for the five scales with counterparts in the FFM: positive emotionality (factor I), negative emotionality (factor IV), agreeableness (factor II), conscientiousness (factor III) and conventionality (factor V). As reported in this table, the five factors are all significantly influenced by genetic variance, with broad-sense heritabilities ranging from 0.33 (agreeableness) to 0.59 (conventionality). Notice that for conscientiousness the nonadditive model provides a statistically improved fit over the purely additive model (tested by fixing the shared environmental parameter to 0.0 and performing a one degree of freedom χ^2 difference test: $\chi^2 = 6.07$, $P \leq .02$). This finding

TABLE 7-3.
Expected covariances among family members for additive and nonadditive biometric models

| Covariance | Random mating | | Expected covariances | | | Assortative mating |
	Additive model	Nonadditive model		Additive model		Nonadditive model
MZ	$Va + Vc$	$Va + Vd$		$Va + Vc$		$Va + Vd$
DZ	$1/2Va = Vc$	$1/2Va + 1/4Vd$		$1/2Va(1 + h^2m) = Vc$		$1/2Va(1 + h^2m) + 1/4Vd$
Spouse	—	—		mVp		mVp

Note. Va, *variance due to additive genetic effects;* Vc, *variance due to shared environmental effects;* Vd, *variance due to genetic dominance;* m, *phenotypic spousal correlation;* Vp, *phenotypic variance.*

TABLE 7–4.

Genetic and environmental variance components for seven natural language personality dimensions

| | Variance components | | | | | |
| | Genetic | | Environmental | | | |
Personality dimensions	Additive (Va)	Nonadditive (Vd)	Shared (Vc)	Nonshared (Ve)	$3\chi^{2a}$	P
Positive valence	0.29	—	0.18	0.53	2.45	0.49
Negative valence	***	***	***	***	***	***
Positive emotionality	0.49	—	0.00	0.51	3.37	0.34
	0.00	0.50	—	0.50	0.71	0.87
Negative emotionality	0.42	—	0.12	0.46	1.67	0.64
Agreeableness	0.33	—	0.00	0.67	3.76	0.29
	0.27	0.06	—	0.67	3.73	0.29
Conscientiousness	0.46	—	0.00	0.54	9.68	0.02
	0.00	0.48	—	0.52	3.61	0.31
Conventionality	0.58	—	0.00	0.42	8.08	0.15
	0.45	0.14	—	0.41	7.39	0.19

Note. N = 313 MZ *pairs; 91 same sex DZ pairs; 149 spouse pairs.* Va, *variance due to additive genetic effects;* Vd, *variance due to nonadditive genetic effects (mostly genetic dominance);* Vc, *variance due to common environmental effects that are shared among family members; and* Ve, *unique or nonshared environmental effects.*
[a]*df = 3, except for conventionality, where df = 5.*

is consistent with results from two studies of twins reared together and apart (Bergeman et al. 1993; Tellegen et al. 1988). Together these replicated findings are heuristic because they potentially speak to the evolutionary significance of conscientiousness; i.e., traits that conferred an adaptive advantage during our evolutionary history are predicted to have a high ratio of nonadditive to additive genetic variance (specifically, directional dominance; Broadhurst and Jinks 1974). This may or may not explain the results for conscientiousness. However, if we suspend our critical faculties for a moment it is easy to imagine a prehistoric scenario in which conscientious parents, hunters, and gatherers enjoyed greater inclusive fitness than their negligent and less industrious neighbors. I will refrain from additional storytelling and note only that our results for the other four dimensions are consistent with behavioral genetic reviews of the Big Five (Bergeman et al. 1993; Loehlin 1992).

There are two reasons for taking a closer look at the biometric findings for positive and negative valence. First, both dimensions fall outside of the Big Five factor space; consequently they have been excluded from behavior genetic reviews of personality (Eaves et al. 1989; Loehlin 1992). Secondly, the genetic and environmental influences on positive and negative valence are structurally different from those of the other five dimensions; thus they deserve special consideration. I will discuss the results for negative valence first.

Notice that the variance components for negative valence are not reported in Table 7–4. They were omitted from the table to emphasize that the previous biometric models failed to account for the pattern of family covariances for negative valence. Not surprisingly, few people in the general population describe themselves as being wicked, evil, or awful. Hence, the factor scores for negative valence are considerably skewed to the right. Biometric methods that rely on maximum likelihood optimization yield biased parameter estimates when data are markedly skewed (Waller and Muthén 1992). It was therefore necessary to use an alternative optimization technique to analyze the negative valence data. The method I used is called genetic Tobit factor analysis (GTFA; Waller and Muthén 1992). Waller and Muthén (1992) have shown that GTFA produces unbiased estimates of behavioral genetic parameters when analyzing skewed data from twins.

Two models were tested in the first set of analyses: the simple additive (Va, Vc, Ve)[3] and nonadditive (Va, Vd, Ve) GTFA models. The additive model failed to converge by 200 iterations. The nonadditive model converged, but yielded a poor fit ($\chi^2 = 12.18$, df $= 3$, $P = .007$; $Va = 0.0$, $Vd = 0.34$, $Ve = 0.66$). Perhaps a different model would fit these data better? An assumption of the previous models is that the observed MZ and DZ variances will not systematically differ by zygosity (Jinks and Fulker 1970). In the present sample, however, the pooled negative valence MZ variance is appreciably *less* than the corresponding DZ variance (the lower triangles of the MZ and DZ [Tobit] covariance matrices are 0.717, 0.242, 0.696 and 0.984, −0.004,

---

[3]See Table 7–4 note (a) for definition of Va, Vc, Vd, and Ve.

and 1.15, respectively). This may indicate that the phenotype of one twin is an important component of the co-twin's environment (and vice versa), a phenomenon known as sibling interaction effects.

Sibling interaction effects are important in quantitative genetic models because they produce systematic differences in twin variances. Biometric models that allow for sibling interactions have been developed by Eaves (1976), Carey (1986, 1992), and others (Neale and Cardon 1992, chap. 10). One model that seems promising for the negative valence data is the sibling competition model (Carey 1986), which predicts a smaller MZ variance than DZ variance. In this model siblings *contrast* rather than *imitate* each other's behavior. Competition effects are specified in the model by adding two equated parameters, labeled *s*, each of which represents the reciprocal influence of one twin's behavior on the other (see Neale and Cardon 1992 for details).

A sibling competition model with additive genetic, dominance genetic, and unique environmental variance components was tested with the negative valence data. The model could not be rejected by the χ^2 significance test ($\chi^2 = 4.212$, df $= 2$, $P = .12$) and it provided a significantly better fit than the model with *s* fixed at 0.00 (i.e., no sibling interactions; $\chi^2 = 7.97$, df $= 1$, $P = .005$). This finding is noteworthy for at least two reasons. First, as pointedly stated by Neale and Cardon: "For I.Q., educational attainment, psychometric assessments of personality, social attitudes, body mass index, heart rate reactivity, and so on, the behavior genetics literature is replete with evidence for the *absence* of the effects of social interaction" (1992, p. 209). Secondly, there are several reasons why negative valence should be influenced by potent social interaction effects.

Developmental psychologists have frequently stressed the importance of within-family social comparisons in the formation of positive and negative self-appraisals. Writing on this issue Dunn and Plomin (1990) have noted that children "show that they are very conscious of differences between themselves and their siblings and that they compare themselves with these different siblings surprisingly early in development" (p. 109). It is also well established that "another person's similarity to oneself (however defined) is a crucial parameter of social comparison" (Kruglanski and Mayseless 1990, p. 195; see also Festinger 1954). Together these findings suggest that twins should be especially prone to making evaluative social comparisons while forming conceptions of self or at least while forming negative self-appraisals. Our data provide no evidence for sibling imitation or contrast effects for the other dimension of self-evaluation: positive valence. The pooled MZ and DZ variances for this trait are virtually identical (0.99 and 0.94, respectively). Nonetheless, there are reasons to suspect that a different form of social interaction is important in the development of positive or grandiose self-evaluations.

The results in Table 7–4 suggest that environmental influences that are shared among siblings account for nearly one-fifth of the variance in the positive valence scores. This is an unusual finding in a domain where shared environmental effects are nonexistent or difficult to detect with the twin design (Plomin and Daniels 1987). By itself, it tells us nothing about which features of the shared environment are important. But it does provide clues concerning where to look for these potent influences. Perhaps supportive and nurturing parents foster positive self-regard in their offspring. Or perhaps through social learning processes children model their parent's positive self-portrayals. Bedner et al. seem to agree with this second position when they suggest that "parent's expression of their own resolution of the self-esteem question is far more influential than what they teach verbally" (1989, p. 257). At moderate levels, positive valence may be related to positive self-esteem because it represents internal evaluations of self-importance and specialness. At more extreme levels it may represent narcissistic and grandiose self-appraisals. If this second idea is true our findings are particularly noteworthy since a review of the DSM-III-R personality disorders concluded that narcissism "has not been assessed in any family, twin, or adoption studies" (Nigg and Goldsmith 1994, p. 47).

Some of these hypotheses can be rigorously tested by a simple extension of the twin design that includes data from parents (Fulker 1982, 1988). The twin-family design used to analyze the positive valence data is called a PE cultural-transmission model (or phenotypic assortment model; Cardon et al. 1991; Eaves et al. 1978). It derives its name from the fact that it quantifies the effect of the parent's phenotype (P) on the child's cultural environment (C). Another strength of this design is that it partitions the shared-environmental component (Vc) of the classical twin design into four related parts—the effects of

1) assortative mating, 2) parental influences, 3) gene-environment co-variance, and 4) the remaining unspecified shared-environmental influences (Fulker 1982). Figure 7–2 illustrates the PE cultural transmission model via a path diagram (Li 1975) using the reversed path notation of Sewall Wright (1968).

The phenotypes of the mother (P_M), father (P_F), and twins (P_{T1}, P_{T2}) are represented in the diagram by the four rectangles. The ovals represent the latent genetic (G), common (shared) environmental (C), and nonshared environmental (E) influences that act on the phenotypes. The model-implied relations between the phenotypes and/or

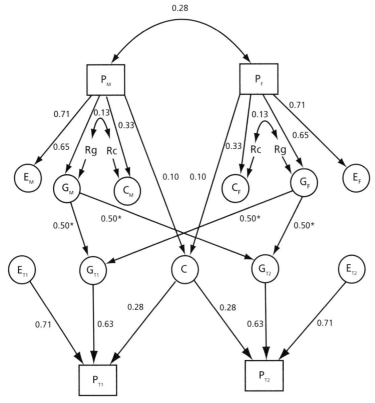

FIGURE 7–2. *A path model of vertical cultural transmission. Subscripts M, F, T1, and T2 denote Mother, Father, Twin1, and Twin2, respectively. P, phenotype; G, additive genetic factor; C, shared-familial or common-environmental factor; and E, nonshared, or unique environmental factor.*

latent variables are denoted in the figure by either single-headed or double-headed arrows. The single-headed arrows represent causal paths whereas the double-headed arrows denote correlations. Notice that two causal paths lead to the genotype of each twin (G_{T1}, G_{T2}). One path originates from the mother's genotype (G_M) and the other from the father's genotype (G_F). The standardized coefficients for these paths, which are fixed parameters given by genetical theory, indicate that children receive one-half of their gene complement from their mother and the remaining half from their father. Notice also that the model allows for assortative mating by connecting the parental phenotypes by a double-headed arrow.

To aid interpretation of Figure 7–2, I have included the standardized path coefficients for the positive valence data. These values were obtained with a program by the author that estimates PE transmission parameters by maximum likelihood methods (the expectations for this model are reported in Neale and Cardon 1992, p. 340). Estimation was carried out with an optimization program written in GAUSS (APTECH 1993). The combined sample included 1,119 twin-family members (80 sets of MZs and their parents, 79 sets of MZs and their mothers, 30 sets of MZs and their fathers, and 157 MZ dyads; 15 sets of DZs with their parents, 21 sets of DZs with their mothers, 7 sets of DZs with their fathers, and 47 DZ dyads). The full model, which estimates 5 free parameters from 50 observed covariances, could not be rejected by the χ^2 significance test ($\chi^2 = 49.98$, df $= 45, P = .28$). A reasonable conclusion is that the model provides a plausible and parsimonious account of the major influences on positive valence.

What are the main findings from this analysis? With regard to genetic influences on positive valence, heritability in the twin-family design is slightly larger ($h^2 = 0.39$) than the estimate in the simple twin design ($h^2 = 0.29$). Shared environmentality is smaller in the extended model ($c^2_{PE} = 0.08$ versus $c^2_{TWIN} = 0.18$). By far the most interesting finding concerns the cultural transmission paths that emanate from the parental phenotypes (P_M, P_F) to the twins' common-environment (C). The standardized coefficients for these paths (constrained to be equal in this analysis) are only 0.10 indicating that less than 3% of the total variance in positive valence is due to vertical cultural transmission. In other words, growing up with parents who believe they are *outstanding*, *superior*, or *remarkable* is not enough to give one an inflated sense of self. Parents contribute to their children's grandiose fantasies by being gene providers rather than narcissistic role models. Of course, other parental dispositions or behaviors may profoundly influence a child's standing on positive valence.

Evaluating the Personality Disorders

The FFM emerged from an assemblage of studies that banished or severely underrepresented trait names from two large classes of personality descriptors: the so-called evaluative terms and the affect-laden state descriptors. Psychologists have since acknowledged the importance of mood terms and temperament indicators in the structure and description of personality (Tellegen 1985; Tellegen and Waller, in press; Watson and Clark 1992). They have yet to recognize the importance of the evaluative terms. Fortunately, other disciplines have been less remiss.

The American Psychiatric Association, for example, in their official nosology: the DSM-III-R (American Psychiatric Association 1987), describes the borderline patient as someone *"characterized by alternation of the extremes of over idealization and devaluation"* (p. 346; high positive and negative valence). Narcissists *"expect to be noticed as 'special' . . . [and] feel that because of their 'specialness', their problems are unique, and can be understood only by other special people"* (p. 349; high positive valence). Avoidant individuals have a *"fear of negative evaluation"* (p. 351), and schizoid and schizotypal persons *"often appear odd or eccentric"* (p. 340; low conventionality). If psychologists are to succeed in describing the personality disorders from the framework of the FFM (Costa and McCrae 1990; Schroeder et al. 1992; Widiger 1993; Widiger and Trull 1992; Wiggins and Pincus 1989) they must first *evaluate the structure of personality*.

References

Allport GW: What units shall we employ?, in Assessment of Human Motives. Edited by Lindzey G. New York, Rinehart, 1958, pp 238–260

Allport GW, Odbert HS: Trait-names: a psycho-lexical study. Psychol Monogr 47(1):1–177, 1936

Angleitner A, Ostendorf F, John O: Towards a taxonomy of personality descriptors in German: a psycholexical study. Eur J Pers 4:89–118, 1990

American Psychiatric Association: Diagnostic and Statistical Manual of Mental Disorders, 3rd Edition, Revised. Washington, DC, American Psychiatric Association, 1987

APTECH: GAUSS User's Manual. Kent, WA, APTECH Systems Inc., 1993

Baumgarten F: Die Charaktereigenschaften. [The character traits], in Beitrage zur Charakter und Persoenlichkeitsforschung. Bern, A. Francke, 1933, pp 1–35

Bedner RL, Wells MG, Peterson SR: Self-Esteem: Paradoxes and Innovations in Clinical Theory and Practice. Washington, DC, American Psychological Association, 1989

Bergeman CS, Chipuer HM, Plomin R, et al: Genetic and environmental effects on openness to experiences, agreeableness and conscientiousness: an adoption/twin study. J Pers 61:159–179, 1993

Briggs SR: Assessing the five-factor model of personality description. J Pers 60:253–293, 1992.

Broadhurst PL, Jinks JL: What genetical architecture can tell us about natural selection of behavioral traits, in The Genetics of Behavior. Edited by van Abeelen JHF. Amsterdam, North-Holland, 1974

Brokken FB: The Language of Personality. Meppel, the Netherlands, Krips, 1978

Cardon LR, Fulker DW, Jöreskog KG: A LISREL model with constrained parameters for twin and adoptive families. Behav Genet 21:327–350, 1991

Carey G: Sibling imitation and contrast effects. Behav Genet 16:319–341, 1986

Carey G: Twin imitation for antisocial behavior: implications for genetic and family environment research. J Abnorm Psychol 101:18–25, 1992.

Cattell RB: The description of personality: basic traits resolved into clusters. J Abnorm Soc Psychol 38:476–506, 1943

Cattell RB: The description of personality: principles and findings in factor analysis. Am J Psychol 58:69–90, 1945

Cattell RB: Description and Measurement of Personality. Yonkers-on-Hudson, World, 1946

Cattell RB: Confirmation and clarification of primary personality factors. Psychometrika 12:197–220, 1947

Cattell RB, Eber HW, Tatsuoka MM: The Handbook for the Sixteen Personality Factor Questionnaire. Champaign, IL, Institute for Personality and Ability Testing, 1970

Chaplin WF, John OP, Goldberg LR: Conceptions of states and traits: dimensional attributes with ideals as prototypes. J Pers Soc Psychol 54:541–557, 1988

Costa PT, McCrae RR: The NEO Personality Inventory Manual. Odessa, FL, Psychological Assessment Resources, 1985

Costa PT, McCrae RR: NEO PI/FFI Manual Supplement. Odessa, FL, Psychological Assessment Resources, 1989

Costa PT, McCrae RR: (1990). Personality disorders and the five-factor model of personality. J Personal Disord 4(4):362–371, 1990

Costa PT, Widiger T (eds): Personality Disorders and the Five-Factor Model of Personality. Washington, DC, American Psychological Association, 1994

Cronbach LJ: Coefficient alpha and the internal structure of tests. Psychometrika 16:297–334, 1951

Darley JM: Social organization for the production of evil. Psychological Inquiry 3:199–218, 1992

DeRaad B, Mulder E, Kloosterman K, et al: Personality descriptive verbs. Eur J Pers 2:81–96, 1988

Digman JM, Takemoto-Chock NK: Factors in the natural language of personality: re-analysis and comparison of six major studies. Multivariate Behavior Research 16:149–170, 1981

Dunn J, Plomin R: Separate Lives: Why Siblings Are So Different. New York, Basic Books, 1990

Eaves LJ: A model for sibling effects in man. Heredity 36:205–214, 1976

Eaves LJ, Last KA, Young PA, et al: Model-fitting approaches to the analysis of human behavior. Heredity 41:249–320, 1978

Eaves LJ, Eysenck HJ, Martin NG: Genes, Culture and Personality: An Empirical Approach. London, Academic Press, 1989

Falconer DS: Quantitative Genetics. Edinburgh, Oliver and Boyd, 1960

Festinger L: A theory of social comparison processes. Hum Relations 7:117–140, 1954

Fisher RA: The correlation between relatives on the supposition of Mendelian inheritance. Trans Royal Soc Edinburgh 52:399–433, 1918

Fiske DW: Consistency of the factorial structures of personality ratings from different sources. J Abnorm Soc Psychol 44:329–344, 1949

Fulker DW: Extensions of the classical twin method, in Human Genetics, Part A: The Unfolding Genome. New York, Alan R Liss, 1982, pp 395–406

Fulker, DW: Genetic and cultural transmission in human behavior, in Proceedings of the Second International Conference on Quantitative Genetics. Edited by Weir BS, Eisen EJ, Goodman MM, Namkoong G. Sunderland, MA, Sinauer, 1988, pp 318–340

Goldberg LR: A historical survey of personality scales and inventories, in Advances in Psychological Assessment, Vol 2. Edited by McReynolds P. Palo Alto, CA, Science and Behavior Books, 1971, pp 293–336

Goldberg LR: Some ruminations about the structure of individual differences: developing a common lexicon for the major characteristics of human personality. Paper presented at the Western Psychological Association, Honolulu, HI, June, 1980

Goldberg LR: Language and individual differences: the search for universals in personality lexicons, in Review of Personality and Social Psychology. Edited by Wheeler L. Beverly Hills, CA, Sage, 1981

Goldberg LR: From ace to zombie: some explorations in the language of personality, in Advances in Personality Assessment. Edited by Speilberger CD, Butcher JN. Hillsdale, NJ, Lawrence Erlbaum Associates, 1982, pp 203–234

Goldberg LR: An alternative "description of personality": the big-five factor structure. J Pers Soc Psychol 59:1216–1229, 1990

Goldberg LR: The development of markers for the big-five factor structure. Psychological Assessment: J Consult Clin Psychol 4:26–42, 1992

Goldberg LR: The structure of phenotypic personality traits. Am Psychol 48:26–34, 1993

Goldberg LR, Kilkowski JM: The prediction of semantic consistency in self-descriptions: characteristics of persons and of terms that affect the consistency of responses to synonym and antonym pairs. J Pers Soc Psychol 48:82–98, 1985

Gough HG, Heilbrun AB Jr: The Adjective Checklist Manual. Palo Alto, CA, Consulting Psychologists Press, 1983

Hamilton DL: Personality attributes associated with extreme response style. Psychol Bull 69:192–203, 1968

Heath AC, Neale MC, Hewitt JK, et al: Testing structural equation models for twin data using LISREL. Behav Genet 19:9–35, 1989

Hogan R: Hogan Personality Inventory Manual. Minneapolis, MN, National Computer Systems, 1986

Jinks JL, Fulker DW: Comparison of the biometrical genetical, MAVA, and classical approaches to the analysis of human behavior. Psychol Bull 73:311–349, 1970

John OP: Towards a taxonomy of personality descriptors, in Personality Psychology: Recent Trends and Emerging Directions. Edited by Buss DM, Cantor N. New York, Springer-Verlag, 1989, pp 261–271

John OP: The "big five" factor taxonomy: dimensions of personality in the natural language and in questionnaires, in Handbook of Personality: Theory and Research. Edited by Pervin LA. New York, Guilford, 1990, pp 66–100

John OP, Goldberg LR, Angleitner A: Better than the alphabet: taxonomies of personality-descriptive terms in English, Dutch, and German, in Personality Psychology in Europe: Theoretical and Empirical Developments. Edited by Bonarius HCJ, van Heck GLM, Smid NG. Lisse, the Netherlands, Swets and Zeitlinger, 1984, pp 83–100

John OP, Angleitner A, Ostendorf F: The lexical approach to personality: a historical review of trait taxonomic research. Eur J Pers 2:171–203, 1988

Klages L: The Science of Character. London, Allen and Unwin, 1932, original work published 1926

Kruglanski AW, Mayseless O: Classic and current social comparison research: expanding the perspective. Psychol Bull 108:195–208, 1990

Leary T: Interpersonal Diagnosis of Personality: A Functional Theory and Methodology for Personality Evaluation. New York, Ronald Press, 1957

Li CC: Path Analysis: A Primer. Pacific Grove, CA, Boxwood Press, 1975

Loehlin JC: Genes and Environment in Personality Development. Newbury Park, CA, Sage, 1992

McCrae RR: Consensual validation of personality traits: evidence from self-reports and ratings. J Pers Soc Psychol 43:293–303, 1982

McCrae RR: Traits and trait names: how well is openness represented in the natural languages? Eur J Pers 4:119–129, 1990

McCrae RR, Costa PT Jr: Clinical assessment can benefit from recent advances in personality psychology. Am Psychol 41:1000–1003, 1986

McCrae RR, John OP: An introduction to the five-factor model and its applications. J Pers 60:175–215, 1992

Murray HA: Explorations in Personality. New York, Oxford University Press, 1938

Neale MC, Cardon LR: Methodology for Genetic Studies of Twins and Families. Dordrecht, the Netherlands, Kluwer Academic, 1992

Nigg JT, Goldsmith HH: Genetics of personality disorders: perspectives from personality and psychopathology research. Psychol Bull 115(3):346–380, 1994

Norman WT: Toward an adequate taxonomy of personality attributes: replicated factor structure in peer nomination personality ratings. J Abnorm Soc Psychol 66:574–583, 1963

Norman T: 2,800 personality trait descriptors: normative operating characteristics for a university population. Department of Psychology, University of Michigan, 1967

Osgood CE, Suci GJ, Tannenbaum PH: The Measurement of Meaning. Urbana, University of Illinois Press, 1957

Peabody D: Trait inferences: evaluative and descriptive aspects. J Pers Soc Psychol Monogr 7(644):1–18, 1967

Peabody D: Evaluative and descriptive aspects in personality perception: a reappraisal. J Pers Soc Psychol 16:639–646, 1970

Peabody D: In search of an evaluative factor: comments on De Boeck. J Pers Soc Psychol 36:622–627, 1978

Peabody D, Goldberg LR: Some determinants of factor structures from personality-trait descriptors. J Pers Soc Psychol 57:552–567, 1989

Peck MS: People of the Lie: The Hope for Healing Human Evil. New York, Simon & Schuster, 1983

Plomin R, Daniels D: Why are children in the same family so different from each other? Behav Brain Sci 10:1–16, 1987

Schroeder ML, Wormworth JA, Livesley WJ: Dimensions of personality disorder and their relationships to the big five dimensions of personality. Psychological Assessment 4:47–53, 1992

Spranger E: Types of Men. Translated by Pigors P. Halle, Niemeyer, 1928

Tellegen A: Structures of mood and personality and their relevance to assessing anxiety, with an emphasis on self-report, in Anxiety and the Anxiety Disorders. Edited by Tuma AH, Maser J. Hillsdale, NJ, Lawrence Erlbaum Associates, 1985, pp 681–706

Tellegen A: Folk concepts and psychological concepts of personality and personality disorder. Psychological Inquiry 4:122–130, 1993

Tellegen A, Waller NG: Reexamining basic dimensions of natural language trait descriptors (abstract). Paper presented at the 95th annual meeting of the American Psychological Association, August, 1987

Tellegen A, Waller NG: Exploring personality through test construction: development of the Multidimensional Personality Questionnaire. In Personality Measures: Development and Evaluation, Vol 1. Edited by Briggs SR, Cheek JM. Greenwich, CT, JAI Press (in press)

Tellegen A, Lykken DT, Bouchard TJ, et al: Personality similarity in twins reared apart and together. J Pers Soc Psychol 54:1031–1039, 1988

Tellegen A, Grove WM, Waller NG: Inventory of Personal Characteristics #7 (IPC7). Minneapolis, University of Minnesota Department of Psychology, 1991

Tupes EC, Christal RC: Recurrent personality factors based on trait ratings. Technical Report, USAF, Lacklund Air Force Base, TX, 1961

Waller NG, Ben-Porath YS: Is it time for clinical psychologists to embrace the five-factor model of personality? Am Psychol 42:887–889, 1987

Waller NG, Muthén B: Genetic Tobit factor analysis: quantitative genetic modeling with censored data. Behav Genet 22:265–292, 1992

Waller NG, Zavala J: Evaluating the Big Five. Psychological Inquiry 4:131–134, 1993

Watson D, Clark LA: On traits and temperament: general and specific factors of emotional experience and their relation to the five-factor model. J Pers 60(2): 441–476, 1992

Webster's New International Dictionary, 2nd Unabridged Edition. Springfield, MA, Merriam, 1925

Webster's New International Dictionary, 3rd Unabridged Edition. Springfield, MA, Merriam, 1961

Widiger TA: The DSM-III-R categorical personality disorder diagnoses: a critique and an alternative. Psychological Inquiry 4:75–90, 1993

Widiger TA, Trull TJ: Personality and psychopathology: an application of the five-factor model. J Pers 60(2):363–393, 1992

Wiggins JS, Pincus AL: Conceptions of personality disorders and dimensions of personality. Psychological Assessment: J Consult Clin Psychol 1:305–316, 1989

Wright S: Evolution and the Genetics of Populations, Vol 1. Genetic and Biometric Foundations. Chicago, University of Chicago Press, 1968

PART III

What Is a Personality Disorder?

CHAPTER 8

Categorical Approaches to Assessment and Diagnosis of Personality Disorders

Armand W. Loranger, Ph.D.

In defense of providing an historical context for this commentary on the categorical approach to the assessment of personality disorders, I will invoke Harry Truman's biographer David McCullough: "History is a guide to navigation in perilous times." (quoted in Klawans 1992, p. 11) And as navigational beacons I will rely on two giants who are no longer with us. They are selected for the acuity of their observations and also because they represent two quite different traditions: psychiatry and psychology.

Aubrey Lewis, psychiatric scholar par excellence, was a dominant figure in British psychiatry for much of this century. In one of his last papers (Lewis 1974) he made the following observation:

> It is plain that Kraepelin found the classification of these conditions defeating, as he frankly admits. Successive editions show him struggling with little success, to cope with the task of shaping categories out of the rich variety of human character and conduct. His efforts and his failures are characteristic examples of the frustration which besets students of personality when they aim at precision. (p. 133)

In a similar vein Lewis (1974) quotes the Harvard psychologist Gordon Allport: "All typologies place boundaries where boundaries do not belong. They are artificial categories . . . each theorist slices nature in any way he chooses, and finds only his cuttings worthy of admiration" (p. 136).

I will not digress to review what Berios (1993) has referred to as the *semantic paleontology* of such terms as character, constitution, temperament, psychopathy, and personality. I will simply note that in the nineteenth century what we now know as personality disorders were included along with many other nonpsychotic conditions under such categories as the *manie sans delire* of Pinel, the *monomania* of Esquirol, the *moral insanity* of Pritchard, the *impulsion* of Dagonet, and the *psychopathic personality* of Koch. I also cannot resist recalling a plea made before the end of the century by Francis Galton (1883): "The subject of character deserves more statistical investigation than it has yet received" (p. 42).

Historically, psychiatry has focused on pathological personality traits and used clinical observation, the mental status examination, and personal history as methods of assessment. It has also embraced a categorical approach to classification. Psychology has centered its interest on normal personality and relied on rating scales and self-administered inventories as the usual methods of assessment. Unlike psychiatry, it has favored a dimensional taxonomy.

The history of medicine is replete with diseases that have shed light on the workings of normal physiology, and discoveries regarding normal physiology have informed and advanced the understanding of pathology. It would be surprising if a similar potential for mutual enrichment were not latent in research on normal and abnormal personality. So far, however, points of contact and the integration and cross-fertilization of ideas have been minimal, partly due to issues of professional identity and partly a "two cultures" syndrome that has left one group largely unfamiliar with or disdainful of the other. This is very likely one of the reasons that progress regarding personality and personality disorders has lagged.

Categories and Dimensions

An ideal categorical classification system should specify the defining features of a disorder, and the category should have points of rarity with normality and other disorders. However, many mental disorders and a considerable number of physical diseases fail to conform to this ideal. Nevertheless, categorical classification has a long clinical tradition and has proved to be a very effective shorthand form of communication. Few would question the utility of such labels as agoraphobia, mania, and schizophrenia.

Critics (Widiger 1992) have noted several disadvantages of applying categorical classification to personality disorders: Personality traits exist on a continuum with normality, some traits may not be specific to a particular category, and some patients belong in more than one category. Advocates of a dimensional approach also argue that dichotomizing behavior that actually exists on a continuum diminishes the reliability of diagnosis.

As already noted, some of these objections to categorical classification are not peculiar to personality disorders and could easily be directed at a number of physical as well as other mental disorders. There is also no inherent reason why one must choose between categories and dimensions. Dimensional information can easily be used to supplement the categorical diagnosis of personality disorders, to the benefit of both clinician and research investigator. In that regard one is reminded of the poet William Blake's comment: "Without contraries there is no progression." Indeed, there are a number of disorders where categories and dimensions harmoniously coexist. Mental retardation and hypertension immediately come to mind.

The use of a categorical system of personality disorders supplemented by dimensions could foster the integration of clinical constructs and those used by students of normal personality. This would facilitate the pursuit of whether normal and maladaptive traits share the same underlying psychological and biological structures. This is not possible with the present classification systems, because they do not describe pathology with the language and traits favored by personality psychologists. An added complication is that the meaning or implication of a particular trait (e.g., introversion or novelty seeking) may be quite different depending on the constellation of traits with which it appears. This could be captured by a profile of traits or typology, but that is essentially a categorical approach. In the meantime, it is possible to convert existing categories (e.g., schizoid, dependent) into dimensions on which everyone might be located, regardless of whether they meet all of the criteria for the diagnosis. This provides valuable information to the clinician, and it adds more power and versatility to the analysis of research findings.

I will show some rather dramatic examples of the favorable effect that dimensions can have on the reliability of personality assessment. First, however, I would like to demonstrate the effect that the introduction of one particular categorical system, DSM-III (American Psychiatric Association 1980), had on the diagnosis of personality disorders in my own institution, the Westchester Division of the New York Hospital-Cornell Medical Center (Loranger 1990). Figure 8–1 compares the rate of personality disorder diagnoses in the last five years of DSM-II (American Psychiatric Association 1968) and the first five years of

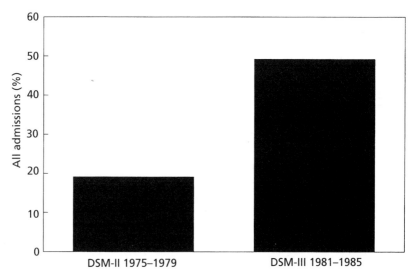

FIGURE 8–1. *A comparison of the rate of personality disorder diagnoses in the last five years of DSM-II and the first five years of DSM-III at the New York Hospital-Cornell Medical Center, Westchester Division.*

DSM-III. The comparison, based on 10,914 admissions, reveals a more than twofold increase in their diagnosis. Figure 8–2 should dispel any suspicions about the possible role of other factors. It compares the rate of personality disorder diagnoses in the first and second halves of 1980, when the transition from DSM-II to DSM-III was made at midyear.

Of course, the $64,000 question is whether personality disorders were previously underdiagnosed or are now overdiagnosed. Could it be that clinicians, enticed by a second axis, confuse personality traits with personality disorders? Could some of the new enthusiasm for personality disorders actually represent a misplaced concern about the role of premorbid personality in creating a vulnerability to some clinical syndromes, or modifying their course, outcome, and response to treatment? In other words, might some patients merely have pathoplastic variants of Axis I disorders? In this regard it is worth recalling that Erik Essen-Moeller, an early advocate of multiaxial psychiatric classification, recommended that a separate axis be devoted to normal personality as well as personality disorders (Essen-Moeller 1961). It

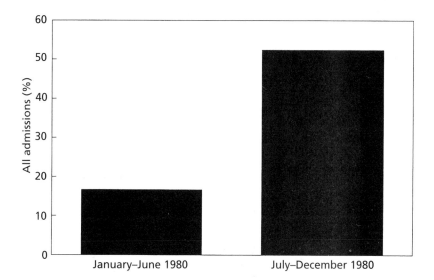

FIGURE 8–2. *A comparison of the rate of personality disorder diagnoses at the New York Hospital-Cornell Medical Center, Westchester Division in the transitional year (1980) from DSM-II (January–June) to DSM-III (July–December).*

TABLE 8–1.

Features of International Personality Disorder Examination (IPDE)

157 items arranged under six headings: Work, Self, Interpersonal Relationships, Affects, Reality Testing, and Impulse Control

Provides diagnoses and dimensional scores for all DSM-III-R and ICD-10 disorders.

Requires administration by experienced clinician, i.e., someone capable of making independent psychiatric diagnoses.

Detailed item-by-item scoring manual defines the scope and meaning of all criteria, and provides anchor points for scoring.

Scoring takes into account age at onset, duration of behavior, and requires substantiation of responses with anecdotes and examples.

Scoring has provision for information from informants.

Final algorithmic integration of scores may be done clerically or by computer.

Available in numerous languages including French, German, Dutch, Norwegian, Danish, Italian, Spanish, Russian, Estonian, Japanese, Swahili, Hindi, Kannada, and Tamil.

Training available worldwide at designated WHO centers.

would be interesting to compare the frequency of personality disorder diagnoses in such a system with that observed with DSM-III.

Reliability

There are data from the pre-DSM-III era (Spitzer and Fleiss 1974) and the field trials of DSM-III and ICD-10 (Sartorius et al. 1993) indicating that clinicians tend to agree less about the diagnosis of personality disorders than they do about many Axis I conditions. Therefore, research investigators may wonder whether some of the new semistructured clinical interviews for personality disorders are as reliable as Axis I instruments. Actually some of the data on this subject, most notably the results of the field trial of the International Personality Disorder Examination (IPDE; Loranger et al. 1994, 1997), are quite encouraging. I developed the IPDE at the request of the World Health Organization (WHO) and the U.S. National Institutes of Health (NIH) as part of the WHO instrumentation package for use in international and transcultural studies. The principal features of the interview are summarized in Table 8–1, and a sample item is displayed in Table 8–2.

The interview was subjected to a worldwide field trial (Loranger et al. 1994, 1997) that involved 716 patients enrolled in 14 clinical facilities in Austria, England, Germany, India, Japan, Kenya, Luxembourg, The Netherlands, Norway, Switzerland, and the United States. Tables 8–3 and 8–4 summarize the interrater reliability data for Axis II of DSM-III-R (American Psychiatric Association 1987), based on independent ratings of the same interview by an examiner and observer. Table 8–4 contains information about the temporal stability of the interview after an average interval of six months.

Note the favorable effect on reliability and temporal stability when one switches from categories to dimensions. This illustrates one of the advantages of supplementing a categorical decision about the presence or absence of a particular personality disorder with dimensional information about the underlying traits. In general, the reliability and stability of the IPDE compare favorably with those reported for semistructured clinical interviews that are used to diagnose the psychotic, mood, anxiety, and substance use disorders (Loranger et al. 1994, 1997). The comparisons, of course, are rough approximations because of differences in the heterogeneity of the patient samples, variations in the base rates of the individual disorders, and the different methods used to determine reliability (examiner-observer vs. test-retest) and temporal stability (same or different interviewer). However, the IPDE field trial was an unusually exacting test, because the interview was administered in numerous languages in North America, Europe, Africa, and Asia by 58 different psychiatrists and clinical psychologists.

Validity

In the absence of an acceptable "gold standard," the problems associated with establishing the validity of personality disorder diagnoses appear intractable. Therefore, some have suggested a less rigorous standard designated by the more base element, LEAD: longitudinal, expert, all data (Spitzer 1983). So far, however, attempts to employ the

TABLE 8–2.
Sample item from the International Personality Disorder Examination (IPDE)

1.   0   1   2   ?   0   1   2   ?   NA

Excessive devotion to work and productivity to the exclusion of leisure activities and friendships (not accounted for by obvious economic necessity)

DSM-III-R Obsessive Compulsive: 4

Undue preoccupation with productivity to the exclusion of pleasure and interpersonal relationships

ICD-10 Anankastic (obsessive compulsive): 5

Do you spend so much time working that you don't have time left for anything else?
If yes: Tell me about it.

Do you spend so much time working that you (also) neglect other people?
If yes: Tell me about it.

208

The examiner should be alert to the use of rationalizations to defend the behavior. The fact that work itself may be pleasurable to the subject should not influence the scoring. The term "devotion" should be taken to mean dedication. There is no requirement that the subject actually enjoy the work, although that is often the case. Personal ambition, high economic aspirations, or inefficient use of time, are also unacceptable excuses. Exoneration due to economic necessity should be extended only when supported by convincing explanations. Allowance should be made for short-term, unusual circumstances (e.g., a physician in training who has little or no control over his work schedule). The same person would not be excused if he persisted in excessive involvement in his work or career. Avoidance of interpersonal relationships or leisure activities for reasons other than devotion to work is not within the scope of the criterion.

2   Dedication to or preoccupation with work that usually prevents any significant pursuit of both leisure activities and interpersonal relationships.

1   Dedication to or preoccupation with work that occasionally prevents any significant pursuit of both leisure activities and interpersonal relationships.

     Dedication to or preoccupation with work that usually prevents any significant pursuit of either leisure activities or interpersonal relationships but not both.

0   Denied or rarely or never leads to exclusion of leisure activities or interpersonal relationships.

TABLE 8–3.

Interrater agreement of IPDE DSM-III-R personality disorder categorical diagnoses (definite or probable) and dimensional scores (N = 141)

Disorder	Diagnostic agreement (k)	Dimensional score agreement (R)
Paranoid	0.51	0.85
Schizoid	0.87	0.86
Schizotypal	—	0.87
Obsessive-compulsive	0.60	0.89
Histrionic	0.66	0.87
Dependent	0.82	0.92
Antisocial	0.73	0.94
Narcissistic	—	0.90
Avoidant	0.78	0.89
Borderline	0.76	0.93
Passive-aggressive	—	0.89
Sadistic	—	0.88
Self-defeating	—	0.79
Any specific PD	0.70	

Note. *Kappa calculated only when base rate is ≥5% according to both raters. Probable diagnosis assigned when patient met one criterion less than required number.*

LEAD standard have revealed its numerous shortcomings. When one considers the practical impediments to a convincing implementation of the method (Loranger 1991), it is difficult to be enthusiastic about it as a solution to the problem of validation. I would suggest a simpler and more pragmatic test: Do the diagnoses provided by a particular semistructured interview provide more replicable and useful answers to questions about etiology, course, and treatment, than those obtained with a different interview or by clinicians in their native habitat?

Obstacles to Validity

Comorbidity

Some of the potential obstacles to the valid assessment of personality disorders deserve additional comment. In most clinical settings the

TABLE 8–4.

Temporal stability of IPDE DSM-III-R personality disorder categorical diagnoses (definite or probable) and dimensional scores (N = 243)

Disorder	Diagnostic stability (k)	Dimensional score stability (R)
Paranoid	0.28	0.68
Schizoid	0.68	0.76
Schizotypal	0.68	0.81
Obsessive-compulsive	—	0.80
Histrionic	0.46	0.78
Dependent	0.43	0.72
Antisocial	0.62	0.92
Narcissistic	—	0.75
Avoidant	0.56	0.77
Borderline	0.72	0.87
Passive-aggressive	0.41	0.78
Sadistic	—	0.76
Self-defeating	0.71	0.75
Any specific PD	0.63	

Note. *Kappa calculated only when base rate is* ≥5% *according to both raters. Average interval between test and retest (temporal stability) was six months. Probable diagnosis assigned when patient met one criterion less than required number.*

majority of patients who receive a diagnosis of personality disorder have other mental disorders. I will demonstrate this by examples from what I believe to be the largest data set yet compiled on the comorbidity of Axis I and Axis II disorders. There are two caveats. First, the data are based entirely on hospitalized cases; and second, all of the diagnoses were made by clinicians without the use of semistructured interviews. However, the size of the sample and the use of a complete set of consecutively admitted patients in the study make the information unique and especially informative. Figures 8–3 and 8–4 illustrate the frequency with which personality disorders were diagnosed in patients with two of the more common Axis I disorders: major depression and anxiety disorders.

The coexistence of personality and other mental disorders is so commonplace that the potential for diagnostic error warrants concern. It probably requires considerable clinical sophistication to distinguish abnormal personality traits from both transient pathological mental

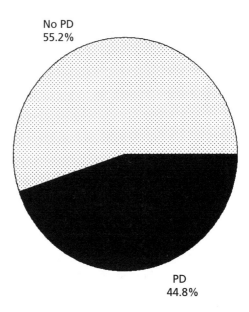

FIGURE 8–3. *The rate of personality disorder diagnoses in 1,684 consecutively admitted patients with a diagnosis of major depression.*

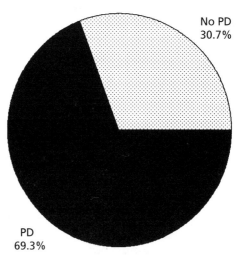

FIGURE 8–4. *The rate of personality disorder diagnoses in 317 consecutively admitted patients with a diagnosis of anxiety disorder.*

states and the manifestations of chronic Axis I disorders. Clinicians may incorrectly ascribe Axis II criteria, including the requisite subjective distress or impairment, to personality traits instead of to the Axis I disorder that is also present. The rather arbitrary assignment of schizotypal to Axis II and dysthymia to Axis I is a reminder of how permeable the membrane between the two axes can be.

Trait-State Issues

Patients in a dysphoric state may also have a selective recall or distorted perception of certain personality traits. The literature on the trait-state problem (Loranger et al. 1991) is virtually unanimous in demonstrating that this is precisely what happens when personality is assessed with self-administered inventories or questionnaires. Figure 8–5 provides a dramatic example in a middle-aged man who took the Minnesota Multiphasic Personality Inventory (MMPI) before and after the successful treatment of a depressive illness. According to the initial profile the patient is distinctly introverted (Scale O). The truth, however, known to family and friends and conveyed by the posttreatment profile, is that in his usual euthymic state he is actually quite extraverted.

We were probably the first to study this phenomenon with a semi-structured clinical interview, a pilot version of the Personality Disorder Examination (PDE) (Loranger et al. 1991). We were relieved to find that we were apparently able to circumvent the trait-state problem in examining predominantly depressed and anxious patients with symptoms of mild to moderate severity. We subsequently replicated the finding in a similar sample with the present version of the interview (A. Loranger and M. Lenzenweger, unpublished data, February 1992). The results thus far are encouraging, but the final verdict is not in on this subject, particularly in patients with severe symptoms. Although one could postpone the personality evaluation until the Axis I condition has remitted, clinicians and research investigators often do not have that luxury. I would also stress the importance of using experienced clinicians to conduct personality disorder assessments. The validity of semi-structured interviews should not be judged independently of the training and clinical sophistication of the interviewer. Regrettably that maxim is too often honored in the breach.

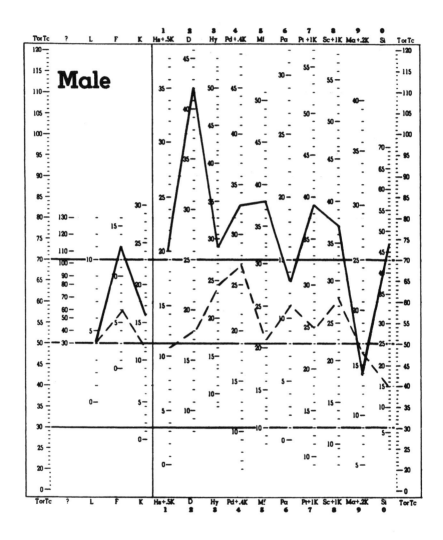

FIGURE 8–5. *An example of a trait-state artifact: the effect of the successful treatment of a pathological mental state (major depression) on an alleged personality trait measure (MMPI O scale, social introversion).*

Dissembling and Lack of Insight

Semistructured interviews assume that patients are aware of their own personality abnormalities. Clinical experience, however, would suggest that such insight is not invariably present. Some patients may also resist acknowledging a behavior because it is socially undesirable or they believe that its disclosure is not in their best interest. Others are inclined to exaggerate their limitations or amplify their distress or impairment due to personality factors, or because they are frantically seeking help or are dissatisfied with the attention or treatment they are receiving.

In clinical practice family members or close friends are frequently used as independent sources of information about patients. Personality disorder interviews like the IPDE provide for informant information. Regrettably, the literature to date would suggest that there is rather poor agreement between patients and informants regarding the information that determines whether a personality disorder is present (Tyrer 1988; Zimmerman et al 1988). One solution, and a not entirely satisfactory one, is to rely on clinical judgment to reconcile the discrepancies. Other options include stratifying research data according to the source of information or assigning only those criteria regarding which the patient and informant agree. These various procedures are not mutually exclusive, and research investigators might wish to use all of them to determine which yields the most replicable findings.

Conclusions

The widespread use of multiaxial classification following the introduction of DSM-III has resulted in an unprecedented interest in personality disorders. There are indications that clinicians make these diagnoses much more frequently than previously. Some of this may be due to a failure to distinguish personality disorders from trait-state artifacts and the pathoplastic influence of premorbid personality on other mental disorders. These potential impediments to valid diagnosis are a source of concern, and they require increased scrutiny by research investigators.

The categorical approach to personality disorder diagnosis remains attractive as an effective shorthand form of communication. Supplementing it with additional dimensional information is desirable for both the clinician and research investigator. Dimensions provide valuable additional information about the patient, enhance the reliability of assessment, and add power and versatility to the analysis of research data.

Some of the new semistructured clinical interviews for personality disorders like the IPDE show diagnostic reliability and temporal stability roughly comparable to those reported with Axis I instruments. The availability of these new interviews should facilitate research on personality disorders in the years to come.

References

Allport GW: Personality: A Psychological Interpretation. New York, Holt, 1937

American Psychiatric Association: Diagnostic and Statistical Manual of Mental Disorders, 2nd Edition. Washington, DC, American Psychiatric Association, 1968

American Psychiatric Association: Diagnostic and Statistical Manual of Mental Disorders, 3rd Edition. Washington, DC, American Psychiatric Association, 1980

American Psychiatric Association: Diagnostic and Statistical Manual of Mental Disorders, 3rd Edition, Revised. Washington, DC, American Psychiatric Association, 1987

Berios GE: European views on personality disorders: a conceptual history. Compr Psychiatry 34:14–30, 1993

Essen-Moeller E: On classification of mental disorders. Acta Psychiatr Scand 37:119–126, 1961

Galton F: Inquiries into Human Faculty. London, Macmillan, 1883

Klawans HL: Life, Death, and In Between. New York, Paragon, 1992

Lewis A: Psychopathic personality: a most elusive category. Psychol Med 4:133–140, 1974

Loranger AW: The impact of DSM-III on diagnostic practice in a university hospital. A comparison of DSM-II and DSM-III in 10,914 patients. Arch Gen Psychiatry 47:672–675, 1990

Loranger AW: Diagnosis of personality disorders: general considerations, in Psychiatry, Vol 1. Edited by Michels R. Philadelphia, Lippincott, 1991, pp 1–14

Loranger AW, Lenzenweger MF, Gartner AF, et al: Trait-state artifacts and the diagnosis of personality disorders. Arch Gen Psychiatry 48:720–728, 1991

Loranger AW, Sartorius N, Andreoli A, et al: The International Personality Disorder Examination (IPDE). The WHO/ADAMHA international pilot study of personality disorders. Arch Gen Psychiatry 51:215–224, 1994

Loranger AW, Sartorius N, Janca A (eds): Assessment and Diagnosis of Personality Disorders. New York, Cambridge University Press, 1997

Sartorius N, Kaelber CT, Cooper JE, et al: Progress toward achieving a common language in psychiatry: results from the field trial of the clinical guidelines accompanying the WHO classification of mental and behavioral disorders in ICD-10. Arch Gen Psychiatry 50:115–124, 1993

Spitzer RL: Psychiatric diagnosis: are clinicians still necessary? Compr Psychiatry 24:399–411, 1983

Spitzer RL, Fleiss JL: A re-analysis of the reliability of psychiatric diagnosis. Br J Psychiatry 125:341–347, 1974

Tyrer P: Personality Disorders: Diagnosis, Management, and Course. Boston, Wright, 1988

Widiger TA: Categorical versus dimensional classification: implications from and for research. J Personal Disord 6:287–300, 1992

Zimmerman M, Pfohl B, Coryell W, et al: Diagnosing personality disorder in depressed patients. A comparison of patient and informant interviews. Arch Gen Psychiatry 45:733–737, 1988

CHAPTER 9

Dimensional Approaches to Personality Disorder Assessment and Diagnosis

Lee Anna Clark, Ph.D.

Researchers in psychology and psychiatry have long recognized that the two domains of personality and psychopathology are closely intertwined, but it is only in recent years that we have developed a sufficient knowledge base in both domains to begin fruitful exploration of their specific interrelations. This chapter discusses dimensional approaches to personality and its psychopathological variant, personality disorder (PD). Whereas dimensional approaches are the norm in research on normal range personality, categorical approaches have predominated in PD research. Therefore, the first issue to be addressed is the advantages of dimensional approaches to PDs—as well as personality—when compared to categorical approaches. Second, two fundamentally different types of dimensional approaches to the study of PDs are dis-

This research was supported in part by National Institute of Mental Health Grant R01-MH43282.

A version of this paper was presented at the 1993 Annual American Psychopathology Association Meeting; New York, NY, March 5, 1993.

The author is indebted to Bruce Pfohl, M.D., for providing data that are included in Tables 9–5 and 9–6.

cussed, and finally evidence for the utility of a trait dimensional approach to the assessment and diagnosis of maladaptive personality is presented.

Advantages of Dimensional Approaches to PDs

It is well known that in establishing the first codified multiaxial system for psychopathology, the framers of DSM-III (American Psychiatric Association 1980) and DSM-III-R (American Psychiatric Association 1987) extended the categorical model that had enjoyed relative success in general medicine and psychiatry to PDs. It is also widely—although certainly not universally—acknowledged that this extension has proven to be somewhat problematic for a variety of reasons. Clark (1992) and colleagues (Clark et al. 1997) have discussed some of the major problems with categorical models of PD, so they are reviewed only briefly here:

1. Such a high degree of comorbidity and mixed diagnoses is observed among PDs that it is difficult to defend the notion of separate diagnostic entities (Clark et al. 1995; Widiger and Rogers 1989).
2. Specific Axis II diagnoses have a high degree of temporal instability compared to both general personality pathology (e.g., Loranger et al. 1991; Pilkonis et al. 1991) and personality traits (e.g., Costa and McCrae 1986; Schuerger et al. 1989).
3. The lack of clear thresholds for distinguishing between patients with and without specific PDs also is difficult to reconcile with discrete categorical entities (Kass et al. 1985).
4. Marked symptom heterogeneity within diagnoses raises questions about the validity and utility of the current diagnoses (Clarkin et al. 1983; Widiger and Frances 1985).
5. The notable lack of agreement on the appropriate conceptualization of the various PDs also raises questions about the validity and

utility of the current diagnoses (Blashfield and Haymaker 1988; Perry 1992).

It is noteworthy that at least some of these problems can be circum-vented—or even solved—through the use of a dimensional rather than categorical approach. Specifically, dimensional approaches: 1) are the-oretically consistent with the complexity of symptom patterns that are observed clinically; 2) increase reliability—both interrater agreement and temporal stability; 3) are theoretically consistent with the observed lack of discrete boundaries between different types of psychopathology and between normality and psychopathology; 4) provide a basis for under-standing symptom heterogeneity within diagnoses by retaining infor-mation about component trait levels; and finally 5) there is a general accord regarding the broad outlines and major divisions of personality trait structure, although the precise topography of the domain is still subject to debate (Watson et al. 1994).

Despite firm evidence of their various strengths, dimensional ap-proaches have failed to be adopted in the official taxonomy. A wide variety of reasons—ranging from the psychological to the anthropolog-ical, not to mention scientific—can be offered to explain this phenom-enon, and Widiger (1991) has written cogently on this topic. That confusion and misunderstanding remain concerning dimensional ap-proaches may be one reason that they have not been more widely accepted. First, there is confusion about what the term "dimensional approach" itself actually connotes; and second, there are widespread beliefs that the field of personality is complex—even chaotic—and that a large number of different dimensional models exist, each of which potentially could be applied to the domain of PDs. One goal of this chapter is to clarify some of this confusion and misunderstanding by addressing 1) the question of what dimensional approaches are and 2) the erroneous belief that the field of personality is still too incoher-ent and unsystematic to be applied usefully to PDs. The high degree of conceptual consensus on the broad outlines of personality trait struc-ture is outlined and evidence is presented that supports the robustness of personality trait structure at more specific levels as well. A second goal is to demonstrate the utility of trait dimensional approaches to the assessment and diagnosis of PDs. To that end, I will present evidence of their predictive power as well as case illustrations.

Two Major Types of Dimensional Approaches to PDs

The term "dimensional approach" has been used in two distinct ways. The first way actually remains rooted firmly in the traditional categorical system and largely accepts the notion of distinct PDs. In this type of dimensional approach, patients are assessed for each of the Axis II disorders, but where this approach differs from the DSM is that each separate disorder is conceptualized as a continuum. Thus, rather than deciding whether a patient is or is not borderline, does or does not meet criteria for paranoid PD, does or does not have an obsessive-compulsive PD, when using this first type of dimensional approach, one would determine the degree to which a patient exhibited borderline traits, the extent to which he or she had a paranoid PD, or the amount of obsessive-compulsivity observed.

Various scales have been used for this type of dimensional assessment. For example, Kass et al. (1985) used a 4-point scale ranging from "no traits," "mild traits," "moderate traits," to "meets DSM criteria." The Personality Assessment Form (Shea et al. 1987), developed for use in the NIMH Treatment of Depression Collaborative Research Project, uses a scale ranging from 1 (not at all) to 6 (to an extreme degree) for each diagnostic dimension. In Loranger's (1988) Personality Disorder Examination (PDE), each criterion is rated on 0 to 2 scale (0 = absent or not clinically significant; 1 = present but of uncertain clinical significance; 2 = present and clinically significant (i.e., at or beyond the DSM threshold), and the ratings are summed to provide a dimensional score for each diagnosis. A similar procedure is used for Pfohl's Structured Interview for DSM-IV Personality (SIDP-IV; Pfohl et al. 1997), except for the number and meaning of the anchor points: 0 = not present; 1 = present, but subthreshold; 2 = moderately present (i.e., at or beyond the DSM threshold); 3 = severely present.

There are also dimensional approaches that derive directly from the DSM-IV criteria (American Psychiatic Association 1994). The User's Guide for the Structured Clinical Interview for DSM-IV Axis II Personality Disorders (SCID-II; First et al. 1997), for example, states that the diagnoses can be scored dimensionally simply by counting the number of criteria met. Similarly, Widiger (1991) has proposed a consistent six-point scale labeled *absent, traits, subthreshold, threshold, moderate,* and *prototypic* based on the number of DSM criteria met for each diagnosis.

Finally, there are number of self-report instruments that provide scores for PD diagnoses. In some, each Axis II criteria is specifically represented by one or more items; examples include the Personality Diagnostic Questionnaire-IV (PDQ-IV; Hyler 1994), Schedule for Nonadaptive and Adaptive Personality (SNAP; Clark 1993), and Wisconsin Personality Inventory (WISPI; Klein et al. 1993). In these instruments, diagnostic scores are obtained either by counting the number of criteria met for each disorder (based on responses to the self-report items) and/or by summing the total number of endorsed items pertaining to a diagnosis. If desired, the DSM cutoffs can be applied to the criterion count to determine presence or absence of a diagnosis. In contrast, the PD scales of the Minnesota Multiphasic Personality Inventory (MMPI-PD; Morey et al. 1985) and those of the Millon Clinical Multiaxial Inventory-III (MCMI-III; Millon et al. 1994) assess the PDs holistically; that is, they provide only a total score for each disorder, without one-to-one matching of items with criteria. For the most part, all of these self-report scales were derived rationally, with an emphasis on the content validity of the items relative to the diagnostic criteria or the diagnostic categories as a whole. For the SNAP diagnostic scales, criterion validity also was considered; that is, scale items were required to be correlated with interview-based ratings of the corresponding criterion and disorder.

In all of these cases—both interview and self-report—the outcome of the assessment process is a complete profile of the degree to which a patient exhibits each PD and not simply a judgment of the presence or absence of each diagnosis, although those judgments also may be available. This type of dimensional approach has some clear advantages over traditional categorical diagnostic procedures. First, as mentioned earlier, ratings of the degree of pathology on a diagnostic dimension are more reliable than categorical judgments. Table 9–1 reports interrater reliabilities for both dimensional and categorical ratings in a heterogeneous sample of 88 patients interviewed using the SIDP-R. In all cases, a knowledgeable informant also was interviewed and both sources of information were used in rating each DSM-III-R Axis II criterion on a 0 to 3 scale: 0 = not present; 1 = present, but subthreshold in severity; 2 = present at or above DSM threshold; 3 = present and severe. A second rater independently scored the protocols using all available information (except self-report test scores). Reliabilities for dimensional scores were computed in two ways: 1) full dimensional scores were obtained by summing all items on a diagnostic scale and 2) criterion dimension scores were obtained by counting the number of criteria met. It is noteworthy that interrater reliabilities are invariably higher for one of the two methods of dimensional scor-

TABLE 9–1.

Interrater reliabilities of Axis II disorders based on the SIDP-R

Axis II disorder	Total score[a]	Number of criteria met[a]	Categorical diagnosis[b]
Paranoid	**0.84**	0.76	.74
Schizoid	**0.77**	0.76	—[c]
Schizotypal	0.80	**0.83**	—[c]
Antisocial	**0.95**	0.94	0.85
Borderline	**0.89**	0.85	0.39
Histrionic	**0.85**	0.76	0.53
Narcissistic	**0.76**	0.67	—[c]
Avoidant	**0.83**	0.75	0.30
Dependent	**0.91**	0.80	0.54
Obsessive-compulsive	**0.76**	0.63	—[c]
Passive-aggressive	**0.83**	0.68	—[c]
Sadistic	**0.76**	0.54	—[c]
Self-defeating	**0.80**	0.58	—[c]
Median	**0.83**	0.76	0.54

Note. N = 88 patients. SIDP-R = Structured Interview for Diagnosing Personality-Revised. (Pfohl et al. 1989). Highest reliability for each diagnosis is shown in boldface.
[a] Pearson's r.
[b] Cohen's kappa statistic.
[c] Base rate too low to calculate.

ing and—with one exception—the reliabilities of the full dimensional scores are higher than those based on the number of criteria met.

Second, from a clinical viewpoint, more information is retained using a dimensional diagnostic approach. This additional information permits identification of patients who are at just-subthreshold levels of disorder, as well as differentiation between patients who are just at threshold versus prototypic cases. Moreover, information about the general "background noise" of PD symptoms (i.e., multiple disorders with one or two symptoms) that is seen in many patients is retained rather than lost in a dimensional diagnosis. All of this information may be useful clinically.

Compare, for example, the dimensional diagnostic profiles shown in Figure 9–1 of two outpatients from a community mental health clinic who were interviewed using the SIDP-R. Subject A is a 27-year-old, single, Caucasian man whose presenting problems were insecurity and concerns about inadequate sexual performance; Subject B is a 38-year-old Caucasian woman, divorced with two children, who sought treatment for depression. Both subjects met full DSM-III-R criteria for avoidant PD on Axis II. However, the dimensional diagnostic assess-

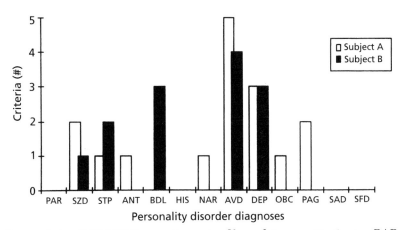

FIGURE 9–1. *DSM-III-R symptom profiles of two outpatients. PAR, paranoid; SZD, schizoid; STP, schizotypal; ANT, antisocial; BDL, borderline; HIS, histrionic; NAR, narcissistic; AVD, avoidant; DEP, dependent; OBC, obsessive-compulsive; PAG, passive-aggressive; SAD, sadistic; SFD, self-defeating.*

ment reveals that both subjects also show symptoms of dependent PD and Subject B additionally met three borderline PD criteria. However useful this information might be clinically, in the typical clinic setting it would neither be preserved in the formal diagnosis nor considered in formulating treatment plans.

Despite good within-method reliabilities and potential clinical utility, however, notable problems remain with this type of dimensional approach. First, Table 9–2 presents convergent validity data for several studies that reported dimensional diagnostic scores. Categorical convergence ranged from 0.09 to 0.50 (median = 0.30), whereas the coefficients for the dimensional scores ranged from 0.19 to 0.77 (median = 0.44). These results are quite discouraging, especially across-methods (i.e., self-report with interviews or structured interviews with the LEAD standard), although again dimensional scores outperform categorical ratings. These data indicate that 1) existing measures of the DSM diagnoses reflect different operationalizations—and perhaps different conceptualizations—of the PDs; and/or 2) various methods of

TABLE 9–2.

Meta-analysis of convergent validates of Axis II disorders

Method (# comparisons)	Categorical[a]	Dimensional[b]
Self-report instruments (4)	—[c]	0.49
Self-report best case:		
MCMI with MMPI-PD (2)	—[c]	0.68
Clinical or structured interview with:		
PDQ (2)	0.09	0.34
PDQ-R (2)	0.35	—[c]
MCMI (2)	0.15	0.26
MMPI-PD (1)[d]	—[c]	0.19
SCID-II with PDE—inpatients (1)	0.50	0.77
SCID-II with PDE—outpatients[e] (1)	0.36	—[c]
Structured interview with LEAD (2)	0.25	—[c]

Note. LEAD = *longitudinal evaluation of all data (Spitzer 1983). Clinical interview data are summarized from Perry 1992, except as noted.*
[a]*Cohen's kappa statistic.*
[b]*Pearson's* r.
[c]*Not reported.*
[d]*Morey et al. (1988).*
[e]*Hyler et al. (1992).*

assessment (self-report vs. structured interview and structured interview vs. clinical case formulation) elicit different types of information from patients so that different conclusions are drawn regarding the nature and degree of their personality pathology. Clearly, a great deal more research is needed in this area.

An important related point is that the validity of the diagnostic dimensional approach depends upon the validity of the PD categories on which the dimensions are based. That is, if the criteria for narcissistic or dependent PD, for example, do not represent a coherent set of symptoms, then nothing is gained by providing a dimensional score rather than a categorical diagnosis. Because it is difficult to develop sound assessment instruments for poorly formulated criteria and incoherent criterion sets, the weak convergent validities shown in Table 9–2 may indicate that the current diagnoses lack construct validity.

Third, viewing disorders on continua rather than categorically does not resolve the problem of within-diagnosis symptom heterogeneity. Two patients at threshold may still have rather different symptom profiles, if one meets criteria 1 through 5, whereas the other meets criteria 5 through 9, for example. Nor does this type of dimensional approach provide a theoretical basis for understanding the high levels of mixed personality pathology that are observed routinely in clinical settings.

Consider, for example, the diagnostic profiles of two state hospital inpatients, shown in Figure 9–2, who were interviewed using the SIDP-R. Subject C is a 34-year-old Caucasian male, separated from his wife, and hospitalized for treatment of depression and substance abuse. Subject D is a single, Caucasian male, age 28, also in treatment for substance abuse. Following the DSM-III-R, both subjects met criteria for paranoid, antisocial, and borderline PD, and Subject D also met criteria for schizotypal PD. Using a dimensional diagnostic approach, we can note potentially important information that typically would be lost in a standard DSM diagnosis. For example, there are differences in the degree of antisocial symptoms (5 vs. 8), and the additional presence of passive-aggressive symptoms in Subject D. In fairness to the DSM, it must be noted that it does provide for the mention of significant but subthreshold "traits"; however, such practice is rare in the typical clinic setting (Spitzer et al. 1982).

Note further that both patients show the same degree of borderline symptomatology. Can we expect they will be similar with regard to their pathology on this dimension? An inspection of their specific symptom pictures reveals that they share only two of the eight borderline criteria, so they actually have rather distinctive profiles with regards to this diagnosis. Failure to provide this potentially important information is a significant weakness of a dimensional diagnostic approach.

Thus, dimensionalizing the DSM diagnoses while still retaining the basic conceptualization of PDs as distinct categorical entities has some practical advantages and does reflect empirical reality more closely, but it is neither a complete nor a theoretically sophisticated solution to a complex set of problems.

Trait Dimensional Approaches to PD Assessment

So what is the alternative? The other major type of dimensional system is a personality trait-based approach. Congruent with the DSM definition of PDs as inflexible and maladaptive personality traits, a trait-based view of PDs maintains that the fundamental dimensions underlying this domain are not the PDs themselves, but the personality traits that compose the disorders. With this concept of dimensions, the outcome of the assessment process is not a profile of diagnoses but a profile of personality traits.

The initial problem with this approach is the question of what dimensions to assess. However, researchers into normal personality structure have been working on this problem for years and, as mentioned earlier, have reached a broad consensus (Watson et al. 1994). Empirically, factor analytic studies repeatedly have identified three to five higher order factors that emerge across a wide variety of multiscale assessment instruments and methods (e.g., Zuckerman et al. 1988); moreover, Eysenck, Tellegen, and others have proposed three-factor theoretical models to explain this robust phenomenon (e.g., Eysenck and Eysenck 1985; Tellegen and Waller, in press). Table 9–3 sum-

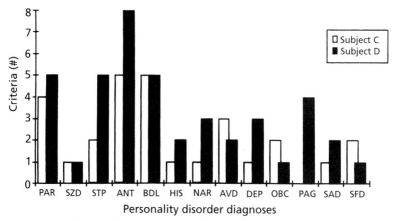

FIGURE 9–2. *DSM-III-R symptoms profiles of two inpatients.* PAR, *paranoid;* SZD, *schizoid;* STP, *schizotypal;* ANT, *antisocial;* BDL, *borderline;* HIS, *histrionic;* NAR, *narcissistic;* AVD, *avoidant;* DEP, *dependent;* OBC, *obsessive-compulsive;* PAG, *passive-aggressive;* SAD, *sadistic;* SFD, *self-defeating.*

marizes the convergent dimensions of the more prominent three-factor models in relation to the well-known five-factor model of personality, which is now identified with a large number of researchers, including Costa and McCrae, Goldberg, John, Peabody, Digman, Hogan, and Widiger, in addition to those initially associated with the model (e.g., Fiske, Tupes and Christal, and Norman). For detailed consideration of these higher order models, both in themselves and also in relation to PDs, the interested reader is referred elsewhere (Clark and Watson, in press; Watson et al. 1994; Widiger 1993).

These robust higher order dimensions represent an important theoretical structure for investigating relations between personality and PDs. However, from the viewpoint of clinical assessment, a more fine-grained analysis may be preferable. Although a number of well-established multiscale inventories exist for assessing normal range personality, only in recent years has progress been made in identifying and assessing replicable trait dimensions in the range of personality pathology. Specifically, two instruments have been developed with a primary focus on lower order traits relevant to PDs: the 15-dimension

TABLE 9–3.

Three robust higher order personality trait dimensions

Author/instrument	Dimension 1	Dimension 2	Dimension 3
Cloninger (TPQ)	Harm avoidance	Reward dependence	Novelty seeking
Eysenck (EPQ)	Neuroticism	Extraversion	Psychoticism
Gough (CPI)	Self-realization (−)	Internality (−)	Norm-favoring (−)
Tellegen (MPQ)	Negative emotionality	Positive emotionality	Constraint (−)
Zuckerman et al. 1988	N-Emotionality	E-Sociability	P-Impulsive, unsocialized sensation seeking
Five-factor model	Neuroticism vs. emotional stability	Extraversion or surgency	Conscientiousness (−) or dependability (−)

Note. The two additional dimensions of the five-factor model are agreeableness and openness to experience (also called culture, intellect, or intellectance).

SNAP (Clark 1993) and the 18-dimension Dimensional Assessment of Personality Pathology-Basic Questionnaire (DAPP-BQ; Livesley 1990).[1]

The development of each of these instruments has been described in detail elsewhere (e.g., Clark 1993; Schroeder et al. 1994), but is summarized briefly here. Livesley first compiled a comprehensive list of trait descriptors and behavioral acts that were characteristic of each of the DSM-III Axis II categories and had clinicians rate the prototypicality of these items for the relevant diagnosis (Livesley 1986). It was found that highly prototypic items for each disorder often referred to the same dimension, so it was possible to characterize each diagnosis using a small number of dimensions each consisting of conceptually related items (Livesley et al. 1989). Self-report items were written to assess each dimension, and following several rounds of data collection using normal and clinical samples, as well as scale refinement based on both factor analytic and clinical considerations, the instrument was finalized at 290 items assessing 18 dimensions. Psychometric analyses showed the scales to be both internally consistent and stable over a six-week retest interval (Schroeder et al. 1992).

Clark (1990) initially identified 22 clusters of PD criteria from the conceptual ratings of clinicians and psychology graduate students. Self-report items were written to assess each symptom cluster and factor analytic methods were used to revise and refine the scales through several rounds of data collection on both normal and patient samples. The final instrument contains 12 primary trait dimensional scales, and 3 somewhat broader temperament scales. The instrument also has 6 validity scales, and dimensional diagnostic scales of the type described earlier, but these will not be discussed.

As with the DAPP-BQ, and consistent with the theoretical notion that personality traits are homogeneous dimensions, the SNAP scales are internally consistent; alpha reliability coefficients ranged from 0.71 to 0.92 (median = 0.81) across six samples, including adolescents,

---

[1]Because they can provide facet or subscale scores, the Tridimensional Personality Questionnaire (TPQ; Cloninger 1987) and the NEO Personality Inventory-Revised (NEO-PIR; Costa and McCrae 1992) also may be considered to assess lower levels of the personality trait hierarchy. They are not included in this discussion, however, because they were designed primarily to assess higher order trait dimensions.

college students, and both inpatients and outpatients (Clark 1993). Moreover, the scales are temporally stable over both short and moderate time spans; retest coefficients averaged 0.81 (range = 0.68 to 0.91) in both a one-week retest of state hospital inpatients and a one-month retest of college students, and 0.79 (range = 0.70 to 0.86) in a two-month college student retest (Clark 1993). It is also noteworthy that the 12 primary trait scales are largely independent: In samples of 804 students and 289 patients, the average scale intercorrelations were |.17| and |.20|, respectively, and all scale pairs were correlated less than 0.60. These results confirm that the scales are assessing more specific, lower order traits rather than broad higher order dimensions.

Returning to the issue of using trait dimensions for assessing PDs, it was noted earlier that personality trait structure has proved highly replicable at the higher order level of three to five broad factors but that these factors may be too general for many clinical purposes. Therefore, it is important to investigate whether personality trait structure is replicable also at the lower order level assessed by the SNAP and DAPP-BQ. Furthermore, it is important to examine whether the traits relevant to personality pathology can be linked with lower order dimensions that have been established for normal range personality. To examine these issues, data will be presented from two large college student samples that completed the SNAP and either the DAPP-BQ or the Multidimensional Personality Questionnaire (MPQ; Tellegen 1993), an instrument developed using factor analytic techniques to assess 11 primary trait dimensions of normal range personality (Tellegen and Waller, in press).

Despite their disparate origins and different processes of development, comparative analyses of these three instruments have revealed a high degree of conceptual convergence (Clark 1993; Clark and Livesley 1994; Harkness 1992). The data presented in Table 9–4 provide support for their empirical convergence as well. An examination of the complete correlation matrices for each pair of instruments is beyond the scope of this chapter (see Clark 1993; Clark et al. 1996 for the complete matrices); accordingly, the strongest convergent correlation for each scale is presented. When scale pairs are perfectly matched (i.e., each correlates most strongly with the other), their correlation is boldfaced. Thus, SNAP Negative Temperament was most strongly cor-

TABLE 9–4.

Convergent validity of three instruments for the assessment of adaptive and maladaptive personality traits

SNAP scale	SNAP–MPQ	SNAP–DAPP-BQ
Negative temperament		
MPQ Stress Reaction	0.88	
DAPP-BQ Anxiety/Affective Instability		0.78/0.69
Mistrust		
MPQ Alienation	0.78	
DAPP-BQ Suspiciousness		0.64
Manipulativeness		
MPQ Aggression	0.62	
DAPP-BQ Interpersonal Disturbance		0.66
Aggression		
MPQ Aggression	0.74	
DAPP-BQ Conduct Problems		0.53
Self-harm		
MPQ Well-being	−0.50	
DAPP-BQ Identity Problems/Self-harm		0.61/0.60
Eccentric perceptions		
MPQ Absorption	0.65	
DAPP-BQ Cognitive Distortion		0.58
Dependency		
MPQ Stress Reaction	0.37	
DAPP-BQ Diffidence/Insecure Attachment		0.50/0.35
Positive temperament		
MPQ Well-being	0.73	
DAPP-BQ Social Avoidance/Identity Problems		−0.51/−0.51
Exhibitionism		
MPQ Social Potency	0.68	
DAPP-BQ Narcissism		0.37
Entitlement		
MPQ Social Potency	0.52	
DAPP-BQ Rejection		0.45
Detachment		
MPQ Social Closeness	−0.84	
DAPP-BQ Restricted Expression/Intimacy Problems		0.58/0.29

(continued)

TABLE 9–4.

Continued

SNAP scale	SNAP–MPQ	SNAP–DAPP-BQ
Disinhibition		
MPQ Control	−0.71	
DAPP-BQ Stimulus Seeking/Conduct Problems		0.68/0.64
DAPP-BQ Passive-opositionality		0.49
Impulsivity		
MPQ Control	−0.84	
DAPP-BQ Stimulus Seeking		0.67
Propriety		
MPQ Traditionalism	**0.73**	
DAPP-BQ Compulsivity		0.42
Workaholism		
MPQ Achievement	**0.79**	
DAPP-BQ Compulsivity		**0.47**

Note. *For SNAP–MPQ correlations, N = 251; for SNAP–DAPP-BQ correlations, N = 164. Correlations are shown in boldface if they were the highest for each of the two scales.*

related with DAPP-BQ Anxiety and vice versa, so this correlation is in boldface; however, DAPP-BQ Affective Instability also correlated most strongly with SNAP Negative Temperament, but not vice versa, so the correlation is listed, but not boldfaced.

Across the two pairs of instruments, the convergent correlations are strong and systematic. Ten of the 15 SNAP scales were perfectly matched, respectively, with the 11 MPQ scales and 18 DAPP-BQ dimensions, with correlations ranging from 0.47 to 0.88. Moreover, most of the convergent correlations were strong even when perfect matches were not achieved (e.g., the SNAP and DAPP-BQ Self-Harm scales correlated 0.60). In only a few instances does one instrument appear to assess a dimension that is not well represented in the others. For example, SNAP Dependency has no clear MPQ counterpart, and DAPP-BQ Insecure Attachment has no strong SNAP correlate. In a few cases, a single MPQ or DAPP-BQ scale maps onto more than one SNAP scale (e.g., MPQ Aggression correlated with both SNAP Manipulativeness and Aggression) or a single SNAP scale was correlated with more than one DAPP-BQ scale (e.g., SNAP Disinhibition was correlated with both DAPP-BQ Stimulus Seeking and Conduct Problems). These kinds of asymmetry, of course, are inevitable given the unequal number of traits assessed across instruments.

These data thus indicate that a reasonably well-defined and systematic structure can be found at lower levels of the hierarchy and not only among the higher order dimensions in personality. These results should be encouraging those clinicians who are uncomfortable reducing the complexity of their patients' personality pathology to three or five broad dimensions. These results also indicate that lower order structure may be highly generalizable, as systematic convergence is found among instruments designed to measure both normal and maladaptive personality. This finding should encourage cross-fertilization across these theoretically related but historically independent research areas.

Relating Diagnostic and Trait Dimensional Approaches to PD Assessment

Part of this cross-fertilization will involve examining relations between the two dimensional approaches to PD assessment described here. That is, what is the relation of trait dimensions to diagnostic dimensions, which are more closely tied to traditional categorical approaches? To answer this question, two patient samples were interviewed with the SIDP-R and also completed the SNAP. Sample 1 is the heterogeneous patient sample described earlier (e.g., see Table 9–1); the Sample 2 data ($N = 47$ for all but three scales, where $n = 40$) were provided by Bruce Pfohl and colleagues and used standard SIDP-R scoring. Ratings for each criterion were summed for each diagnosis to yield total diagnostic scores.

First, it is worthwhile examining the overall degree of overlap between these two assessment methods. Table 9–5 presents multiple correlations between the SNAP scales and the diagnostic interview scores; the two methods can be seen to share a great deal of common variance. In sample 1, multiple correlations ranged from 0.51 (obsessive-compulsive and passive-aggressive) to 0.82 (antisocial) with a median

TABLE 9–5.

Predicting diagnostic dimensions from personality trait profiles in two samples

Diagnostic dimensions	Multiple R	
	Sample 1	Sample 2
Paranoid	0.75	0.57
Schizoid	0.54	0.62
Schizotypal	0.63	0.73
Antisocial	0.82	0.85
Borderline	0.79	0.84
Histrionic	0.62	0.75
Narcissistic	0.62	0.73
Avoidant	0.66	0.77
Dependent	0.65	0.83
Obsessive-compulsive	0.51	0.69
Passive-aggressive	0.51	0.73
Sadistic	0.65	0.65
Self-defeating	0.55	0.79
Median	**0.63**	**0.73**

Note. *Sample 1, N = 88 patients; Sample 2, N = 40 patients. Diagnostic scores are derived from the Structured Interview for DSM-III-R Personality (Pfohl et al. 1989).*

value of 0.63. In sample 2, the association was even stronger, with multiple correlations ranging from 0.62 (schizoid) to 0.85 (antisocial) with a median value of 0.73. Thus, using all of the information in a SNAP profile, one can predict between approximately one-quarter and three-quarters (median = 42% in sample 1, 55% in sample 2) of the variance in interview-based diagnostic ratings. These data indicate that the trait dimensions assessed by this self-report measure also underlie clinical ratings of personality pathology; thus, joint study of these two assessment methods can further our understanding of both personality traits and diagnoses.

It is also instructive to examine the first-order correlations between specific traits and diagnoses; these are presented in Table 9–6. Although there are some sample-based differences, for the most part the observed relations generally are both systematic and in accord with theoretical predictions about the traits comprising each diagnosis. For example, across both samples, SNAP Manipulativeness and Disinhibition cor-

TABLE 9–6.

Convergent validity of personality traits with diagnostic dimensions in two samples

| SNAP scale | Diagnostic scale | Multiple R | |
		Sample 1	Sample 2
Negative temperament[a]	Borderline	**0.48**	0.40
	Dependent	0.43	**0.57**
Mistrust	Paranoid	**0.56**	0.30
	Dependent	0.21	**0.60**
	Schizotypal	0.43	0.45
Manipulativeness	Antisocial	**0.57**	0.41
Aggression	Antisocial	**0.62**	0.36
	Passive-aggressive	0.31	**0.47**
	Borderline	0.52	0.44
Self-harm	Borderline	0.65	0.70
	Antisocial	0.42	0.42
Eccentric perceptions	Schizotypal	0.33	0.36
	Borderline	0.33	**0.43**
Dependency	Dependent	0.52	0.50
Positive temperament[a]	Antisocial	**0.32**	0.06
	Histrionic	0.25	0.28
Exhibitionism	Histrionic	**0.39**	−0.04
	Dependent	0.10	**−0.55**
Entitlement	Paranoid	**0.32**	0.10
	Self-defeating	−0.05	**−0.48**
Detachment	Avoidant	**0.50**	0.38
	Obsessive-compulsive	0.08	**0.52**
Disinhibition[a]	Antisocial	**0.67**	0.59
Impulsivity	Antisocial	**0.45**	0.39
	Borderline	0.32	**0.41**
Propriety	Antisocial	**−0.28**	−0.19
	Obsessive-compulsive	0.04	**0.40**
Workaholism	Self-defeating	0.20	0.34
	Obsessive-compulsive	0.18	**0.40**

Note. *Sample 1, N = 88 patients; Sample 2, N = 47 patients, except as noted. Diagnostic scores are derived from the Structured Interview for DSM-III-R Personality (Pfohl et al. 1989). Included are the highest correlation for each scale in each sample and also any scale-diagnosis correlations that were ≥0.40 in both samples. The stonger correlation for each scale is in boldface if significantly different.*
[a]*N = 40.*

related most strongly with ratings of antisocial PD, self-reported dependency was related to clinically rated dependent PD, and Self-harm predicted ratings of borderline PD. Some scales appear to "work better" in one sample or the other. For example, SNAP Exhibitionism is associated with ratings of histrionic PD only in sample 1, whereas Workaholism correlates with ratings of obsessive-compulsive PD only in sample 2. The sample-based inconsistencies require further research.

Other correlations are consistent but lower than would be expected theoretically; for example, Eccentric Perceptions related to ratings of schizotypal PD in both samples, but only at a moderate level. Moreover, a few relations are conspicuous by their absence; for example, Entitlement was not strongly correlated with narcissistic PD in either sample. Perhaps persons who are rated clinically as narcissistic are unable or unwilling to endorse feelings and acts of entitlement on a self-report inventory. These unexpected findings also require further research. Nevertheless, it is interesting to compare these trait-diagnostic correlations to those between self-report and interview scores that each targeted specific diagnoses (see Table 9–2). In brief, scales that attempt to operationalize diagnoses in self-report may capture *less* of the diagnostic variance than do these scales, which focus on the basic traits comprising the disorders.

Taken together, these data indicate that trait dimensions are related systematically to clinically rated personality pathology not only in a broad and general sense, but also at the level of specific scale-diagnosis relations, although some inconsistent and unexpected findings require further exploration. More broadly, these findings suggest that personality trait measures, which normally are associated with normal-range personality assessment, also can play a valuable role in the assessment of pathological personalities.

Clinical Application of a Trait Dimensional Approach

Figure 9–3 presents the SNAP profiles of the two patients with avoidant PD whose diagnostic profiles were shown earlier (see Figure 9–1). As would be expected from the correlational analyses, both profiles show an elevation on the Detachment scale, indicating withdrawal from interpersonal relations. In addition, Subject B shows marked potential for self-harm and a low tolerance for the attention of others (low Exhibitionism). Recall that this subject additionally met three borderline PD criteria: affective instability, suicidal behavior, and feelings of emptiness. The SNAP profile of Subject A indicates that he has an anti-traditional, impulsive behavioral style (low propriety, high impulsivity) which simply was not reflected in his DSM-III-R symptom picture. It would be useful to explore the meaning of this scale elevation further. These trait profiles, therefore, have important similarities that reflect the DSM categorization of avoidant PD, but they also suggest impor-

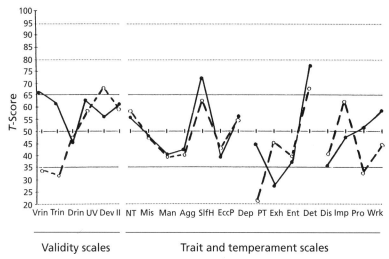

FIGURE **9–3.** SNAP *personality trait profiles of the two outpatients whose DSM-III-R symptoms profiles are shown in Figure 9–1. Subject A (open circles, broken line): 27-year-old Caucasian male; Subject B (filled circles, solid line): 38-year-old Caucasian female. Vrin, Variable Response Inconsistency; Trin, True Response Inconsistency; Drin, Desirability Response Inconsistency; UV, Unlikely Virtues; Dev, Deviant Responding; II, Index of Invalidity Responding; NT, Negative Temperament; Mis, Mistrust; Man, Manipulativeness; Agg, Aggression; SlfH, Self-harm; EccP, Eccentric Perceptions; Dep, Dependency; PT, Positive Temperament; Exh, Exhibitionism; Ent, Entitlement; Det, Detachment; Dis, Disinhibition; Imp, Impulsivity; Pro, Propriety; Wrk, Workaholism.*

tant differences in the personalities of these subjects that go beyond
the DSM categorization. These differences may prove as useful in
formulating treatment plans as the similarities.

Figure 9–4 presents the SNAP profiles of the two inpatient subjects
whose DSM-III-R profiles were shown in Figure 9–2. Important points
of similarity between them that would be expected from the correlational data are again seen: Both subjects met criteria for borderline,
paranoid, and antisocial PD; concomitantly, both subjects report a
strong potential for Self-harm, marked Mistrust, and Aggression on the
SNAP. Subject D who additionally met criteria for schizotypal and
passive-aggressive PD shows corresponding elevations on the eccentric

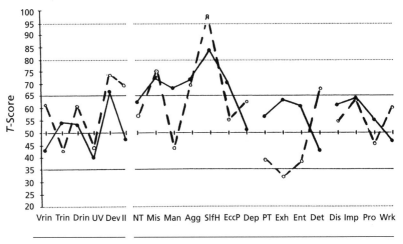

FIGURE 9–4. *SNAP personality trait profiles of the two inpatients whose
DSM-III-R symptom profiles are shown in Figure 9–2. Subject C (open
circles, broken line): 34-year-old Caucasian male; Subject D (filled cir-
cles, solid line): 28-year-old Caucasian male. Vrin, Variable Response
Inconsistency; Trin, True Response Inconsistency; Drin, Desirability Re-
sponse Inconsistency; UV, Unlikely Virtues; Dev, Deviant Responding;
II, Index of Invalidity Responding; NT, Negative Temperament; Mis,
Mistrust; Man, Manipulativeness; Agg, Aggression; SlfH, Self-harm;
EccP, Eccentric Perceptions; Dep, Dependency; PT, Positive Tempera-
ment; Exh, Exhibitionism; Ent, Entitlement; Det, Detachment; Dis,
Disinhibition; Imp, Impulsivity; Pro, Propriety; Wrk, Workaholism.*

perceptions and manipulativeness scales. What the trait profile reveals that is not obvious in the DSM-III-R symptom picture is the interpersonal difficulties of Subject C; he reports feeling simultaneously detached from others (high Detachment), intolerant of others' attention (low Exhibitionism), and yet dependent (high Dependency). Moreover, this subject's depression is also indicated in his personality profile by low scores on scales measuring energy and positive emotions (low Positive Temperament) and positive self-presentation (Entitlement). Again, in treatment planning, knowledge of these personality characteristics provides useful information beyond that supplied by the DSM-III-R symptom picture.

In conclusion, it should be clear that a trait dimensional approach is not incompatible with categorical diagnoses. Indeed, if the relation between traits and disorders is well understood—and our understanding of those relations is far from complete—then the information derived from a trait dimensional analysis can be used rather directly for diagnostic purposes. Thus, the study of PD will be enhanced by basic research into the fundamental trait dimensions of personality, first because these are the units that theoretically are used to formulate PD diagnoses, and second, because of the tremendous opportunity that such research provides for developing a unified theory of normal and maladaptive personality.

References

American Psychiatric Association: Diagnostic and Statistical Manual of Mental Disorders, 3rd Edition. Washington, DC, American Psychiatric Association, 1980

American Psychiatric Association: Diagnostic and Statistical Manual of Mental Disorders, 3rd Edition, Revised. Washington, DC, American Psychiatric Association, 1987

American Psychiatric Association: Diagnostic and Statistical Manual of Mental Disorders, 4th Edition. Washington, DC, American Psychiatric Association, 1994

Blashfield RK, Haymaker D: A prototype analysis of the diagnostic criteria for DSM-III-R personality disorders. J Personal Disord 2:272–280, 1988

Clark LA: Toward a consensual set of symptom clusters for assessment of personality disorder, in Advances in Personality Assessment, Vol 8. Edited by Butcher JN, Spielberger CD. Hillsdale, NJ, Lawrence Erlbaum Associates, 1990, pp 243–266

Clark LA: Resolving taxonomic issues in personality disorders: the value of large-scale analyses of symptom data. J Personal Disord 6:360–376, 1992

Clark LA: Manual for the Schedule for Nonadaptive and Adaptive Personality. Minneapolis, University of Minnesota Press, 1993

Clark LA, Livesley WJ: Two approaches to identifying the dimensions of personality disorder: convergence on the five-factor model, in Personality Disorders and the Five-Factor Model of Personality. Edited by Costa PT Jr, Widiger TA. New York, American Psychological Association, 1994, pp 261–278

Clark LA, Watson D: Temperament: a new paradigm for trait psychology, in Handbook of Personality, 2nd Edition. Edited by Pervin L, John O (in press)

Clark LA, Watson D, Reynolds S: Diagnosis and classification in psychopathology: challenges to the current system and future directions. Annu Rev Psychol 46:121–153, 1995

Clark LA, Livesley WJ, Schroeder ML, Irish S: The structure of maladaptive personality traits: convergent validity between two systems. Psychological Assessment 8:294–303, 1996

Clark LA, Livesley WJ, Morey L: Personality disorder assessment: the challenge of construct validity. J Personal Disord 11:205–231, 1997

Clarkin JF, Widiger TA, Frances A, et al: Prototypic typology and the borderline personality disorder. J Abnorm Psychol 92:263–275, 1983

Cloninger CR: Tridimensional Personality Questionnaire, Version iv. St. Louis, MO, Department of Psychiatry, Washington University School of Medicine, 1987

Costa PT Jr, McCrae RR: Personality stability and its implications for clinical psychology. Clin Psychol Rev 6:407–423, 1986

Costa PT Jr, McCrae RR: Revised NEO Personality Inventory (NEO-PI-R) and NEO Five-Factor Inventory (NEO-FFI) Professional Manual. Odessa, FL, Psychological Assessment Resources, 1992

Eysenck HJ, Eysenck MW: Personality and Individual Differences. New York, Plenum, 1985

First M, Gibbon M, Spitzer RL, et al: User's Guide for the Structured Clinical Interview for the DSM-IV Axis II Personality Disorders. Washington, DC, American Psychiatric Press, 1997

Harkness A: Fundamental topics in the personality disorders: candidate trait dimensions from lower regions of the hierarchy. Psychological Assessment 4:251–259, 1992

Hyler SE: PDQ-IV: Personality Diagnostic Questionnaire-IV/(PDQ-IV). New York, New York State Psychiatric Institute, 1994

Hyler SE, Skodol AE, Oldham JM, et al: Validity of the Personality Diagnostic Questionnaire-Revised (PDQ-R): a replication in an outpatient sample. Compr Psychiatry 33:73–77, 1992

Kass F, Skodol AE, Charles E, et al: Scaled ratings of DSM-III personality disorders. Am J Psychiatry 142:627–630, 1985

Klein MH, Benjamin LS, Rosenfeld R, et al: The Wisconsin Personality Disorders Inventory: development, reliability, and validity. J Personal Disord 7:285–303, 1993

Livesley WJ: Trait and behavioral prototypes of personality disorder. Am J Psychiatry 143:728–732, 1986

Livesley WJ: Dimensional Assessment of Personality Pathology-Basic Questionnaire. Unpublished manuscript, University of British Columbia, 1990

Livesley WJ, Jackson DN, Schroeder ML: A study of the factorial structure of personality pathology. J Personal Disord 3:292–306, 1989

Loranger AW: Personality Disorder Examination (PDE) Manual. Yonkers, NY, DV Communications, 1988

Loranger AW, Lenzenweger MF, Gartner AF, et al: Trait-state artifacts and the diagnosis of personality disorders. Arch Gen Psychiatry 48:720–728, 1991

Millon T, David R, Millon C: Manual for the Millon Clinical Multiaxial Inventory-III (MCMI-III). Minneapolis, MN, National Computer Systems, 1994

Morey LC, Waugh MH, Blashfield RK: MMPI scales for DSM-III personality disorders: their derivation and correlates. J Pers Assess 49:245–256, 1985

Morey LC, Blashfield RK, Webb WW, et al: MMPI scales for DSM-III personality disorders: a preliminary study. J Clin Psychol 44:47–50, 1988

Perry C: Problems and considerations in the valid assessment of personality disorders. Am J Psychiatry 149:1645–1653, 1992

Pfohl B, Blum N, Zimmerman M, et al: Structured Interview for DSM-III-R Personality (SIDP-R). Iowa City, University of Iowa, Department of Psychiatry, 1989

Pfohl B, Blum N, Zimmerman M, et al: Structural Interview for DSM-IV Personality (SIDP-IV). Washington, DC, American Psychiatric Press, 1997

Pilkonis PA, Heape CL, Ruddy J, et al: Validity in the diagnosis of personality disorders: the use of the LEAD standard. Psychological Assessment 3:46–54, 1991

Schroeder ML, Wormworth JA, Livesley WJ: Dimensions of personality disorder and their relationships to the big five dimensions of personality. Psychological Assessment 4:47–53, 1992

Schroeder ML, Wormworth JA, Livesley WJ: Dimensions of personality disorder and their relationships to the Big Five dimensions of personality, in Personality Disorders and the Five-Factor Model of Personality. Edited by Costa PT Jr, Widiger TA. Washington, DC, American Psychiatric Press, 1994, pp 117–127

Schuerger JM, Zarrella KL, Hotz AS: Factors that influence the temporal stability of personality by questionnaire. J Pers Soc Psychol 56:777–783, 1989

Shea MT, Glass DR, Pilkonis PA, et al: Frequency and implications of personality disorders in a sample of depressed outpatients. J Personal Disord 1:27–42, 1987

Spitzer RL: Psychiatric diagnosis: are clinicians still necessary? Compr Psychiatry 24:399–411, 1983

Spitzer RL, Skodol AE, Williams JBW, et al: Supervising intake diagnosis: a psychiatric "Rashomon." Arch Gen Psychiatry 39:1299–1305, 1982

Tellegen A: Multidimensional Personality Questionnaire. Minneapolis, University of Minnesota Press, 1993

Tellegen A, Waller NG: Exploring personality through test construction: development of the Multidimensional Personality Questionnaire, in Personality Measures: Development and Evaluation, Vol 1. Edited by Briggs SR, Cheek JM. Greenwich, CT, JAI Press (in press)

Watson D, Clark LA, Harkness A: Structures of personality and their relevance to the study of psychopathology. J Abnorm Psychol 103:18–31, 1994

Widiger TA: The DSM-III-R categorical personality disorder diagnoses: a critique and an alternative. Psychological Inquiry 4:75–90, 1993

Widiger TA: Personality disorder dimensional models proposed for DSM-IV. J Personal Disord 5:386–398, 1991

Widiger TA, Frances A: The DSM-III personality disorders: perspectives from psychology. Arch Gen Psychiatry 42:615–623, 1985

Widiger TA, Rogers JH: Prevalence and comorbidity of personality disorders. Psychiatr Ann 19:132–136, 1989

Zuckerman M, Kuhlman DM, Camac C: What lies beyond E and N? Factor analyses of scales believed to measure basic dimensions of personality. J Pers Soc Psychol 54:96–107, 1988

CHAPTER 10

Emotional Traits and Personality Dimensions

Dragan M. Svrakic, M.D., Ph.D.
Thomas R. Przybeck, Ph.D.
Cynthia Whitehead, B.A.
C. Robert Cloninger, M.D.

The study of the relationship between emotionality and personality is tied to the theoretical model one chooses to represent these phenomena and the methods one chooses to measure the constructs adumbrated by theory. One productive conceptualization of mood and personality and their relationship is that of the trait or psychometric tradition, in which both mood and personality are viewed as consisting of a limited number of basic aspects or dimensions, each of which is amenable to measurement.

Even though emotionality can be distinguished to some extent from personality by the element of behavior (emotionality refers to internal mental or cognitive states, or dispositions, whereas personality also includes external styles of behavior in addition to internal mental states), emotionality and personality are closely related and difficult to

This research was supported in part by Grant MH31302 from the National Institute of Mental Health, Grants AA07982 and AA08028 from the National Institute of Alcoholism, and a pilot research grant from the MacArthur Foundation Mental Health Research Network I (Psychobiology of Depression).

separate for observation and study. The concepts overlap from both psychometric and neuroadaptive perspectives. For example, personality is observed as individual differences in motivated behavior and emotionality (Cloninger 1987). Likewise, temperament is defined as early developing personality traits (Buss and Plomin 1984) manifested as emotionality (Goldsmith 1987) or as individual differences in emotionality, sociability, and activity (Buss and Plomin 1984). From a neurobiological perspective, Panksepp (1982) maintained that key emotions arise ultimately from "hardwired" neural circuits in the limbic brain that facilitate diverse and adaptive behavioral and physiological responses to major classes of environmental challenges. These circuits, and their corresponding emotions, arose early in mammalian brain evolution and remain similar in humans and other mammals. The "basic" emotions are considered critical motivational phenomena that have had adaptive function at all evolutionary levels (Izard 1977).

Several lines of evidence suggest that basic emotions critically determine both normal and deviant personality development and contour. It has been repeatedly shown, for example, that a limited number of emotions (three to five) portray individual differences in personality in children (Ainsworth et al. 1978; Maziad et al. 1986) and adults (Lang 1985; Tellegen 1985). Likewise, in the domain of deviant personality, personality disorders seem to reflect behavioral expression of three deviant emotional types (American Psychiatric Association 1987). Accordingly, authors may see personality as directly deriving from basic emotions (Tellegen 1985), or define individual differences in personality and behavior as reflecting differences in patterns of discrete emotions across individuals (Maziad et al. 1986), or consider emotions as central organizing axes for personality (Malatesta 1988).

However, more recent advances in personality theory suggest that there are authentic and meaningful distinctions between personality dimensions and mood traits. More informatively, personality can be naturally decomposed into distinct psychobiological dimensions of temperament and character. Temperament (or the "emotional core" of personality) is postulated (Cloninger et al. 1993) to be related to a perceptual memory system involving corticostriatal projections underlying the processing of visuospatial information, affective valence, and unconscious habit formation. Character (or the "conceptual core" of personality) is postulated (Cloninger et al. 1993) to be related to a conceptual memory system involving cortico-limbo-diencephalic projections underlying conscious processing of symbolic meaning and insight learning of concepts. Cloninger (1991) developed a psychometric instrument, the Temperament and Character Inventory (TCI), that evaluates four temperament and three character higher-order traits. The basic temperament and character traits are discussed in more detail in the method section. Briefly, Cloninger (1987) describes temperament in terms of four dimensions which reflect brain systems for inhibition, activation, and maintenance of behavior, and underlie preconceptual biases in patterns of adaptive response to experience. In addition to understanding personality as being tied to specific brain structures, Cloninger (1987) views emotionality as a critical component in the brain systems that guide learning processes and regulate motivated behavior. In other words, Cloninger (1987) proposes that key temperament dimensions can be systematically associated with basic mood traits.

In this chapter we empirically test the hypothesis that the higher-order temperament traits of novelty seeking (NS), harm avoidance (HA), and reward dependence (RD) are related to the basic emotions of anger and impulsivity, fear and anxiety, and love and attachment, respectively (Cloninger 1987; Cloninger et al. 1993). We also test the hypothesis that these basic emotions tend to influence the character traits of self-directedness (SD) and cooperativeness (CO). To that end we analyze the relationship between temperament and character traits assessed by the TCI (Cloninger 1991) and enduring moods traits assessed by the Multiple Affective Adjective Checklist—Revised (MAACL R) trait form (Zuckerman and Lubin 1985). In addition to evaluating the relationship between personality and emotionality, this design offered a chance to assess the construct validity of the TCI relative to the previously validated MAACL R.

Methods

Subjects

As a part of a larger project studying effects of personality and mood on learning, 100 college students (53 men and 47 women) completed the TCI and the MAACL R. The instruments were given at the same time, and the order of administration was alternated. The mean age was 23.7, ranging from 16 to 60. We collected basic demographic information and interviewed each subject with respect to family and personal psychiatric history, presence or absence of mental and/or physical disorders. No subjects reported any diagnosed or treated mental disorder or any significant physical disorder.

Instruments

The TCI

Initially, Cloninger's (1987) biosocial model of personality described three higher-order temperament dimensions of NS, HA, and RD, each composed of four lower-order traits (Table 10–1). The Tridimensional Personality Questionnaire (TPQ) was developed to measure these temperament traits (Cloninger 1987). The postulated structure of temperament and the heritability of the temperament dimensions have been supported in normative, twin, and clinical samples (with the exception that persistence (P), originally thought to be a component of RD, emerged as a distinct fourth temperament dimension) (see Cloninger et al. 1991 and Heath et al. 1994 for details). Conceptual refinements of the biosocial personality model and substantial revisions of the TPQ have since been introduced (Cloninger et al. 1993; Cloninger and Svrakic 1992). The revisions were designed to improve self-report evaluation of personality and its disorders in clinical and general population samples. In addition to four basic temperament traits of NS, HA, RD, and P, the TPQ has been expanded to include three higher-order character traits of SD, CO, and self-transcendence (ST). These character dimensions are defined in terms of three aspects of self-concept, including conceptualization (or identification) of the self as an autonomous individual (i.e., SD), as an integral part of human society (i.e., CO), and as an integral part of the universe (i.e., ST) (Cloninger et al. 1993). The seven basic higher-order scales for temperament and character consist of 25 subscales for 12 temperament and 13 character

TABLE 10–1.

TCI scales and subscales

I Temperament

Novelty seeking (NS) (40 items)
NS1: exploratory excitability vs. stoic rigidity (11 items)
NS2: impulsiveness vs. reflection (10 items)
NS3: extravagance vs. reserve (9 items)
NS4: disorderliness (10 items)

Harm avoidance (HA) (35 items)
HA1: worry and pessimism vs. uninhabited optimism (11 items)
HA2: fear of uncertainty (7 items)
HA3: shyness vs. gregariousness (8 items)
HA4: fatigability vs. vigor (9 items)

Reward dependence (RD) (30 items)
RD1: sentimentality (9 items)
RD3: attachment vs. detachment (8 items)
RD4: dependence vs. independence (5 items)

Persistence (8 items)

II Character

Self-directedness (SD) (21 items)
SD1: responsibility vs. blaming (8 items)
SD2: purposefulness vs. lack of goal direction (8 items)
SD3: resourcefulness (5 items)

Cooperativeness (CO) (25 items)
CO1: social acceptance vs. social intolerance (8 items)
CO2: empathy vs. social disinterest (8 items)
CO3: helpfulness vs. unhelpfulness (9 items)

traits. In other words, the revised model describes 7 higher-order and 25 primary or lower-order traits of temperament and character.

The TCI (Table 10–1) was rationally derived based on an explicit psychobiological model of personality to measure the temperament and character dimensions. In this study we use version 7 of the TCI, which evaluates three temperament dimensions of NS, HA, and RD, and two character dimensions of SD and CO. This version is a 151-item, self-report, true-false questionnaire that takes about 30 minutes to complete.

The temperament dimensions of NS, HA, and RD are described

elsewhere (Cloninger 1987). In brief, the structure of temperament was inferred largely from psychometric and genetic studies of personality in humans, and neurobiological studies of the functional organization of brain networks underlying classical and operant learning responses to simple appetitive or aversive stimuli in humans and mammals. Behaviorally, the temperament dimensions were defined in terms of individual differences in associative learning in response to novelty, danger or punishment, and reward, respectively. NS is viewed as a heritable bias in the activation or initiation of behaviors such as frequent exploratory activity in response to novelty, impulsive decision making, extravagance in approach to cues of reward, quick loss of temper, and active avoidance of frustration. HA is viewed as a heritable bias in the inhibition or cessation of behaviors, such as pessimistic worry in anticipation of future problems, passive avoidant behaviors (such as fear of uncertainty and shyness of strangers), and rapid fatigability. RD is viewed as a heritable bias in the maintenance or continuation of ongoing behaviors, and is manifest as sentimentality, social attachment, and dependence on approval by others.

As already noted, Cloninger et al. (1993) conceptualizes character as the conceptual core of personality, which is closely related to a conceptual memory system involving cortico-limbo-diencephalic projections underlying conscious processing of symbolic meaning and insight learning of concepts. The SD character dimension consists of three subscales: Responsibility versus blaming (SD1) distinguishes persons who accept responsibility for how they choose to act from persons who blame other people and external circumstances for what is happening to them. Purposefulness versus lack of goal direction (SD2) distinguishes people who have a clear sense of meaning and direction in their lives from those who are uncertain of their long-term goals and feel driven to react to current circumstances and immediate needs. Resourcefulness versus resourcelessness (SD3) describes persons who show initiative in identifying opportunities to solve problems rather than feeling unable to overcome obstacles they encounter.

The CO character dimension has three subscales as well: Social acceptance versus social intolerance (C1) measures the extent to which individuals accept and tolerate other people who have different opinions and behavior. Empathy versus social disinterest (C2) measures the extent to which individuals try to consider the feelings of other people as much as their own. Helpfulness versus unhelpfulness (C3) describes persons who enjoy being of service to others versus those who always seek their own profit.

The TCI has been tested in college students, clinical samples, and general population samples (Cloninger and Svrakic 1992; Cloninger et al. 1993; Svrakic et al. 1993).

The MAACL R

The MAACL R is a 132-item test that takes 5–10 minutes to administer and measures five lower-order mood traits (anxiety, depression, hostility, positive affect, and sensation seeking). These mood traits reflect two higher-order mood dimensions of positive affect plus sensation seeking and dysphoria (encompassing anxiety, depression, and hostility).

Each of the mood traits is measured by a series of adjectives. Subjects are asked to check "present" adjectives and to skip "absent" ones (Zuckerman and Lubin 1985).

The MAACL R is distributed in two forms, a state form and a trait form. The trait form (used in this study) asks subjects to check adjectives describing how they "generally" feel.

Normative values for the trait version of the MAACL R were established in a national area probability sample of 1543 adults (Zucker and Lubin 1985). The psychometric properties of the MAACL R are summarized in the MAACL R manual (Zuckerman and Lubin 1985).

The MAACL R (trait form), with five mood dimensions, seemed appropriate for a study addressing the issue of the relationship between enduring moods and five personality dimensions assessed by the TCI.

In this study we used a computer to administer the MAACL R. The adjectives were presented one at the time and the subject had to respond with "yes" or "no" to each adjective in order to get the next one. This was intended to eliminate acquiescence response set (the tendency to endorse many or few items regardless of content). Also, the MAACL R manual (Zuckerman and Lubin 1985) does not report scores for college students. Hence, we based our analyses on the raw MAACL R scores (rather than using the T scores). Also, a sentence reminding subjects to describe the way they "generally feel" appeared on the screen with each adjective. This was intended to reduce the effect of current mood state on the subjects' performance on the MAACL R.

Self-report versus interview ratings of personality and behavior.
The reliability of self-report measures is a major concern in any study that relies heavily on such instruments. The TPQ and the TCI (i.e., expanded TPQ) provide reliable descriptions of personality traits that correspond well to expert ratings and evaluation by clinicians. In a clinical sample of psychiatric patients (Brown et al. 1992), the TPQ self-report evaluation of the three temperament dimensions was correlated moderately to highly with interviewer's assessment of the same dimensions. The latter was obtained using a semistructured interview called the Tridimensional Inventory of Personality Style (TIPS) (Cloninger 1987). The TIPS measures seven aspects of NS, HA, and RD (a total of 21 aspects) on a scale of -3 to $+3$ (0 is considered average). Each aspect has a behavioral summary to help the interviewer to select those that fit best the subject's character traits. The total of the seven aspects for each dimension (ITOT) was then added, with a possible range of from -21 to $+21$. A summary score was also determined by the interviewer (ISUM) which consisted of paragraph summaries from -3 to $+3$ on each dimension of NS, HA, and RD. The paragraph that best fit the subject's personality determined his or her score. The same summary scale was completed for each dimension by each subject's physician and called the MD score. Physicians were blind to the TPQ and TIPS interview results (Table 10–2).

The correlations were quite high between the self-administered TPQ and ratings obtained by the interviewer (ITOT and ISUM), suggesting that the TPQ can be used as a valid self-report measure of the three higher-order temperament traits. Agreement between the physician's assessment (MD) and the TPQ was much lower. This may reflect the physicians' lack of training in the various dimensions, compounded by the use of a single summary scale for comparison of the physician's assessment to the self-report. Although the same summary scale was

TABLE 10–2.

Correlations between self-report and interview measures of personality

	TPQ	ITOT	ISUM	MD
Novelty seeking				
TPQ	—	0.76	0.78	0.51
ITOT		—	0.89	0.47
ISUM			—	0.50
MD				—
Harm avoidance				
TPQ	—	0.65	0.69	0.41
ITOT		—	0.91	0.58
ISUM			—	0.56
MD				—
Reward dependence				
TPQ	—	0.60	0.62	0.53
ITOT		—	0.92	0.63
ISUM			—	0.60
MD				—

Note. TPQ = Tridimensional Personality Questionnaire; ITOT = The interviewer's assessment of the components for each dimension in the TPQ added with a possible range of from −21 to +21; ISUM = a summary score determined by the interviewer, which consisted of paragraph summaries for each dimension in the TPQ; MD = This same summary scale was completed for each dimension by each subject's physician.

also used by the interviewer, it was completed after conducting a more detailed semistructured interview.

Analyses.   Before comparing the results on the two instruments, we examined each test relative to established standards to be confident that each performed as expected. We assessed means, scale reliability, interscale correlations, and factor structure of each test. We next analyzed the correlations between the MAACL R and the TCI scores, after which we performed stepwise multiple regression analyses of the MAACL R and the TCI scales.

Statistical analyses were carried out using Version 6.0 of the SAS statistical software (SAS Institute 1989).

Results

The TCI scores (Table 10–3) were similar to those obtained in a sample of 300 adults (Cloninger and Svrakic 1992; Cloninger et al. 1993). The higher NS scores in the college group reflect the lower age of the sample. This is a postulated feature of the NS dimension (Cloninger 1987).

As shown in Table 10–3, the Cronbach's alphas for the TCI dimensions were moderate to high. The alpha coefficients for the temperament scales were higher than those previously reported for version 5 of the TPQ (Cloninger et al. 1991; Svrakic et al. 1991), reflecting changes made to the temperament scales. The alphas for the MAACL R were somewhat lower, but generally corresponded to those reported in the manual (Zuckerman and Lubin 1985).

The MAACL R manual does not report scores for college students. The mean scores and standard deviations in this sample corresponded to those reported for adolescents in the manual (p. 6), except that positive affect was much higher (17.1) than in adolescents (7.4 males, 11.0 females), whereas hostility was somewhat lower (1.5) than in adolescents (2.5 males, 2.8 females). These differences may reflect a social desirability effect due to the requirement that each adjective be scored "like me" or "not like me."

The TCI interscale correlations were low to moderate. Among the temperament scales there was a weak correlation between HA and NS ($r = -0.18$). SD was negatively correlated with HA ($r = -0.44$) while the CO scale was related to RD ($r = 0.48$). SD and CO were moderately correlated ($r = 0.32$).

The MAACL R mood dimensions were moderately correlated with each other. The r's for anxiety, depression and hostility ranged from 0.38 to 0.65. The same holds for sensation seeking and positive affect (0.49). The only unrelated scales were sensation seeking and hostility (0.09). The three negative mood traits (anxiety, depression, and hostility) correlated inversely with positive mood traits (positive affect and sensation seeking) ($-0.20 \geq r \geq -0.53$). This pattern of the MAACL R interscale correlations corresponds to that reported in the manual (Zuckerman and Lubin 1985).

TABLE 10–3.

Mean scores and Cronbach's alphas for TCI and MAACL R

	Sample 1		Sample 2		
	Mean	SD	Mean	SD	alpha
Novelty seeking	21.5	(6.4)	19.2	(6.0)	0.82
NS1	7.3	(2.3)	6.3	(2.3)	0.67
NS2	3.8	(2.7)	3.7	(2.2)	0.76
NS3	5.3	(2.4)	5.0	(2.3)	0.79
NS4	5.1	(1.9)	4.3	(2.1)	0.42
Harm avoidance	13.8	(7.1)	12.6	(6.8)	0.88
HA1	3.8	(2.8)	3.2	(2.4)	0.80
HA2	3.5	(2.0)	3.6	(2.0)	0.73
HA3	3.8	(2.3)	3.3	(2.3)	0.79
HA4	2.6	(2.2)	2.5	(2.2)	0.76
Reward dependence	21.3	(4.3)	20.0	(4.6)	0.72
RD1	6.6	(1.8)	6.6	(1.9)	0.54
RD2	6.0	(1.8)	5.6	(1.9)	0.66
RD3	5.3	(2.5)	4.7	(2.3)	0.82
RD4	3.4	(1.3)	3.0	(1.4)	0.52
Self-directedness	15.7	(4.6)	15.2	(4.3)	0.86
SD1	6.1	(2.3)	5.8	(2.0)	0.83
SD2	5.7	(1.9)	5.5	(1.8)	0.64
SD3	4.0	(1.4)	4.0	(2.0)	0.75
Cooperativeness	21.1	(3.2)	19.4	(3.9)	0.74
CO1	7.2	(1.2)	6.7	(1.5)	0.58
CO2	6.1	(1.8)	5.5	(1.5)	0.63
CO3	7.8	(1.4)	7.2	(1.7)	0.52
Anxiety	2.6	(2.3)			0.76
Depression	1.8	(2.4)			0.84
Hostility	1.5	(1.9)			0.76
Positive affect	17.1	(4.3)			0.88
Sensation seeking	6.9	(2.6)			0.73

Note. *Sample 1*, N = *100; Sample 2*, N = *300 adult subjects. NS1, exploratory excitability; NS2, impulsiveness; NS3, extravagance; NS4, disorderliness. HA1, anticipatory worry; HA2, fear of uncertainty; HA3, shyness with strangers; HA4, fatigability. RD1, sentimentality; RD2, persistence; RD3, attachment; RD4, dependence. SD1, responsibility; SD2, purposefulness; SD3, resourcefulness; CO1, social acceptance; CO2, empathy; CO3, helpfulness.*

The pattern of results described so far for the two instruments indicates that performance on each was generally consistent with previous reports and provided substantiation for the meaningfulness of a comparison of the two.

Table 10–4 presents the correlations between the TCI personality traits and the MAACL R mood traits. On the scale level, NS was related to hostility (0.23). RD was positively related to positive affect (0.27), and negatively to hostility (-0.20). HA was related to anxiety (0.54) and depression (0.39), and negatively to sensation seeking (-0.53) and positive affect (-0.44).

As noted, psychometric (Cloninger et al. 1991) and twin data (Heath et al. 1994) suggest that RD consists of two separate factors, the first including RD1, RD3, and RD4 (sentimentality, attachment, and dependence), the second including RD2 (persistence). Correlations between RD1, RD3, RD4, and the MAACL R mood traits corresponded to those for the full RD dimension (see Table 10–4).

If the lower-order traits of temperament and character (i.e., the TCI subscales) are considered (see Table 10–4), a more complicated set of relationships between the two instruments emerges. Among the NS subscales, two were related to the MAACL R scales: NS1 (exploratory excitability) was related to sensation seeking (0.31), NS2 (impulsivity) to hostility (0.27) and negatively to positive affect (-0.22). NS3 (extravagance) and NS4 (disorderliness) have no significant correlation with any MAACL R scale.

No HA subscale was related to hostility. All HA subscales have significant correlations with anxiety ($0.24 \leq r \leq 0.61$), positive affect ($-0.47 \leq r \leq -0.26$) and sensation seeking ($-0.47 \leq r \leq -0.34$), and all except shyness (HA3) are correlated with depression ($0.24 \leq r \leq 0.44$) (see Table 10–4).

Among the RD subscales, RD1 (sentimentality) was related to depression (0.22), RD3 (attachment) to positive affect (0.31) and to hostility (-0.20), and RD4 (dependence) negatively to hostility (-0.27) (see Table 10–4).

With respect to the TCI character dimensions (see Table 10–4), SD was related to sensation seeking (0.42), positive affect (0.37), depression (-0.56), anxiety (-0.54), and hostility (-0.29). The SD subscales all show a similar pattern with the exception of SD2 (pur-

TABLE 10–4.

Correlations (r) between MAACL R and TCI scales (×100)

	Host	SenSk	Anx	Depr	PosAff
NS	23[c]	09	04	13	−06
NS1	11	31[c]	−03	−05	08
NS2	27[c]	−08	19	18	−22[c]
NS3	04	00	00	16	09
NS4	18	05	−08	02	−11
HA	04	−53[a]	54[a]	39[a]	−44[a]
HA1	15	−34[b]	61[a]	44[a]	−47[a]
HA2	−12	−47[a]	36[b]	24[c]	−27[c]
HA3	05	−37[b]	35[b]	17	−26[c]
HA4	00	−45[a]	24[c]	28[c]	−28[c]
RD	−20[c]	07	02	00	27[c]
RD1	−01	−02	13	22[c]	16
RD2	00	18	−19	−19	01
RD3	−20[c]	10	−01	−07	31[c]
RD4	−27[c]	−18	15	−06	06
SD	−29[c]	42[a]	−54[a]	−56[a]	37[a]
SD1	−31[c]	29[a]	−48[a]	−57[a]	35[b]
SD2	−17	39[a]	−40[a]	−40[a]	27[c]
SD3	−21[c]	39[a]	−47[a]	−37[a]	29[c]
CO	−56[a]	09	−24[c]	−19	26[c]
CO1	−39[a]	01	−17	−06	09
CO2	−46[a]	17	−26[c]	−24[c]	29[c]
CO3	−41[a]	−01	−11	−10	19

Note. NS1, *exploratory excitability;* NS2, *impulsiveness;* NS3, *extravagance;* NS4, *disorderliness.* HA1, *anticipatory worry;* HA2, *fear of uncertainty;* HA3, *shyness with strangers;* HA4, *fatigability.* RD1, *sentimentality;* RD2, *persistence;* RD3, attachment; RD4 dependence. SD1, *responsibility;* SD2, *purposefulness;* SD3, resourcefulness. CO1, *social acceptance;* CO2, *empathy;* CO3, helpfulness. Host, Hostility; SenSk, Sensation seeking; Anx, Anxiety; Depr, Depression; PosAff, Positive affect.

[a]P < .0001.
[b]P < .001.
[c]P < .05.

posefulness), which is not correlated with hostility. CO was related to positive affect (0.26) and to hostility (-0.56). All three CO subscales were inversely related to hostility ($-0.39 \geq r \geq -0.46$). Also, empathy (CO2) was related to anxiety (-0.26), depression (-0.24), and positive affect (0.29).

Stepwise multiple regressions of the TCI personality dimensions on the MAACL R mood traits are summarized in Table 10–5.

HA was predicted by high anxiety and low sensation seeking. RD was predicted by positive affect. NS was predicted weakly by hostility. SD was primarily predicted by low depression, and by low anxiety and high sensation seeking. CO was predicted by low hostility.

The MAACL R predicted these NS subscales: NS1 (exploratory excitability) by sensation seeking ($R^2 = 0.10$); NS2 (impulsivity) by hostility ($R^2 = 0.08$); NS3 (extravagance) by positive affect ($R^2 = 0.04$). The MAACL R predicted these HA subscales: HA1 (anticipatory worry) was predicted by high anxiety ($R^2 = 0.38$) and low positive affect ($R^2 = 0.06$); HA2 (fear of uncertainty) by low sensation seeking ($R^2 = 0.22$), high anxiety ($R^2 = 0.07$), and hostility ($R^2 = 0.04$); HA3 (shyness with strangers) by low sensation seeking ($R^2 = 0.12$), high anxiety ($R^2 = 0.08$), and depression ($R^2 = 0.04$); HA4 (fatigability) by low sensation seeking ($R^2 = 0.20$). The MAACL R predicted these RD subscales: RD1 (sentimentality) was predicted by positive affect

TABLE 10–5.

MAACL R mood traits predicting TCI personality dimensions

	HA	RD	NS	SD	CO
Hostility			22[c]		($-$)56[a]
Positive affect		26[b]			
Sensation seeking	($-$)44[a]			24[a]	
Anxiety	54[a]			($-$)24[b]	
Depression				($-$)56[a]	
Multiple R	69[a]	26[b]	22[c]	66[a]	56[a]

Note. ($-$) *signifies "low," all other data are "high."*
[a]P < .0001.
[b]P < .01.
[c]P < .05.

($R^2 = 0.09$) and depression ($R^2 = 0.05$); RD2 (persistence) by low depression ($R^2 = 0.04$): RD3 (attachment) by positive affect ($R^2 = 0.10$); RD4 (dependence) by high anxiety ($R^2 = 0.07$) and by low hostility ($R^2 = 0.07$).

For the CO subscales, social acceptance, empathy, and helpfulness (CO1–CO3) were predicted by low hostility ($0.17 \leq R^2 \leq 0.26$). Among the SD subscales, SD1 (responsibility) was predicted by low depression ($R^2 = 0.32$), SD2 (purposefulness) by sensation seeking ($R^2 = 0.07$) and low anxiety ($R^2 = 0.03$), and SD3 (resourcefulness) by sensation seeking ($R^2 = 0.10$) and low anxiety ($R^2 = 0.22$).

Stepwise multiple regressions of the MAACL R moods on the TCI temperament and character traits are presented in Table 10–6. The TCI scales explained between 40% and 49% of the variance in each of the five MAACL R scales.

Hostility was predicted by low empathy (CO2), low social acceptance (CO1), high exploratory excitability (NS1), low responsibility (SD1), and low helpfulness (CO3). Sensation seeking was predicted by low fear of uncertainty (HA2), high purposefulness (SD2), low fatigability (HA4), and high exploratory excitability (NS1). Anxiety was primarily predicted by high anticipatory worry (HA1), low responsibility (SD1), and high impulsivity (NS2). Depression was predicted by low responsibility (SD1), high anticipatory worry (HA1), and high extravagance (NS3). Positive affect was predicted by low anticipatory worry (HA1), high attachment (RD3), low impulsivity (NS2), high sentimentality (RD1), and high responsibility (SD1).

Discussion

This study extends our previous work in the field of mood and personality. In prior work (Svrakic et al. 1992) we have shown that *mood states* affect personality domains differentially: Some aspects of personality, such as the temperament dimensions of NS and RD, were largely independent from current depression and anxiety, as measured by the Profile of Mood States (POMS; Lorr and McNair 1984/1988). In contrast, the temperament dimension of HA was highly sensitive to these

TABLE 10–6.

TCI personality traits predicting MAACL R mood traits

	Host	SenSk	Anx	Depr	PosAff	(−)Dysph
NS1	22[c]	17[d]				14[d]
NS2			20[c]		(−)24[b]	26[b]
NS3				20[d]		
NS4						
HA1			62[a]	24[b]	(−)47[a]	33[a]
HA2		(−)47[a]				
HA3						
HA4		(−)24[b]				
RD1					17[d]	
RD2						
RD3					32[b]	
RD4						
SD1	(−)20[d]		(−)28[b]	(−)56[a]	17[d]	(−)57[a]
SD2		33[a]				
SD3						
CO1	(−)24[b]					
CO2	(−)46[a]					
CO3	(−)17[d]					
Multiple R	63[a]	65[a]	70[a]	65[a]	66[a]	73[a]

Note. (−) *signifies "low," all other data are "high."*

NS1, exploratory excitability; NS2, impulsiveness; NS3, extravagance; NS4, disorderliness. HA1, anticipatory worry; HA2, fear of uncertainty; HA3, shyness with strangers; HA4, fatigability. RD1, sentimentality; RD2, persistence; RD3, attachment; RD4, dependence. SD1, responsibility; SD2, purposefulness; SD3, resourcefulness. CO1, social acceptance; CO2, empathy; CO3, helpfulness. Host, Hostility; SenSk, Sensation seeking; Anx, Anxiety; Depr, Depression; PosAff, Positive affect; Dysph, Dysphoria (anxiety, hostility, and depression).

[a]$P < .0001$.
[b]$P < .005$.
[c]$P < .01$.
[d]$P < .05$.

mood states (Svrakic et al. 1992). However, HA was related to *a wide variety* of mood states measured by the POMS; this was easily interpretable with respect to some of the mood states (e.g., composed-anxious), but enigmatic for others (e.g., clearheaded-confused).

In this study, enduring *mood traits* and personality dimensions were related in a meaningful and predictable way. Note that the observed *pattern* of this relationship was striking. Some of the observed correlations and regressions were lower than expected. This is, however, partly due to the sample size of 100 subjects.

The results presented in this article correspond to theoretical predictions (Cloninger 1987; Cloninger et al. 1993) and support the construct validity of the TCI temperament and character dimensions. NS was predicted by high hostility, HA primarily by anxiety, and RD with positive affect. This supports the hypothesis (Cloninger 1987; Cloninger et al. 1993) that the higher-order temperament traits are related to the basic emotional traits of anger and impulsivity, fear and anxiety, love and attachment.

With respect to character, CO and its subscales (social acceptance, empathy, helpfulness) were primarily affected by hostility. SD and its subscales (responsibility, purposefulness, resourcefulness) were primarily affected by depression.

Cloninger (Cloninger 1987; Cloninger and Svrakic 1992; Cloninger et al. 1993) postulates that basic temperament traits represent heritable emotional dispositions manifested as specific behavioral patterns early in life. Through the interaction between these emotionally ridden traits and environment, individually specific character traits develop. In environments that do not modify extreme expressions of temperament, the latter may interfere with the development of character. For example, in the present study impulsive and hostile individuals manifested high scores on the temperament trait of NS. Moreover, impulsive and hostile individuals also manifested low scores on CO and its lower-order traits, notably social acceptance, empathy, and helpfulness, supporting the hypothesis (Cloninger et al. 1993) that extreme temperament traits tend to interfere with optimal character development.

The relationship among chronic depression, personality, and personality disorders seems very complicated. In the present study, chronic depression was related to low SD. We have shown elsewhere (Svrakic et al. 1993) that low SD also represents a core feature determining the presence or absence of any personality disorder. It is reasonable to assume that certain personality factors, such as low SD, that increase susceptibility to deviant behaviors may also increase susceptibility to chronic mood disorders and vice versa. In other words, low SD appears to be a common denominator for personality disorders and chronic depression. This shared dimension may explain the clinical observation that mood syndromes and personality disorders can be interwoven to the extent that no meaningful distinction between them can be made, as implied in concepts of depressive personality, hysteroid dysphoria, and characterological depression.

It should be emphasized here that character traits are expected to be influenced to some extent by a spectrum of mood states and situations. Character is the "code" of direct behavior observed as relatively stable but flexible patterns of behavioral adjustment and idiosyncratic social, ethical, religious, and spiritual attitudes. The term *flexible* as used here emphasizes that these relatively stable patterns of behavioral adjustment are expected to reflect to some extent current mood and/ or current circumstances. Hence, the expression of character traits of SD and CO is expected to be state and/or context dependent to a larger extent than that of temperament traits of NS, RD, and P.

Traditionally, it has been difficult to define personality correlates of mood and anxiety disorders. For example, both depression and anxiety correlate highly with neuroticism (Eysenck and Eysenck 1968). In this study, correlation and regression analyses demonstrated that HA was primarily related to anxiety whereas SD was primarily related to depression. In addition to providing a guideline for future neurobiological studies of temperament and character, the observed relationship suggests that these personality traits may be used as discriminators between depression and anxiety in clinical practice.

In the present study the relationship between HA and the MAACL R mood traits was nonspecific to some extent (i.e., HA correlated more broadly with mood traits than NS, RD, SD, and CO [see Table 10–4]). This might reflect the fact that the MAACL R includes more mood scales that emphasize various aspects of affect and are conceptually related to HA, than those conceptually related to NS and RD. This emphasis is further reflected by the fact that only relatively small portions of the variance in NS and RD can be explained from the MAACL R scales (see Table 10–5).

This study demonstrates that the MAACL R is a solid measure of emotionality. However, the TCI explains more variance in the MAACL R then vice versa (see Tables 10–5 and 10–6). While only

5% and 7% of the variance in NS and RD can be explained from the MAACL R, the TCI subscales predict at least 40% of the variance in each of the MAACL R scales. Apparently, personality is a more efficient predictor of mood than vice versa. This may partly reflect the structure of the two instruments (the version 7 of the TCI consists of 18 subscales evaluating highly specific behaviors, whereas the MAACL R consists of five scales evaluating relatively broad mood dimensions). As illustrated in Table 10–6, one enduring mood predicts on average four different behaviors. In other words, a limited number of basic mood traits is expressed as a fairly large number of distinct behaviors (e.g., anger can be expressed as crime, hostility, physical or mental cruelty, passive-aggression, etc.). Hence, tests measuring personality and behavior are expected to be more specific than tests measuring emotionality.

According to this study, sensation seeking and NS have an intricate relationship. The MAACL R sensation seeking scale seems to be a composite measure of high NS (i.e., high exploratory excitability), low HA (i.e., low fear of uncertainty and fatigability), and high SD (i.e., high purposefulness) (see Table 10–6). The 40-item version of the Zuckerman's Sensation Seeking—form V (Zuckerman et al. 1978) consists of four subscales (thrill and adventure seeking, experience seeking, disinhibition, and boredom susceptibility). This version with four subscales is even more likely to be factorially manifold with no simple relationship to the personality dimension of NS (Cloninger 1988).

The DSM-III-R classifies personality disorders into three clusters: Cluster A (aloof) personality disorders (schizoid, schizotypal, and paranoid), Cluster B (impulsive) personality disorders (narcissistic, borderline, antisocial, and histrionic), and Cluster C (fearful) personality disorders (obsessive-compulsive, avoidant, passive-aggressive, and dependent). In prior work we (Svrakic et al. 1993) have shown that low RD predicts Cluster A (aloof) personality disorders, high NS predicts Cluster B (impulsive) personality disorders, and high HA predicts Cluster C (fearful) personality disorders. In this study, RD was correlated with positive affect, NS with anger and impulsivity, and HA with fear and anxiety, supporting the construct validity of the three clusters. However, even though each of the three major temperament dimensions corresponds to one of the DSM-III-R clusters, specific combinations of temperament dimensions (i.e., combinations of traits described as typical of separate clusters) define clinical subtypes of individual personality disorders. In other words, each of the personality disorders has a unique profile of high and low scores on the three temperament dimensions. For example, antisocial personality disorder is characterized by high NS, low HA, and low RD. This suggests that discrete personality disorders have features that characterize more than one cluster.

References

Ainsworth MDS, Blehar MC, Waters E, et al: Patterns of Attachment: A Psychological Study of the Strange Situation. Hillsdale, NJ, Lawrence Erlbaum Associates, 1978

American Psychiatric Association: Diagnostic and Statistical Manual of Mental Disorders, 3rd Edition, Revised. Washington, DC, American Psychiatric Association, 1987

Brown S, Svrakic DM. Przybeck TR, et al: The relationship of personality to mood and anxiety states: a dimensional approach. J Psychiatr Res 26(3):197–211, 1992

Buss A, Plomin R: Temperament: Early Developing Personality Traits. Hillsdale, NJ, Lawrence Erlbaum Associates, 1984

Cloninger CR: A systematic method for clinical description and classification of personality variants. Arch Gen Psychiatry 44:573–588, 1987

Cloninger CR: Sensation seeking and behavior disorders: a reply to M. Zuckerman. Arch Gen Psychiatry 45:502–504, 1988

Cloninger CR: The Temperament and Character Inventory. St. Louis, MO, Washington University School of Medicine, 1991

Cloninger CR, Svrakic D: Personality dimensions as a conceptual framework for explaining variations in normal, neurotic, and personality disordered behavior, in Handbook of Anxiety, Vol 5. Edited by Burrows GD, Roth M, Noyes R. Netherlands, Elsevier, 1992, pp 79–104

Cloninger CR, Przybeck TR, Svrakic DM: The Tridimensional Personality Questionnaire: U.S. normative data. Psychol Rep 69:1047–1057, 1991

Cloninger CR, Svrakic DM, Przybeck TR: A psychobiological model of temperament and character. Arch Gen Psychiatry 50:975–990, 1993

Eysenck HJ, Eysenck S: Manual for the Eysenck Personality Inventory, San Diego, CA, EdiTS, 1968

Goldsmith H: Roundtable: what is temperament? Four approaches. Child Dev 58:505–529, 1987

Heath AC, Cloninger CR, Martin NG: Testing a model for the genetic structure of personality. J Pers Soc Psychol 66:762–775, 1994

Izard C: Human Emotions. New York, Plenum, 1977

Lang P: The cognitive psychophysiology of emotion, in Anxiety and Anxiety Disorders. Edited by Tuma H, Masser J. Hillsdale, NJ, Lawrence Erlbaum Associates, 1985, pp 131–170

Lorr M, McNair D: Manual. Profile of Mood States. San Diego, CA, Educational and Industrial Testing Service, 1984/1988.

Malatesta CZ: The role of emotions in the development and organization of personality. Nebraska Symp Motivation 36:1–57, 1988

Maziade M, Boutin P, Cote R, et al: Empirical characteristics of the NYLS temperament in middle childhood: congruities and incongruities with other studies. Child Psychiatry Hum Dev 17:38–52, 1986

Panksepp J: Toward a general psychobiological theory of emotions. Behav Brain Sci 5:407–467, 1982

SAS Institute: SAS System for Statistical Analysis. Release 6.0. Cary, NC, SAS Institute, 1989

Svrakic DM, Przybeck TR, Cloninger CR: Further contribution to the conceptual validity of the tridimensional personality questionnaire: Yugoslav and US data. Compr Psychiatry 32:195–209, 1991

Svrakic DM, Przybeck TR, Cloninger CR: Mood states and personality traits. J Affective Disord 24:217–226, 1992

Svrakic DM, Whitehead S, Przybeck TR, et al: Differential diagnosis of personality disorders by the seven factor model of temperament and character. Arch Gen Psychiatry 50:991–999, 1993

Tellegen A: Structures of mood and personality and their relevance to assessing anxiety, with an emphasis on self-report, in Anxiety and Anxiety Disorders. Edited by Tuma H, Maser J. Hillsdale, NJ, Lawrence Erlbaum Associates, 1985, pp 681–706

Zuckerman M, Lubin B: Manual for the MAACL-R. San Diego, CA, Educational and Industrial Testing Service, 1985

Zuckerman M, Eysenck S, Eysenck HJ: Sensation seeking in England and America: cross-cultural, age, and sex comparisons. J Consult Clin Psychol 46:139–149, 1978

PART IV

What Causes Good and Bad Personality Development?

CHAPTER 11

Biological and Cultural Inheritance of Stature and Attitudes

Lindon J. Eaves, Ph.D., D.Sc., Andrew C. Heath, D.Phil.,

Nicholas G. Martin, Ph.D., Michael C. Neale, Ph.D.,

J. M. Meyer, Ph.D., J. L. Silberg, Ph.D.,

Linda A. Corey, Ph.D., Kimberley Truett, M.S., Ellen Walters, M.S.

Almost a century ago, Karl Pearson (1904) concluded one of the earliest attempts to compare the inheritance of physical and behavioral traits with a generalization that appears, at best, Promethean and, at worst, an example of egregious scientific hubris. He wrote, "the mental characters are not features which differentiate man from the lower types of life. If they are inherited like man's physical characters, if they are inherited even as the protopodite of the water flea, what reason is there for demanding a special evolution for man's mental and moral side?"

Pearson shared with Galton and Darwin the view that the "mental and moral" (Pearson 1904) characters of humans could be detached neither from the evolutionary history of the human species nor from the biological ancestry of the individual. The intervening decades, however, have made it clear that Pearson's claim, even if it should turn out to be true, was premature given the state of knowledge. As Galton

This research is supported by Grants GM-30250, AG-04954, AA-06781, MH-40828, and HL-48148 from the National Institutes of Health and a gift from RJR Nabisco.

himself was aware, the early studies of hereditary genius (Galton 1869) may have established a prima facie case for the biological transmission of abilities, but in truth the effects of biological and social factors were confounded. Galton's solution to the problem was to study "the history of twins" (Galton 1883) but in this field his seminal studies were largely anecdotal. Pearson and Lee's (1903) quantitative studies of familial correlations for stature and other physical measures, partly through the genius of Ronald Fisher (1918) have achieved the status of classics of the genetic literature. Even today, their data provide preliminary an-swers to questions about the role of nonadditive genetic effects and various types of nonrandom mating to quantitative inheritance in man.

Even with respect to human stature, however, Fisher noted that Pearson and Lee's landmark study, based as it was on remarkably large samples, left some questions unanswered. Notably, Fisher pointed out that he was still unsure about the contribution of nonadditive genetic effects to variation in stature and that still larger samples of sibling pairs would be desired. He pointed out that some of the data available (not gathered by Pearson and Lee) for more distant relationships, such as those on first cousins, were inconsistent with the model he had pro-posed and may point to problems of sampling in more remote rela-tionships. He argued that Pearson and Lee's data were probably more consistent with "genotypic" rather then "somatic" assortative mating (i.e., mate selection was based not on the phenotype for stature per se but on a correlated variable that was a more perfect index of the genotype.

By contrast, Pearson's studies of the "mental and moral" charac-teristics of humans have been virtually ignored. They are fraught with problems of rater bias because Pearson used ratings of students by their teachers. Furthermore, these studies were confined to a small range of relationships. As a result, resemblance between the findings for physi-cal and behavioral traits could well be coincidental.

Since these early studies, theoretical and empirical developments in social psychology, cultural anthropology, and population genetics have drawn attention to the phenomena of learning, cultural diversity, and nongenetic evolution. Behavioral correlations between nuclear family members, even though they may *look* similar to those for phy-sique cannot now be used by themselves to support genetic theories.

The fact that, with very few exceptions, the linguistic map of human subpopulations can be superimposed on a genetic map (see for example Cavalli-Sforza 1991) confirms that, at the level of the cultural group, the effects of genes and culture are highly correlated. At the level of the human family, Cavalli-Sforza and Feldman (1973, 1981) have developed a variety of nongenetic transmission models in which the mathematical constraints of Mendelian inheritance and evolution no longer apply. These models have been applied to nuclear family resemblance in social attitudes (e.g., Cavalli-Sforza et al. 1982). Recognizing the limitation of the classical genetic theory of family resemblance led, in the 1970s and 1980s, to a flurry of quantitative models for the joint effects of biological and cultural inheritance that differed in their assumptions about the mechanisms of nongenetic inheritance and assortative mating (Cattell 1960, 1963; Cloninger et al. 1979; Eaves 1976; Heath 1983; Heath and Eaves 1985; Morton 1974; Rao et al. 1974, 1977).

Studies of the inheritance of normal behavior have focussed mainly on cognitive and personality variables. Studies of social attitudes have largely been adjuncts to the measurement of personality without any explicit theoretical justification in their own right. However, attitudes may be singled out on a priori grounds as a model system for the study of *non*genetic inheritance in humans (see for example Cavalli-Sforza and Feldman 1981; Cavalli-Sforza et al. 1982). Although no set of "scales" can capture all the nuances of differences within a culture, attitudes could not exist apart from a species that had evolved an extended matrix of social structures and interactions. It thus appears that social attitudes provide one avenue into quintessentially *human* characteristics.

Published studies show substantial parent-offspring resemblance for attitude variables (Feather 1978; Insel 1974) and some evidence of heterogeneity across sexes in parent-offspring correlation. Insel argued that his data supported a significant role of maternal inheritance. A number of large studies of twins reared together (Eaves and Eysenck 1974; Eaves et al. 1989; Loehlin and Nichols 1976; Martin and Jardine 1986; Martin et al. 1986) have generally shown that MZ twins are more similar than DZ twins and have given some support to the view that genetic factors play at least some role in the transmission of social attitudes. However, these studies have also shown consistently that DZ twin resemblance in attitudes is too high to be explained simply by the usual assumption of additive gene action and random mating. The twin studies have thus established a prima facie case for a significant contribution of the shared family environment, explaining as much as 30% of the total variation in measured attitudes. Many of these authors have noted, however, that the contribution of the family environment is confounded with the genetic consequences of assortative mating in studies of twins reared together. Indeed, Martin et al. (1986) suggested that the spousal correlations for social attitudes were sufficiently high (see for example Eaves et al. 1989; Feather 1978; Insel 1974) to explain virtually *all* of the apparent shared environmental effect in twin studies. The Minnesota studies of separated twins (e.g., Tellegen et al. 1988; Waller et al. 1990) add some weight to this interpretation because they show that the correlations of twins separated at birth do not differ significantly from those of twins reared together. Compelling though such reports are, their relatively small sample sizes inevitably mean, however, that quite large shared environmental effects could still be present yet missed for want of statistical power. Eaves et al. (1978) report correlations in conservatism for a small volunteer sample of adult adoptees and their relatives that are consistent with the overall finding that the shared family environment has little impact. However, the small sample and the possibility of serious volunteer bias do not give us much confidence in these findings. Other adoption studies, notably the Texas Adoption Study (e.g., Loehlin et al. 1985), do not use instruments specifically to assess "social attitudes" in young adults but a wide variety of factors from broadly based personality tests all yield very small correlations for nonbiological relatives. These results are consistent with a very small contribution of the shared family environment. Scarr (1981) arrived at similar conclusions on the basis of a comparison of the correlations for authoritarianism in biological and adoptive families.

Apart from the larger twin studies, few studies have had the power to detect or analyze sex differences in the expression of genetic and environmental effects on social attitudes. This becomes critical for our understanding of the social environment since cultural expectations may differ for men and women, and mothers may play a different role from fathers in shaping the behavior of their male and female offspring.

At present, a researcher who wishes to gain a picture of the role of biological and cultural inheritance in humans is forced to piece together a picture from a variety of different studies conducted with different restricted designs, in different target populations, and using different instruments. Few studies have the power to address the heterogeneity of biological and social effects over sexes. It is sometimes difficult to decide whether inconsistencies between studies reflect differences between samples, populations, or measurements. Sometimes it is hard to decide, given the small sample sizes available, whether similarities with the findings of smaller studies point to anything more significant than a lack of power.

Design and Rationale
of the Virginia 30,000

The Virginia 30,000 study was conceived in the mid-1980s as an attempt to generate a data base sufficiently broad in measurements, rich in relationships, and large in samples, that it might be possible to obtain clearer answers to lingering questions about the role of biological and cultural transmission in human differences. A study was needed that could give estimates of both genetic and nongenetic components of family resemblance without recourse to the dwindling population of adoptees while also allowing for tests of additive and nonadditive genetic effects, sex differences in the expression of genes and environment, resolution of alternative models of assortative mating, and tests of the consistency of any "model" across a broad range of relationships.

Long experience with data analysis and simulation studies (e.g., Eaves 1972; Heath et al. 1985; Martin et al. 1978) had shown that very large samples were likely to be needed to test many hypotheses, especially those about sex differences in genetic and environmental effects. Thus, many of the designs that had obvious intuitive appeal, such as the various adoption designs and the study of separated twins, required populations that were likely to be too small to yield answers to some of the questions we were asking. Nuclear families and extended pedigrees were easily obtained, but these groups left genetic and social factors as confounded as they were in Galton's original studies of hereditary genius and Pearson's studies of "mental and moral" traits.

Theoretical analyses and simulations in the early 1980s (Eaves 1980; Heath 1983; Heath and Eaves 1985; Heath et al. 1985) suggested that the "extended twin-kinship design" could, with sufficiently large samples, provide adequate tests of many features of the transmission of human differences in a single study.

We illustrate the value and flexibility of the Virginia 30,000 study by outlining some early results that reexamine the early claims of Galton, Pearson, and Fisher about the causes of family resemblance in measures chosen a priori to reflect distinct mechanisms of biological and cultural inheritance in humans. *Stature* is chosen to represent a physical variable, height, that is usually regarded as unquestionably genetic. As a measure most likely to reveal the impact of nongenetic inheritance, we follow the proposal of Cavalli-Sforza and his colleagues (1981, 1982) and study a measure of social attitudes. In this first report, we explore the transmission of individual differences in *conservatism*, a composite measure emerging from the joint analysis of a large number of individual attitudes.

An idealized pedigree for the Virginia 30,000 study is illustrated in Figure 11–1. Each pedigree starts with a pair of adult twins. Twins may be either identical (monozygotic, MZ) or fraternal (dizygotic, DZ). MZ pairs may be male or female. DZ pairs may be male, female, or of opposite sex. There are thus five basic kinds of pedigree depending on the zygosity and sex of the twins. The pedigree is then augmented by tracing outward from the twins to include as many living parents, spouses, siblings, and children of twins as may be ascertained. Typically, we were unable to ascertain many pedigrees in which we could contact all three generations. Most pedigrees comprised either twins with their collateral relatives and parents or twins with their collateral relatives and children.

As Francis Galton himself suggested (1883), twins reared together provide a powerful and easily accessible starting point for the resolution

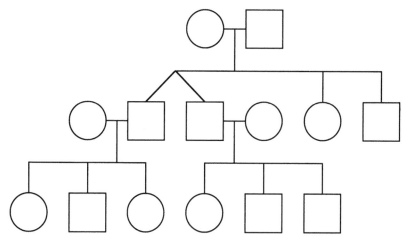

FIGURE 11–1. *Idealized family structure for the Virginia 30,000 study. Standard conventions are used for drawing pedigrees: Circles denote women and squares denote men. Horizontal bars between circles and squares denote spouses. Offspring from a mating are indicated by vertical lines connected by horizontal bars. Twins are connected by diagonal lines.*

of biological and cultural inheritance and thus comprise the core of the present study. However, twins have the weakness that the genetic consequences of assortative mating are confounded with the effects of the shared environment (e.g., Eaves 1970) so we included the parents and spouses of twins to allow us to estimate and analyze the causes and effects of assortative mating (see for example Eaves and Heath 1981; Heath and Eaves 1985) and social interaction between spouses (Heath 1987). Furthermore, since studies of twins alone are always subject to the criticism that twins are not typical of the genetic and environmental effects in the population, we included the siblings of twins in the design to allow for tests of additional environmental similarity in twins. Following Young et al. (1980), we noted that the study of twins and their parents provided a powerful extension of the nuclear family design that allowed some resolution of the additive and non-additive effects of genes from those of the shared family environment and assortative mating contributed by parents. With Nance and Corey (1976; see also Haley et al. 1981) we recognized that the children of MZ twins are socially cousins but genetically half siblings. The MZ twin of a parent may be called "uncle" or "aunt" but, at least under random mating, shares the same genetic relationship as a biological parent. These novel relationships exploit the genetic similarity of MZ twins to generate a number of additional relationships involving individuals who share comparable biological relationships to those in the nuclear family without entering into the standard social relationships of the nuclear family.

Ascertainment of the Virginia 30,000 was conducted in two stages. Twin pairs were recruited from the Virginia Population-based Twin Registry (Corey et al. 1991) and from the American Association of Retired Persons (AARP) as a result of a letter of invitation published in the AARP newsletter. Twins were mailed the "twin" version of a 16-page "Health and Lifestyle Survey" (HLS). The survey was compiled to assess a number of aspects of physique, personality, lifestyle, environment, life events, and personal history related to health. Respondents were asked to supply names, addresses, and telephone numbers of their living parents, spouses, siblings, and children. The relatives of twins were then contacted to complete their own version of the HLS, which secured identical self-report data for the items analyzed in this report.

The final sample comprised 29,691 individuals. Table 11–1 summarizes the composition of the sample by sex and relationship to the twins. A few other relationships (e.g., half-siblings, adoptees) are also represented in the sample but their numbers are generally too small

TABLE 11–1.

Sample sizes of twins and the principal adult relatives of twins in the Virginia 30,000 study

	Males	Females	Total
Twins	5,325	9,436	14,761
Parents of twins	913	1,447	2,360
Spouses of twins	2,515	1,876	4,391
Children of twins	1,890	2,910	4,800
Siblings of twins	1,260	1,924	3,184
Other	67	128	195
Total	11,970	17,721	29,691

to have a significant impact on the analysis, and these individuals are not included in these numbers.

If, on account of relatively small numbers, we ignore relationships across three generations, but take into account the sex of the relatives and whether avuncular relationships are defined through paternal or maternal siblings, there are 80 unique biological and social relationships in the Virginia 30,000 (see Table 11–3). This contrasts with only 5 relationships in the classical twin study, 8 in the conventional nuclear family study, and 10 in the "twin-parent" design. Thus, the Virginia 30,000 design provides a rich variety of biological and social relationships that may be used to test the generalizability of explanations of family resemblance across a wide range of circumstances.

Measures Chosen for Analysis

Stature was obtained by self-report. Subjects were asked "How tall are you?" and gave their height in feet and inches. A small handful of outliers whose reported heights were less than 4' or greater than 7' were excluded from the analysis.

The HLS yields a variety of behavioral measures. This chapter considers a single composite measure of *conservatism* derived from a 28-item social attitudes inventory modeled after the Wilson-Patterson Conservatism Scale (Wilson 1973; Wilson and Patterson 1970) that had been used in several earlier twin studies (see for example Eaves et al. 1989). In these earlier studies, measures of social attitudes were found to be surprisingly reliable and showed patterns of twin and family resemblance that were quite distinct from those widely replicated in studies of the major dimensions of personality (see Eaves et al. 1989 for examples of typical findings for personality measures).

The instrument devised for our study (Table 11–2) comprised selected reliable items from the original inventory supplemented by several experimental items chosen to reflect issues that were controversial in the United States in the late 1980s, when the study was conducted. Items consisted of a single word or phrase (see Table 11–2) to which

TABLE 11–2.

Key to scoring social attitude items for conservatism

Item		Key
(1)	Death penalty	+
(2)	Astrology	−
(3)	X-rated movies	−
(4)	Modern art	−
(5)	Women's liberation	−
(6)	Foreign aid	−
(7)	Federal housing	−
(8)	Democrats	−
(9)	Military drill	+
(10)	The draft	+
(11)	Abortion	−
(12)	Property tax	−
(13)	Gay rights	−
(14)	Liberals	−
(15)	Immigration	−
(16)	Capitalism	+
(17)	Segregation	+
(18)	Moral Majority	+
(19)	Pacificism	−
(20)	Censorship	+
(21)	Nuclear power	+
(22)	Living together	−
(23)	Republicans	+
(24)	Divorce	−
(25)	School prayer	+
(26)	Unions	−
(27)	Socialism	−
(28)	Busing	+

Note. *Subjects are asked to indicate agreement or disagreement by circling "Yes" or "No" as appropriate, or to indicate uncertainty by circling "?." A "+" indicates "Yes" is the keyed direction of response.*

subjects responded in one of three categories ("Yes," "?," "No") to rate the agreement or disagreement with the topic.

Preliminary factor analyses showed that five correlated factors, grouping the items roughly according to major content areas, were probably sufficient to account for the pattern of interitem correlations.

However, the dominant eigenvalue and its associated vector justified a first approximation in terms of a single "radicalism-conservatism" dimension. A scale was constructed (see Table 11–2) that gave equal positive or negative weight to the items based on the sign of salient loadings on the first general factor. Items were scored 0, 1, or 2 giving a possible raw score range of 0 to 56. Scores were imputed for subjects having more than 75% valid responses by taking the average score obtained using the valid responses multiplied by the total number of items in the full scale (28). Subjects with 75% or fewer valid responses were omitted.

Regression analyses were conducted using the SAS regression procedure for both stature and conservatism to examine mean score differences associated with sex, source of data (Virginia Twin Registry vs. AARP), twin vs. nontwin, age and age^2. The corresponding interaction terms were also included in the analysis. The normalized residuals from the full regression model were computed for both stature and conservatism and used to compute product-moment correlations between relatives. Correlations were based on every possible pair belonging to a particular relationship. The same individual may contribute more than once to a given correlation. As a result, the sampling errors of the observed correlations may be larger than expected on the basis of the raw sample sizes. Furthermore, the same individual may contribute to several correlations resulting in correlations among some of the estimated correlation coefficients. Simulation studies have shown (e.g., McGue et al. 1987) that treating such correlations as independent in analyses of family resemblance tends not to bias parameter estimates but may lead to the attribution of too much precision to the analytical results. Current computational methods make a full maximum-likelihood solution impracticable with a data set of this size and number of relationships.

Correlations Between Relatives

Table 11–3 gives the correlations for the residual stature and conservatism scores for all 80 relationships included in this analysis.

TABLE 11–3.

Correlations between relatives for stature and conservatism in the Virginia 30,000

Relationship	Stature		Conservatism	
	N (pairs)	r	N (pairs)	r
Nuclear family				
Spouses	4,751	0.223	4,915	0.619
Male siblings	1,493	0.432	1,551	0.341
Female siblings	3,524	0.429	3,643	0.405
Opposite-sex siblings	4,255	0.411	4,395	0.328
Father-son	2,160	0.439	2,247	0.410
Father-daughter	2,971	0.411	3,095	0.397
Mother-son	3,035	0.446	3,138	0.369
Mother-daughter	4,476	0.430	4,667	0.456
Twins				
Dizygotic male	573	0.483	579	0.379
Dizygotic female	1,164	0.502	1,142	0.432
Opposite-sex dizygotic	1,307	0.432	1,312	0.319
Monozygotic male	775	0.850	790	0.593
Monozygotic female	1,847	0.855	1,839	0.637
Avuncular with sibling of parent				
Paternal uncle-nephew	92	0.427	100	0.334
Paternal uncle-niece	155	0.228	156	0.324
Maternal aunt-nephew	402	0.185	405	0.200
Maternal aunt-niece	536	0.314	547	0.226
Paternal aunt-nephew	131	0.275	133	0.264
Paternal aunt-niece	196	0.231	200	0.112
Maternal uncle-nephew	236	0.253	235	0.175
Maternal uncle-niece	284	0.230	297	0.166
Avuncular with dizygotic twin of parent				
Paternal uncle-nephew	105	0.369	110	0.107
Paternal uncle-niece	137	0.077	144	0.108
Maternal aunt-nephew	345	0.260	332	0.200
Maternal aunt-niece	525	0.239	516	0.250
Paternal aunt-nephew	118	0.242	114	0.282
Paternal aunt-niece	188	0.244	180	0.314
Maternal uncle-nephew	150	0.288	154	0.185
Maternal uncle-niece	202	0.271	206	0.225

(*continued*)

TABLE 11–3.

Continued

Relationship	Stature		Conservatism	
	N (pr)	r	N (pr)	r
Avuncular with monozygotic twin of parent				
Paternal uncle-nephew	217	0.529	221	0.428
Paternal uncle-niece	337	0.444	341	0.315
Maternal aunt-nephew	673	0.458	661	0.367
Maternal aunt-niece	1,040	0.377	1,035	0.318
Cousins related through monozygotic twin parents				
Male pairs related through MZ male parents	39	0.406	40	0.564
Female pairs related through MZ male parents	92	0.271	95	0.265
Male-female pairs related through MZ male parents	107	0.351	107	0.264
Male pairs related through MZ female parents	153	0.279	158	0.238
Female pairs related through MZ female parents	340	0.215	339	0.287
Male-female pairs related through MZ female parents	449	0.274	459	0.309
Cousins related through dizygotic twin parents				
Male pairs related through DZ male parents	19	0.788	19	0.091
Female pairs related through DZ male parents	41	0.559	42	0.339
Male-female pairs related through DZ male parents	52	0.550	52	0.173
Male pairs related through DZ female parents	52	0.185	53	−0.117
Female pairs related through DZ female parents	138	0.156	141	0.275
Male-female pairs related through DZ female parents	159	0.232	163	0.240
Male pairs with male-female twin parents	38	0.113	39	0.242
Female pairs with male-female twin parents	71	0.343	70	0.227
Male-female pairs with male-female twin parents	51	0.091	52	0.066
Male-female pairs with female-male twin parents	72	0.264	70	0.112
Relationships by marriage				
Siblings-in-law				
Wife of twin with nontwin brother of twin	337	0.092	371	0.386
Husband of twin with nontwin sister of twin	728	0.116	745	0.219
Husband of twin with nontwin brother of twin	422	0.101	443	0.222
Wife of twin with nontwin sister of twin	447	0.069	486	0.175
Wife of twin with husband's DZ male co-twin	387	0.125	417	0.263
Husband of twin with wife's DZ female co-twin	603	0.166	618	0.310
Husband of twin with wife's DZ male co-twin	353	0.155	363	0.202
Wife of twin with husband's DZ female co-twin	458	0.218	455	0.290
Wife of twin with husband's MZ male co-twin	589	0.252	625	0.490
Husband of twin with wife's MZ female co-twin	1,139	0.207	1,153	0.409

(continued)

TABLE 11–3.
Continued

	Stature		Conservatism	
Relationship	N (pr)	r	N (pr)	r
Parents-in-law				
Father-in-law/daughter-in-law	205	0.170	208	0.312
Father-in-law/son-in-law	188	−0.016	211	0.219
Mother-in-law/daughter-in-law	293	−0.013	311	0.250
Mother-in-law/son-in-law	338	0.140	360	0.308
Affine avuncular				
Nephew with wife of father's DZ twin	54	0.483	57	−0.048
Niece with wife of father's DZ twin	80	0.356	82	0.159
Nephew with husband of mother's DZ twin	126	0.196	128	0.158
Niece with husband of mother's DZ twin	169	−0.010	179	0.166
Nephew with husband of father's DZ twin	36	−0.029	38	0.015
Niece with husband of father's DZ twin	68	−0.003	70	0.055
Nephew with wife of mother's DZ twin	64	−0.210	71	0.230
Niece with wife of mother's DZ twin	95	−0.033	99	0.195
Nephew with wife of father's MZ twin	129	0.154	134	0.366
Niece with wife of father's MZ twin	213	0.194	224	0.276
Nephew with husband of mother's MZ twin	342	0.147	353	0.239
Niece with husband of mother's MZ twin	502	0.194	511	0.222
Twin's spouses				
Wives of male DZ twins	100	0.066	104	0.212
Husbands of female DZ twins	120	0.130	129	0.325
Spouses of male-female DZ twins	167	0.008	172	0.185
Wives of male MZ twins	172	0.199	188	0.378
Husbands of female MZ twins	300	0.231	304	0.267

Before embarking on any more rigorous analysis, it is helpful to study some of the correlations between relatives to obtain an overall perspective on family resemblance and its likely causes. Figure 11–2 summarizes the correlations for nuclear family members. We note remarkable uniformity at a little over 0.4 between the various parent-offspring and sibling correlations for stature. The correlations for conservatism also hover around 0.4 but are more heterogeneous. The average parent-offspring correlation for conservatism is a little larger than that for siblings. The correlations for conservatism are more het-

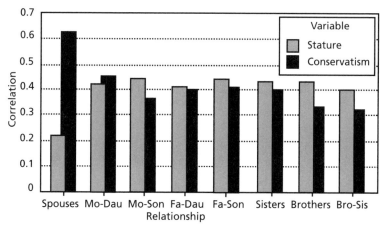

FIGURE 11–2. *Nuclear family correlations for stature and conservatism.*

erogeneous across sexes and are marginally lower for pairs of opposite sex. Thus, our self-report data for conservatism reveal marked family resemblance of the order that Pearson had claimed for his ratings of siblings. The lower correlations for opposite-sex pairs for conservatism, together with the higher correlation for female pairs compared with male pairs, indicates that some modest sex differences may be expected in either the genetic or social transmission of attitudes. However, all the nuclear family correlations are quite large and positive regardless of sex. This finding precludes two common myths about parent-offspring relationships for social variables: that children "react against" their parents (which would produce negative correlations) and that children model on their same-sex parent (because there would be far greater differences between same and opposite-sex parent-offspring correlations). Such effects are not precluded by the data as modest factors in the transmission of attitudes, but clearly the Virginia 30,000 data preclude these effects playing an overwhelming role.

The major contrast between the nuclear family correlations for stature and conservatism is that between spouses. For conservatism, the observed correlation of 0.62 is as great as that for MZ twins and almost three times as large as that for stature. The small spousal correlation for stature may be sufficient to have detectable genetic consequences for such a heritable trait. If the large correlation between mates for conservatism is due to like marrying like ("assortative mating") rather than spousal convergence due to social interaction, it would have very marked effects on the correlations for other relationships whether these be caused genetically, environmentally, or both. In our data, the Spearman correlation between absolute intrapair differences and duration of marriage for spouse pairs was −0.0298 ($P = .04$, $N = 4,884$ pairs). The fact that this correlation is small and barely significant suggests that either convergence has all occurred prior to marriage, or that the large spousal correlation is due to assortative mating. In general (see Heath 1987), spousal interaction will tend to result in disproportionately high correlations between spouses compared with those for other relationships by marriage including the spouses of twins and siblings.

Correlations for nuclear families establish a baseline for the degree of family resemblance but contribute little to the resolution of biological from cultural inheritance. Figure 11–3 summarizes the correlations for MZ and DZ twins. Barring mutations, the genetic effects of MZ twins are perfectly correlated. When mating is random and genetic effects are additive (i.e., there is no dominance or epistasis) the genetic effects of DZ twins (and siblings) are expected to correlate only 0.5. Thus, in the simplest of all worlds in which mating is random, gene effects are additive, and the only environmental effects are uncorrelated between relatives, the correlation for DZ twins is expected, within

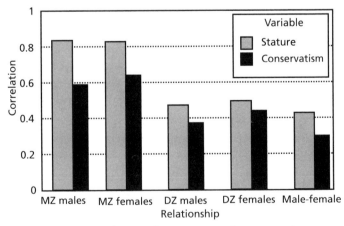

FIGURE 11–3. *Twin correlations for stature and conservatism.*

sampling error, to be one-half of that between MZ twins. DZ corre-lations in excess of one-half the MZ correlation may point directly to the genetic and environmental consequences of assortative mating, or to effects of the shared family environment. If DZ correlations are less than one-half those for MZ it is possible that the genetic effects are not additive (see for example Jinks and Fulker 1970). If the twin cor-relations are both significant but equal, there can clearly be no genetic effects but there must be substantial effects of the shared environment. A significant excess of the MZ over the DZ correlations establishes a prima facie case (though not incontrovertible evidence) for the con-tribution of genetic factors.

For both stature and conservatism, the Virginia 30,000 data con-firm the well-documented excess of the MZ correlations over those for DZ. Thus, genetic factors appear to play a role. In the case of stature, it comes as no surprise. For those who are unaware of the twin literature on social attitudes, the findings may be more disconcerting because they appear to challenge commonly held theoretical and philosophical suppositions that humans are largely immune from the effects of their biological inheritance once we transcend the purely physical domain.

The broad trend for DZ correlations is close to that for siblings. The differences across sexes are more marked for conservatism than stature, and the ordering of the three DZ correlations for conservatism mirrors perfectly that for siblings. There is a slight excess of the DZ correlations over those for siblings with respect to stature, but barely so for conservatism.

We note that the correlations for same-sex DZ twins (and siblings) are greater than one-half the corresponding MZ correlations. This ex-cess is present for both stature and conservatism, but more marked for conservatism. This result implies either that the genetic correlation for DZ twins is greater than 0.5 due to assortative mating or population stratification, or that there are significant effects of the shared family environment, or both. It is conceivable that the excess may have dif-ferent causes in the two variables.

Figure 11–4 presents correlations for 16 of the most salient rela-tionships pooled over sexes. The sample sizes for many of these cor-relations are extremely large (over 8,000 sibling pairs, and 12,000 parent-offspring pairs) but significant heterogeneity between sexes for

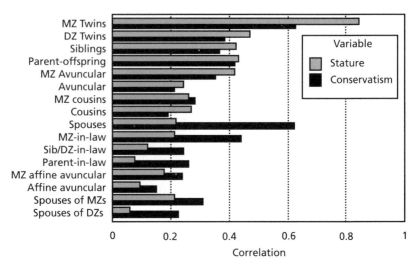

FIGURE 11–4. *Principal correlations between relatives for stature and conservatism pooled over sexes.*

some of the relationships (compare Table 11–4 and Figures 11–2 and 11–3) is ignored so the figure is primarily to assist the visualization of trends.

Considering first the biological relationships, Figure 11–4 reveals the marked similarity in the pattern of correlations for stature and conservatism. There is a striking linear relationship between the observed correlation and the degree of genetic relatedness. The high correlation between cousins related through DZ twins for stature is a marked and inexplicable exception to this pattern. The correlations for stature illustrate as clearly as possible the pattern to be expected for a variable in which there is a large additive genetic component of variance. We note especially that there is no difference between the parent-offspring correlation for stature and the avuncular correlation involving MZ co-twins of parents. Nongenetic explanations of the excess similarity of MZ twins become increasingly strained as we confirm that other biological relationships derived from MZ twins fit closely the predictions of a genetic model when compared with those for other relationships. The correlations for conservatism show a similar pattern, with the lower MZ correlation noted earlier. However, the parent-offspring correlation is slightly higher than the MZ avuncular correlation suggesting that some of the parent-offspring resemblance may have a nongenetic component (e.g., phenotypic assortative mating).

The pooled correlations also demonstrate clearly the impact of assortative mating on the correlations between relatives. Both stature and conservatism show evidence of assortative mating. However, the spousal correlations for conservatism are very much larger than those for stature. The effect of assortment for conservatism pervades all the correlations by marriage for our data. On closer examination, the comparative data for stature and conservatism show some important similarities and differences. For both traits, the correlations by marriage involving DZ twins are lower than those involving MZ twins. This finding does not favor the view advanced by Morton and his colleagues (Morton 1974; Rao et al. 1974) that assortment is based primarily on the *social*, rather then genetic components, of the phenotype. If spouses select one another primarily for aspects of the environment they share, such as the socioeconomic status of their parents, then we would predict no difference between correlations for in-laws of MZ and DZ twins. Our data thus suggest mate selection also involves genetic aspects of the phenotype.

A Model for Family Resemblance in Extended Twin Kinships

The previous discussion provides a preliminary sense of the main features of family resemblance for a physical and behavioral trait. However, it does not provide quantitative estimates of the various social and biological factors contributing to individual differences. Neither does it yield any analysis of how sex affects the transmission and expression of genetic and environmental effects. This goal can only be realized by formulating, fitting, and testing a mathematical model for family resemblance in the 80 correlations. One such model, described in detail by Truett et al. (1994) is presented in Figure 11–5 as a path diagram (see Li 1976, Neale and Cardon 1992; Wright 1921). We stress at the outset that this is not the only model that could be devised, but it represents a good place to start because it allows for additive and

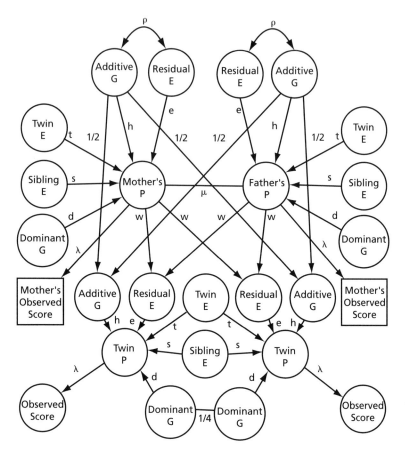

FIGURE 11–5. *Path model for biological and cultural inheritance in the absence of sex-dependent effects.*

The "latent" phenotypes of mothers, fathers, and children on which assortment and cultural inheritance are based are indicated by circles and the observed scores by squares.

Single-headed arrows represent the hypothesized direction of causation. Correlations which have an extraneous cause, such as that between genetic and environmental effects in parents, are denoted by double-headed arrows. A bar with no arrows ("co-path," Cloninger 1980) denotes the correlation between mates whose cause is extraneous to the diagram but which induces correlations between other causal factors in the model (e.g., between the genetic effects of husbands and wives).

Legend: G, genes; E, environment; P, phenotype; h, additive genetic effects; d, genetic dominance; e, path from environment to phenotype; w, path from parental phenotype to offspring environment; μ, phenotypic correlation between mates; s, path from residual sibling shared environment to phenotype; t, path from additional twin shared environment to phenotype; ρ, correlation between genotype and environment; λ, regression of observed score on the latent phenotype.

dominant genetic effects, nongenetic inheritance from parents to child, some forms of assortative mating, sex differences in genetic and environmental effects, and some additional nongenetic sources of family resemblance including the shared sibling and twin environments. There is no one "right" way to write the model. Other investigators may choose to devise alternative models or parametrizations.

The model assumes, initially that assortative mating, if present, is based on the measured phenotype, P ("primary phenotypic assortative mating," Heath and Eaves 1985). Similarly, it is assumed that vertical cultural transmission from parent to offspring is based on the measured phenotype of the parents rather than on some latent or correlated variable ("P to E" vertical cultural inheritance). The effects of the sibling and twin shared environments are assumed to contribute to variation among individuals regardless of relationship. However, the sibling environment is perfectly correlated in sibling and twin pairs, and the twin environment is perfectly correlated in twin pairs. Thus, the model assumes that twins and siblings will differ in correlation, but not in variance, as a result of how they are influenced by their shared environment. That is, twins and siblings are assumed to sample the same marginal distribution of environmental effects as other individuals but they differ in the environmental correlation. The genotype-environment correlation, ρ, occurs when the parental phenotype, which contributes to the offspring's environment through parent-offspring transmission, is partly genetic in origin. This results in a correlation between the offspring's environment and genes. The process of transmission and assortment is assumed to be in equilibrium, and thus, ρ is constant between generations. That is, ρ is constrained to be same in parents and offspring. Since models are fitted to correlations, the scale of measurement has unit variance; therefore, we impose the further constraint that the sum of all sources of variation is unity.

As already noted, the measured trait may not correlate perfectly with the trait for which mate selection and cultural transmission are actually occurring. Morton (1974) argued for a model of "social homogamy" in which assortment and cultural transmission are based on a correlated latent variable to which genes make no contribution. Another mechanism of assortment (proposed by Heath and Eaves 1985) presents a model for mixed homogamy in which mate selection on both the social background of the spouses and the phenotype of the mate. We have used "phenotypic assortment plus error" (Heath 1983) in which the actual measurement is considered a more or less unreliable index of the latent score on which assortment is based. In this model, all expected correlations were multiplied by the square of the path from "true" (or latent) score to "observed" score (the reliability [λ]). When there is significant assortative mating or cultural inheritance, there is sufficient information in the extended twin-kinship design to estimate λ without repeted measurements.

Allowing for Sex Differences in Model Parameters

One of the principal advantages of a study involving large samples of relatives is the opportunity to test a variety of models of sex-dependent etiology and transmission. For the simple case of randomly mating populations, a model for sex differences in gene action was specified by Eaves (1977) that allowed for the same genes to have different magnitudes of effect on males and females. This model allows for estimation of separate genetic variances for males and females and a correlation between gene effects in males and females. The genetic correlation between the sexes will be unity if the effects of all autosomal loci on one sex are constant multiples of their effects on the other sex. In this case, we speak of "scalar sex-limitation of the gene effects."

Analogous definitions may be given for the "sex-limited" effects of the shared environment. If the magnitudes of the loci or, by analogy, "environmental effects" on one sex are not constant multiples of their effects on the other sex, then we speak of nonscalar sex limitation of genetic (or environmental) effects. The present model extends the analysis of sex-dependent effects to the more difficult cases of combined assortative mating and cultural inheritance. In the path diagram (Figure 11-6) we employ the following notation for the effects of dominance, sibling enironment, and special twin environment: d_m, s_m, and t_m in males respectively, and d_f, s_f, and t_f for their counterparts in fe-

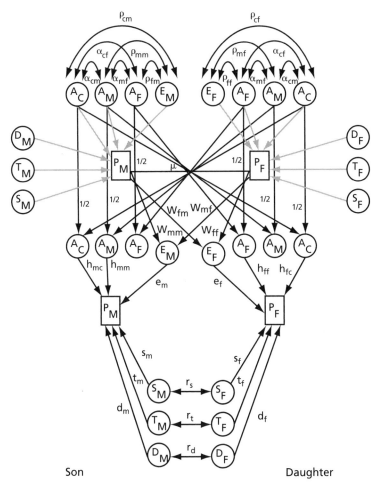

Son   Daughter

FIGURE 11–6. *Path model for biological and culture inheritance when genetic and environmental effects depend on sex. Note. For simplicity, the figure only presents the biological and cultural effects on the* reliable *variance in the phenotype. If assortment and cultural transmission are based on a latent trait then paths from true scores to observed scores may be included for males and females, λ_m and λ_f, respectively, as in Figure 11–5.*

males; and r_d, r_s, and r_t, for the correlations across sexes of the dominant, sibling environmental, and twin environmental effects.

Since vertical cultural transmission is assumed under this model to be based on the parental phenotype for the trait under investigation, the question of "nonscalar" vertical cultural transmission does not apply. However, the cultural impact of mothers may differ from that of fathers and may further depend on the sex of the offspring. In the model for sex differences, therefore, we require four cultural parameters: w_{mm}; w_{mf}; w_{fm}; w_{ff}. The first subscript denotes the sex (m = male) of the offspring and the second denotes the sex of the parent.

Specification of sex-limited additive genetic effects is more difficult when there is assortative mating that induces correlations between loci that would otherwise be independent (see for example Fisher 1918). We have adopted one of several formally equivalent ways of parameterizing the additive sex-limited effects. Recognizing that the additive genetic variances in the two sexes and the genetic covariance between them require three free parameters for their complete specification, we assume that one set of genes explains all the genetic variance in females and the genetic covariance between the sexes. The paths from this "common" set of genes to the male and female phenotypes are denoted by h_{mc} and h_{fc}, respectively. A second set of genes has effects specific only to males, and the path from these genes to the male phenotype is specified by h_{mm}. Although the "male-specific" genes are not expressed in females, they are still present in females and correlated, through phenotypic assortment, with the "common genes." We denote the induced correlation between the two sets of additive genetic effects by α_{cm}.

The joint effects of assortment and vertical cultural transmission induce four genotype-environment correlations: two between the "common" additive genetic effects and the environments of males and females, ρ_{cm} and ρ_{cf}, respectively; two between the "male-specific" additive genetic effects and the environments of males and females, ρ_{mm} and ρ_{mf}, respectively. These genotype-environment correlations are estimated as constrained parameters when fitting the model (i.e., they are functions of other parameters). Separate parameters are required to specify the path from male environment to phenotype (e_m) and female environment to phenotype (e_f). Under the simple model for "phenotypic assortment with error," the paths from true score to observed score, λ_m and λ_f, may differ between males and females.

Since the total phenotypic variance is standardized to unity in both sexes, two further constraints are required to enforce these conditions. Thus, seven constraints are imposed on parameter values under the full model. The full model for sex-limited effects is given for pairs of opposite-sex DZ twins in Figure 11–6.

Fitting the Model

The method of iterative constrained diagonal weighted least squares was used to fit the full (nonlinear) model to the 80 correlations for each personality and social attitude variable in turn. The model is fitted to the z-transforms of the raw correlations to improve the approximation to normality (see Rao et al. 1977). Truett et al. (1996) give further details of the model fitting method. The expected correlations between relatives may be derived algebraically from the path model. These are extremely complex and are not reproduced here. The Numerical Algorithms Group's FORTRAN subroutine E04UEF was used for constrained numerical minimization of the residual sum of squares (Numerical Algorithms Group 1990).

The full model, involving 19 free parameters, was fitted first. The weighted residual sum of squares for $80 - 19 = 61$ df is employed as a guide to the overall goodness-of-fit of the model. The false assumption of independence in the observed correlations is likely to result in our rejecting the model too often if we treat this statistic uncritically as χ^2. However, the implications of this strategy for comparisons of alternative models based on examination of changes in χ^2 associated with reductions in the full model are less predictable (McGue et al. 1987).

In order to test the significance of combinations of effects having particular theoretical importance, a series of reduced models was fitted in every case and the increase in the residual sum of squares noted as a guide to the deterioration in fit associated with deleting specific effects from the model. Reduced models were fitted to test the following specific hypotheses: 1) that all genetic and environmental effects were homogenous over sexes; 2) that there were no genetic effects ($h = 0$, $d = 0$ in both sexes); 3) that there were no nonadditive (dominant) genetic effects ($d = 0$ in both sexes); 4) that there were no effects of the shared environment of any kind ($s = t = w = 0$ in both sexes); 5) that there was no vertical cultural inheritance ($w = 0$ in both sexes); 6) that assortment and cultural inheritance were based on the measured phenotype rather that a latent "true" phenotype ($\lambda = 1$ in both sexes). These tests do not exhaust all the possibilities. However, in view of the danger of capitalizing on chance with multiple tests it is more appropriate to restrict testing to a few major effects of a priori importance.

Results

Table 11–4 presents the weighted least squares estimates of the parameters of the full model for family resemblance in stature and conservatism. Table 11–5 gives χ^2 statistics testing approximate goodness-of-fit of the model and for testing the major hypotheses enumerated previously. We note that large numerical estimates of the cultural transmission parameters, w, nevertheless may imply a relatively small contribution to the total environmental variance because the path e may itself be small.

Using the parameter values from the full model in Table 11–4, the contributions of the different genetic and environmental sources to variation in the two traits were computed using the formulae given by Truett et al. (1994). The tabulated parameter values, and Truett's formulae, refer only to the *reliable* variance. Hence, for example, the value of 0.012 for the environmental path coefficient for stature in males does not imply that the environment plays no role in creating differences in stature. It does, however, imply that the environment plays little role in creating those differences that contribute to the choice of spouse. Table 11–6 summarizes the estimated contributions of the major sources of variation to differences in stature and conservatism for males and females.

TABLE 11–4.

Results of model-fitting to correlations in stature and conservatism

Parameter	Estimate	
	Stature	Conservatism
Genetic		
h_{fc}	0.940	0.580
h_{mc}	0.921	0.866
h_{mm}	0	0
d_f	0.282	0.360
d_m	0.333	0.295
r_d	−0.063	−0.002
Assortment		
μ	0.275	0.720
μ_{cm}	0	0
Cultural transmission		
w_{ff}	0.280	0.172
w_{mf}	−1.000	−0.368
w_{fm}	0.296	0.026
w_{mm}	−0.135	0.208
Other shared environment		
s_f	0.136	0.233
s_m	0	0
r_s	—	—
t_f	0.295	0.210
t_m	0.235	0.036
r_t	0.505	1
Unique environment		
e_f	−0.145	0.493
e_m	0.012	0.592
Genotype-environment correlations		
ρ_{cf}	0.332	0.124
ρ_{cm}	−0.649	−0.094
ρ_{mf}	0	0
ρ_{mm}	0	0
Latent variable		
λ_f	0.932	0.979
λ_m	0.921	0.878

TABLE 11-5.

Tests of significance and summary statistics from model-fitting analysis of stature and conservatism

Item	χ^2	df	AIC	SS%	χ^2	df	P%
Stature							
Full model	127.02	61	4.90	98.85	—	—	<.01
Sex differences	163.15	73	17.15	98.52	36.13	12	.03
Shared environment	139.21	71	−2.79	98.73	12.19	10	27.25
Vertical cultural inheritance	128.01	65	−1.98	98.84	0.09	4	99.90
Genetic effects	711.66	67	577.66	93.53	524.64	6	<.01
Dominance	140.48	64	12.48	98.72	13.46	3	.37
Assortative mating	600.91	62	476.91	97.53	473.89	1	<.01
Latent assortment	135.93	63	9.93	98.76	8.91	2	1.16
Conservatism							
Full model	65.51	61	−59.49	99.37	—	—	42.23
Sex differences	279.17	73	133.17	97.20	213.66	12	<.01
Shared environment	83.25	71	−58.75	99.17	17.74	10	5.95
Vertical cultural inheritance	79.26	65	−50.74	99.21	9.75	4	4.48
Genetic effects	507.44	67	373.46	94.92	441.93	6	<.01
Dominance	336.28	64	208.28	96.63	270.77	3	<.01
Assortative mating	3,661.04	62	3,537.01	63.33	3,595.53	1	<.01
Latent assortment	88.92	63	−37.08	99.11	23.41	2	<.01

Note. χ^2 = Chi-square testing goodness-of-fit; AIC = Akaike Information Criterion; SS% = percentage of sum of weighted squared raw z statistics explained by parameters of model; χ^2 = Chi-square testing effects removed from model; P% = significance level (%).

TABLE 11–6.

Estimated contributions of sources of variation to differences in stature and conservatism

| | Proportion of total variation (%) | | | |
| | Stature | | Conservatism | |
Source	Males	Females	Males	Females
Genetic				
Additive	55.8	59.6	35.5	19.8
Assortment	16.1	17.2	22.2	12.4
Dominance	9.4	6.9	6.7	12.5
"Total genetic"	83.9	86.7	64.4	44.7
Environment				
Maternal	0.0	0.2	1.5	1.0
Paternal	0.0	0.2	0.0	0.1
Twin	4.7	7.6	0.1	4.2
Sibling	0.0	1.6	0.0	5.2
Within-family	0.0	1.4	17.5	32.4
"Error"	15.3	13.1	22.9	4.1
G-E covariance	− 1.2	− 7.9	− 6.2	8.1

Discussion

The overall fit of the model for conservatism is surprisingly good ($P >$ .4). The fit for stature is relatively poor; some of the largest individual contributions to the highly significant weighted residual sum of squares come from male cousins (13.02), opposite-sex cousins (10.48), and female cousins (8.87) (all related through male DZ twins), The fit for 300 other relationships, including those for twins and nuclear families, is quite close given the very large sample sizes. In this respect, our study seems to suffer from similar problems to those reviewed by Fisher (1918) who remarks:

> In general, the hypothesis of cumulative Mendelian factors seems to fit the facts very accurately. The only marked discrepancy from ex-

isting published work lies in the correlation for first cousins. . . . The values found . . . are certainly extremely high, but until we have a record of complete cousinships without selection, it will not be possible to obtain satisfactory numerical evidence on this question. (p. 433)

Comparison of the results for the two variables reveals similarities and differences in the transmission of stature and attitudes. Both have genetic components. The genetic variation of both stature and conservatism is inflated by assortative mating and nonadditive genetic effects ("dominance" in our model). For stature, Fisher (1918) estimates that about 14% of the total variance is attributable to dominance effects. Our values for both sexes are somewhat lower but significantly greater than zero. The effects of dominance may obscure other nonadditive effects including the interaction of genetic differences with the effects of age and secular trends in the data. The contribution of assortative mating to the genetic variation in stature reflects a relatively low marital correlation operating on a trait that, after correction for errors of measurement, is almost completely heritable. Fisher (1918) observes "some ambiguity still remains as to the causes of marital correlations: our numerical conclusions are considerably affected according as this is assumed to be of purely somatic [phenotypic] or purely genetic origin" (p. 33) but then remarks that his results are in close agreement with partial genetic origin of assortment. Our results for stature agree with this view insofar as our data require us to exclude some of the measured effects on stature from those affecting assortment. In our model, these are referred to as "error." In contrast, the pervasive effects of assortment on family resemblance for conservatism reflect a much higher degree of phenotypic ("somatic") assortment for a trait that is affected significantly less by additive genetic effects. Nongenetic differences within MZ twin pairs are seen to have an impact on the choice of mate for conservatism.

Fisher (1918) notes that most of the evidence for dominance, in Pearson and Lee's data, comes from the sibling correlation. He ignores the possibility that nongenetic effects may also be correlated between relatives. Our design includes MZ twins and their relatives, which provides additional tests for the effects of nonadditive genetic factors and allows a more subtle analysis of the environment. For stature, Fisher notes (1918, p. 433) that "examination of the best possible available figures for human measurements shows that there is little or no evidence of nongenetic causes." Our data give little reason to disagree with this early finding as far as stature is concerned once we allow for the effects of errors of measurement in our self-reported observations. Our data include MZ twins, which give a more direct measure of nongenetic effects. The results for the Virginia 30,000 also give little reason to infer a marked role for nongenetic inheritance for human stature.

How far is Pearson's attempt to universalize these findings to human behavior justified? By assessing human attitudes we have attempted to operationalize those essentially "human" characteristics that, unlike cognition and personality, defy attempts to develop convincing animal models. Social attitudes cannot exist without culture. Normative attitudes change continually. Yet there are enormous individual differences that we have attempted to quantify in our survey. Pearson's early claim that the inheritance of human behavior owed nothing to any characteristically "human" principle was overstated but not unfounded. It is certainly the case that nuclear family resemblance in conservatism is almost as great as that for stature (see Figure 11–2). However, it is misleading to assert that this result points to an equivalent genetic contribution because the effects of assortative mating on the correlations for conservatism are considerably greater than those for stature. The total environmental variance for conservatism is approximately twice that for stature. Most of the environmental effect, however, is due to differences within families and fluctuations within individuals over time that contribute to greater differences within MZ twin pairs. Although conservatism indeed differs from stature in showing a significant effect of vertical cultural inheritance from parent to child, the contributions of parent-offspring social transmission to adult attitude differences are relatively small compared with other genetic and environmental effects.

There are significant differences between the sexes in the relative contributions of genes and environment. These effects were ignored in the early studies. We believe our study is the first to attempt an empirical resolution of all the different genetic and environmental sources of sex differences in the expression of genetic and environmental effects. These effects are greater for conservatism than stature and are consistent with women being somewhat more influenced by environmental factors than men. The effects of vertical cultural inheritance, though contributing only a relatively small amount to sibling resemblance, appear to depend slightly more on mothers than fathers.

By focusing on those characteristics that attitudes have in common, as we have done by using a scale score based on a large number of items that are only weakly correlated, it might be argued that we have ignored those idiosyncrasies of style that might be more sensitive to social learning than overall tendencies. Furthermore, the general "conservatism" factor is only a first approximation to a more complex factor structure underlying these items. Any heterogeneity in the causes of variation in among the primary factors will be obscured in this broader analysis.

The similarities in the pattern of family resemblance for stature and attitudes point to important communality between the origins of physique and behavior. They suggest that there is no "sacred territory" in human behavior that can be delineated simply by virtue of its immunity from the effects of genes. The effects of genes reach the highest points of culture. In this respect, Pearson was probably correct in regarding biological inheritance as the theme that unified the "mental and moral" characteristics of humans with "[even] the protopodite of the water flea." This conclusion has important cultural implications for how humans perceive themselves. It is probably for this reason that many critics have resisted it with a zeal that has sometimes precluded creative reflection. Clearly, our findings and others like them have within themselves the seeds of hubris. We may not conclude too hastily that humans are "nothing but" their genes or that because thought and feeling cannot directly alter stature they have no effect on behavior. Behavior-genetic studies like the Virginia 30,000 are still blunt instruments. Within the range of possible pathways from genotype to phenotype there remain a number of radically different alternatives, all of which would lead to patterns of family resemblance suggesting the importance of genetic factors. Cross-sectional studies of family resemblance do not have much power to resolve the ontogenetic role of the individual as "actor" in the creation of his or her phenotype. The process of human development and adaptation has been committed by evolution to an organism that engages in more or less continual dialogue with the ecosystem. The individual behavioral phenotype at any moment is a selective record of this conversation. If the findings of behavioral genetics are to be believed, the dialogue between the individual and the ecosystem does not begin at birth with a blank tape but with some of the experiments, successes, and failures of previous generations encoded in the genetic material. In humans, these are not primarily the stereotyped patterns of other species but rather clues about salient features of the environment and strategies for dealing with novelty and change. The fact of genetic diversity yields individuals whose conversations with the environment take on different shapes ontogenetically. Different individuals attend somewhat differently to the features of their environment, try different experiments, and respond differently to the answers. The result is not pure "chaos," however, as would be the case if the genotype set only the initial conditions of the ontogenetic dialogue. Rather, the outcome is an ordered set of correlations between relatives, which follow more closely the pattern of biological rather than purely cultural inheritance. Thus, we conclude that the genotype is at the center of human action, even of human creativity, by virtue of setting the basic parameters of the organism's continual adaptation by selecting, assimilating, and transforming information derived from the environment.

The path from gene to behavior is long and complex, involving the nonrandom selection of the environment by individuals of different genetic liability or the nonrandom imposition of environmental treatments on individuals, even within the family, as a consequence of perceived genetic differences. Insofar as inherited differences bias the individual toward different features of the environment, we expect a correlation between the effects of genes and environment on the phenotype ("genotype-environment correlation," Cattell 1960, 1963; Eaves et al. 1977; Jinks and Fulker 1970; Plomin et al. 1977). The type of genotype-environment correlation generated by the individual as "actor" will lead, in cross-sectional studies, to environmental effects that cannot be separated from other genetic effects (Jinks and Fulker 1970). Indeed, in one sense they are "genetic" effects since they arise because genetic differences between individuals have resulted in the differential selection and elicitation of particular environmental effects. Such genotype-environment correlations constitute one aspect of what Richard Dawkins (1982) has called the "extended phenotype."

Insofar as genetically different individuals respond differently to changes in their environment we expect, in the statistical sense, "genotype × environment interaction." Such interactions were termed "plasticity" in the early work of Cavalli-Sforza and Feldman (1973) on the theme of cultural inheritance. The consequences of the interaction of genotype and environment for family resemblance have been traced theoretically by Jinks and Fulker (1970). Interactions between genetic effects and environmental differences *within* families will be confounded with the effects of the within-family environment in cross-sectional studies. Interactions between genetic effects and environmental differences *between* families (such as those created by vertical cultural inheritance) will, in our types of families, be divided between genetic effects and those of the family environment. Thus, our cross-sectional study gives little leverage on the precise way in which genes and environment correlate and interact during development.

The fact that our study is cross-sectional and limited to adults implies a relatively simple-minded and "static" conception of the role of the family environment and parental treatment in behavioral development. It has commonly been assumed that the effects of parental treatment are additive to those of the genes and persistent throughout life. The primary adaptive role of parents may, however, be to support the organism during development so that it survives long enough with the cognitive and social skills necessary to adapt freely to the niches available to it as an adult. Long-term reliance on parents as sources of specific values in a rapidly changing environment may be maladaptive. Thus, it may be naive to expect a large persistent direct nongenetic effect of parents on the adult attitudes of their children. The study of attitude development in younger people, especially among adolescent twins and adoptees, may tell a different story and reveal a large but transient effect of the shared environment on the attitudes of younger people. On the other hand, if the large spousal correlations for attitudes are any criterion, spouses invest a lot of their resources in choosing a partner for life and reproduction of very similar attitudes. Explanations of the kind "people who have similar attitudes tend to get on better" beg the more fundamental question of why they should care so much about attitudes and invest so little in other aspects of personality such as extraversion and neuroticism (see for example Eaves et al. 1989) for which spousal correlations are consistently zero.

We caution that the results for social attitudes cannot be generalized to the point where it is assumed that *all* differences in behavior have a genetic component. An analysis of religious affiliation in twins and their parents, for example (Eaves et al. 1990), shows that genes play little or no role in determining whether or not children follow in the religious traditions of their parents. Such counterexamples lead us to give even more credence to our current findings because we are compelled to conclude that the finding that nongenetic effects play such a small part in the transmission of social attitudes cannot simply be explained away by a philosophical prejudice of the researchers or by the inherent bias of the research design.

We have stressed that our use of a single general conservatism factor is an oversimplification of the structure of social attitudes. Truett et al. (1992) show that there are several correlated primary factors underlying the general conservatism factor that show differential patterns of association with indices of religiosity and education. Further analysis of the Virginia 30,000 will clarify these complex relationships.

No human science, genetic or social, is wholly free from the problems inherent in the epistemic distance demanded by scientific "objectivity." Paul Ricouer has observed (1967) that there is no platform from which all human diversity can be viewed with absolute detachment, "the objectivity of science, without a point of view and without a situation, does not equalize cultures except by neutralizing their value; it cannot think the positive reasons for their equal value." As culture tries to deal with the new insights of human genetics, particularly behavioral genetics, humans need to be clear about what is offensive to their humanity. The offense lies not in whether human behavior is conceived in "genetic" or "environmental" terms, or some combination of both. The scientific "facts" do not disengage humans from the moral imperatives that constitute the wellsprings of social action and even of science itself. Genetic *and* environmental explanations both become offensive at the point where they attribute more or less worth to individuals by the circumstances and gifts of their birth. Critics of too close an alliance between "science" and "state" can point to the historical abuses of the scientific cores of both Marxist and Darwinian theories (see for example Popper 1960).

The impetus to genetic research and technology provided by the human genome initiative has resulted (e.g., Duster 1990; Kevles and Hood 1992) in the resurrection of the specter of "genetic determinism" and the non sequitur that behavioral genetics is inherently a reactionary science that threatens the freedom and dignity of humans. Such views are superficial, scientifically and philosophically. Genetic models are no more nor less "deterministic" than environmental models. Neither are they any more or less "materialistic." They are no more nor less a "threat to humanity" than any other branch of the human sciences. Both seek to analyze the complexity of human behavior in terms of more abstract principles that are conceived as "causes." Whether these causes are genetic or environmental makes little logical or practical difference. We note that one of the most rigorous proponents of "determinism" was a psychologist who set little store by the role of genes in behavior (e.g., Skinner 1971). What genetic studies may have done is to temporarily "disenfranchise" a series of vaguer social paradigms for the understanding of behavior. Among "deterministic" models, genetic models have become serious contenders for the elucidation of "cause." Among "materialistic" models, genetic models have offered a prime candidate for the material ground of behavior in the shape of the double helix.

The human sciences have to be judged by how well they deal with the "*humanum.*" Scientifically speaking, this success does not depend, initially, on whether the underlying principles of explanation are genetic or environmental but on how far such principles render intelligible the most characteristic qualities of the organism. Thus, a model that takes into account the role of genes in the ontogeny and identity of humans who show initiative, creativity, and even "freedom" is, at one level, paying greater tribute to humanity than an "environmental" one that denies the individual any active role in shaping his or her destiny. Our data on social attitudes do not preclude nongenetic effects but they do make it increasingly difficult to discount the role of genes in shaping the developmental trajectory of humans at the level of traits, such as social attitudes, that have little meaning outside the human domain.

The broader cultural and philosophical implications of genetic studies of human behavior are far from clear. Studies such as the Virginia 30,000 strongly suggest that human's understanding of their humanity will require that they deal at every level with the relationship between the human genome and the highest faculties of affect and cognition with which they have been gifted by natural selection. Legitimate scientific criticism of careless research will continue to play an important part in this process. It is no less urgent that philosophers, historians, sociologists, and other commentators start to engage the findings of behavioral genetics positively in ways that owe more to ingenuity and less to panic.

References

Cattell RB: The multiple abstract variance analysis equations and solutions for nature-nurture research on continuous variables. Psychol Rev 67:353–372, 1960

Cattell RB: The interaction of hereditary and environmental influences. Br J Stat Psychol 16:191–210, 1963

Cavalli-Sforza LL: Genes, people and languages. Sci Am 265:104–110, 1991

Cavalli-Sforza LL, Feldman MW: Cultural versus biological inheritance: phenotypic transmission from parents to offspring (a theory of direct effects of parental phenotypes on children's phenotypes.) Am J Hum Genet 25:618–637, 1973

Cavalli-Sforza LL, Feldman MW: Cultural Transmission and Evolution: A Quantitative Approach. Princeton, NJ, Princeton University Press, 1981

Cavalli-Sforza LL, Feldman MW, Chen KH, et al: Theory and observation in cultural transmission. Science 218:19–27, 1982

Cloninger CR: Interpretation of intrinsic and extrinsic structural relations by path analysis: theory and applications to assortative mating. Genet Res 36:135–145, 1980

Cloninger CR, Rice J, Reich T: Multifactorial inheritance with cultural transmission and assortative mating. Am J Hum Genet 31:178–188, 1979

Corey LA, Berg K, Pellock JM, et al: The occurrence of epilepsy and febrile seizures in Virginian and Norwegian twins. Neurology 41:1433–1436, 1991

Dawkins R: The Extended Phenotype: The Gene as the Unit of Selection. Oxford, England, Oxford University Press, 1982

Duster TS: Backdoor to Eugenics. New York, Routledge & Kegan Paul, 1990

Eaves LJ: Aspects of Human Psychogenetics. University of Birmingham, Ph.D. Thesis, 1970

Eaves LJ: Computer simulation of sample size and experimental design in human psychogenetics. Psychol Bull 77:144–152, 1972

Eaves LJ: The effect of cultural transmission on continuous variation. Heredity 37:41–57, 1976

Eaves LJ: Inferring the causes of human variation. J Royal Stat Soc, Series A 140:324–355, 1977

Eaves LJ: The use of twins in the analysis of assortative mating. Heredity 43:399–409, 1980

Eaves LJ, Eysenck HJ: Genetics and the development of social attitudes. Nature 249:288–289, 1974

Eaves LJ, Heath AC: Detection of the effects of asymmetric assortative mating. Nature 289:205–206, 1981

Eaves LJ, Last KA, Martin NG, et al: A progressive approach to non-additivity and genotype-environmental covariance in the analysis of human differences. Br J Math Stat Psychol 30:1–42, 1977

Eaves LJ, Last KA, Young PA, et al: Model-fitting approaches to the analysis of human behavior. Heredity 41:249–320, 1978

Eaves LJ, Eysenck HJ, Martin NG: Genes, Culture and Personality: An Empirical Approach. London, Academic Press, 1989

Eaves LJ, Martin NG, Heath AC: Religious affiliation in twins and their parents: testing a model of cultural inheritance. Behav Genet 20:1–22, 1990

Feather NT: Family resemblance in conservatism: are daughters more similar to parents than sons are? J Pers 46:260–278, 1978

Fisher RA: On the correlation between relatives on the supposition of Mendelian inheritance. Trans Royal Soc Edinburgh 52:399–433, 1918

Galton F: Hereditary Genius: An Inquiry into Its Laws and Consequences. London, Macmillan, 1869

Galton F: Inquiry into Human Faculty. London, Macmillan, 1883

Haley CS, Jinks JL, Last KA: The monozygotic twin half-sib method for analyzing maternal effects and sex linkage in humans. Heredity 46:227–238, 1981

Heath AC: Human Quantitative Genetics: Some Issues and Applications. University of Oxford, D.Phil dissertation, 1983

Heath AC: The analysis of marital interaction in cross-sectional twin data. Acta Genet Med Gemellol (Roma) 36:41–49, 1987

Heath AC, Eaves LJ: Resolving the effects of phenotype and social background on mate selection. Behav Genet 15:15–30, 1985

Heath AC, Kendler KS, Eaves LJ, et al: The resolution of cultural and biological inheritance: informativeness of different relationships. Behav Genet 15:439–465, 1985

Insel P: Maternal effects on personality. Behav Genet 4:133–144, 1974

Jinks JL, Fulker DW: Comparison of the biometrical genetical, MAVA and classical approaches to the analysis of human behavior. Psychol Bull 73:311–349, 1970

Kevles DJ, Hood L: The Code of Codes: Scientific and Social Issues in the Human Genome Project. Cambridge, MA, Harvard University Press, 1992

Li CC: First Course in Population Genetics. Pacific Grove, CA, The Boxwood Press, 1976

Loehlin JC, Nichols RC: Heredity, Environment and Personality: A Study of 850 Sets of Twins. Austin, University of Texas Press, 1976

Loehlin JC, Willerman L, Horn JM: Personality resemblances in adoptive families when children are late adolescent or adult. J Pers Soc Psychol 48:376–392, 1985

Martin NG, Jardine R: Eysenck's contributions to behavior genetics, in Hans Eysenck: Consensus and Controversy. Edited by Modgil S, Modgil C. Philadelphia, Falmer Press, 1986

Martin NG, Eaves LJ, Kearsey MJ, et al: The power of the classical twin study. Heredity 40:97–116, 1978

Martin NG, Eaves LJ, Jardine R, et al: Transmission of social attitudes. Proc Natl Acad Sci U S A 83:4364–4368, 1986

McGue M, Wette R, Rao DC: A Monte-Carlo evaluation of three statistical methods used in path analysis. Genet Epidemiol 4:129–156, 1987

Morton NE: Analysis of family resemblance. I. Introduction. Am J Hum Genet 26:318–330, 1974

Nance WE, Corey LA: Genetic models for the analysis of data from the families of identical twins. Genetics 83:811–825, 1976

Neale MC, Cardon LR: Methodology for Genetic Studies of Twins and Families. Dordrecht, the Netherlands, Kluwer Academic, 1992

Numerical Algorithms Group: NAG FORTRAN Library Manual: Mark 14. Oxford, Numerical Algorithms Group, 1990

Pearson K: On the laws of inheritance in man. II. On the inheritance of the mental and moral characters in man, and its comparison with the inheritance of the physical characters. Biometrika 3:131–190, 1904

Pearson K, Lee A: On the laws of inheritance in man. I. Inheritance of physical characters. Biometrika 2:357–462, 1903

Plomin R, DeFries JC, Loehlin JC: Genotype-environment interaction and correlation in the analysis of behavior. Psychol Bull 84:309–322, 1977

Popper KR: The Poverty of Historicism, 2nd Edition. London, Routledge & Kegan Paul, 1960

Rao DC, Morton NE, Yee S: Analysis of family resemblance, II. A linear model for family correlation. Am J Hum Genet 26:331–359, 1974

Rao DC, Morton NE, Elston RC, et al: Causal analysis of academic performance. Behav Genet 7:147–159, 1977

Ricoeur P: The Symbolism of Evil. New York, Harper & Row, 1967

Scarr S: Race, Social Class and Individual Differences in I.Q.: New Studies of Old Issues. Hillsdale, NJ, Lawrence Erlbaum Associates, 1981

Skinner BF: Beyond Freedom and Dignity. New York, Knopf, 1971

Tellegen A, Lykken DT, Bouchard TJ, et al: Personality similarity in twins reared apart and together. J Pers Soc Psychol 54:1031–1039, 1988

Truett KR, Eaves LJ, Meyer JM, et al: Religion and education as cultural mediators of attitudes: a multivariate analysis. Behav Genet 22:43–62, 1992

Truett KR, Eaves LJ, Heath AC, et al: A model system for analysis of family resemblance in extended kinships of twins. Behav Genet 1994

Waller NG, Kojetin BA, Bouchard TJ, et al: Genetic and environmental influences on religious interests, attitudes, and values: a study of twins reared apart and together. Psychol Sci 10:138–142, 1990

Wilson GD (ed): The Psychology of Conservatism. London, Academic Press, 1973

Wilson GD, Patterson JR: Manual for the Conservatism Scale. London, Academic Press, 1970

Wright S: Correlation and causation. J Agriculture Res 20:557–585, 1921

Young PA, Eaves LJ, Eysenck HJ: Intergenerational stability and change in the causes of variation in personality. Personality and Individual Differences 1:35–55, 1980

Psychosocial Factors in the Development of Personality Disorders

Lorna Smith Benjamin, Ph.D.

Psychoanalytic methods, which emphasize the role of developmental factors in psychopathology, have receded in importance since the appearance of modern psychotropic medications. It is widely accepted now that biological psychiatry has better credentials as a science than does psychoanalysis. However, the present emphasis on "biological" methods may have introduced an imbalance in the ancient controversy between nature (genetic factors) and nurture (developmental factors). This chapter suggests that a better balance could be achieved if results from recent methodological advances in behavioral science are taken into account. The new evidence comes from 1) epidemiological tal-

Many thanks are expressed to friends and colleagues who made very helpful comments on an earlier version of this chapter: Donna Gelfand, Bill Henry, Marjorie Klein, Tim Smith, and Hans Strupp. Analyses of inpatients are based on a project supported by a grant to the author from the National Institute of Mental Health (grant MH-33604). Analyses of mother-infant interactions are based on a project supported by a pilot grant from the MacArthur Research Network, l. That project drew on a data bank gathered by Donna Gelfand, PI and Douglas Teti, CO-PI on NIH grant MH41474. Special thanks are expressed to Professors Gelfand and Teti for sharing their videotapes of the mother-infant interactions, and to Kelly Schloredt and Karen Callaway, who generated the SASB codes.

lies that establish strong associations between traumatic experiences in childhood and adult psychopathology; 2) genetic studies that carefully assess the contributions of environment as well as consanguinity; 3) applications of multivariate correlational models; and 4) interpersonal circumplex models that can quite precisely link perceptions of social events during childhood to adult social behavior and symptoms. This chapter develops this fourth approach by offering illustrative data based on Structural Analysis of Social Behavior (SASB), a circumplex model.

Recent Psychoanalytic Hypotheses About Developmental Factors

For decades the classical psychoanalytic view prevailed that psychopathology in adulthood stems from unconscious conflict among warring unconscious forces named the id, ego, and superego. Destructive patterns observed in adult personality were believed to arise from untoward childhood experiences misshaping these forces. In recent years, the classical psychoanalytic view has shifted away from theory that invokes abstract forces toward more concretely interpersonal formulations. The Sullivanian school in the United States (Sullivan 1953) and the Object Relations School in Britain (reviewed by Ornstein and Kay 1990) are pivotal examples. An illustrative summary of the new perspective was offered by Gunderson (1992):

> In this framework, the dependent personality evolves from parental deprivation; obsessive-compulsive traits are created from control struggles; and hysteric traits derive, in part, from parental seduction and competition. The object relations perspective also prompted the development of two other personality types, whereby traumatically unstable parental attachments became the pivotal precursors to developing a borderline type of personality, and grossly unempathic parental attachments became critical to the development of the narcissistic personality type. (p. 9)

Gunderson illustrates how object relations revisionists retain the classical psychoanalytic idea that unconscious motivations and patterns developed during childhood can determine personality and psychopathology. This assumption forms the basis of *dynamic psychotherapies*, which are distinguished from many other therapies by the belief that unconscious wishes and fears generated during childhood must be addressed in the treatment process.

The Scientific Evidence

Neither the classical psychoanalytic nor the object relations perspective has proved amenable to validation by scientific methods. Gunderson (1992) continued:

> The data on which all of these dynamically based personality categories have been identified come from within intensive psychoanalytic therapies. Because of the inferential nature of these data and the absence of empirical verification for the constructs derived from the data, this model is subject to heavy criticism from all who favor scientifically replicable data sources. More far reaching is the criticism that the dynamically based topologies reflect epiphenomena that obscure more basic biologically determined ways to classify personality types. (p. 10)

The Rise of Psychotropic Medications and the Fall of the Practice of Dynamic Psychotherapy

Toward the end of the 1950s, when psychoanalysis dominated American psychiatry, neuroleptic and antidepressant medications first appeared. Because of their efficacy, the drugs provided an attractive treatment alternative. As this so-called biological psychiatry ascended, the theoretical and practical importance of dynamic psychotherapy diminished. The "chemical imbalance" and "brain disease" models now hold that many mental problems arise more from biochemical and neurological defects than from remarkable childhood or current social experiences. This perspective has characterized clinical practice and research in recent years. Schizophrenia, bipolar disorder, and autism are offered as examples of severe mental disorders for which there are known effective medical treatments (National Advisory Mental Health Council 1993). It is often reasoned that if such clinical syndromes are effectively addressed by medication, then they must be based on biological factors transmitted in the genes. One theoretical contingent believes some DSM Axis II personality disorders also are primarily determined by genetic factors (e.g., Lowing et al. 1983; Schulz et al. 1989). Personality disorders often are accompanied by comorbid clinical syndromes (e.g., Oldham and Skodol 1992). Such concurrence suggests that hypotheses about causes of personality (e.g., borderline personality disorder) also have implications for causes of clinical syndromes (e.g., anxiety or depressive disorders).

In the matter of causes of mental disorder, the nurture side of the ancient nature-nurture controversy is represented by developmental learning experiences. The nature side is represented by the idea that mental disorder is based on faulty genes. Psychoanalysis may have overemphasized the nurture side during the decades of the 1940s and 1950s. Now, some advocates biological psychiatry may be creating an imbalance on the nature side. Dynamic psychotherapy is given relatively minor emphasis in many residency programs (American Psychiatric Association 1993, pp. 3–4). Instead, training is more focused on diagnosis and on treatments by pharmacological, electroshock, and behavioral methods.

Even the most compelling data in support of nature show that genetic factors contribute no more than 50% of the variance. It is reasonable to argue that nurture probably has at least as much influence as nature. If the scientific merits of the developmental side could be better recognized now, perhaps a more appropriate middle ground could be defined in current research and practice. This chapter reviews some methods that might help to strike a proper balance. There are at least four lines of inquiry that make important contributions to the goal of restoring balance to the nature-nurture equation.

Epidemiological Studies That Suggest Childhood Experiences Affect Personality

The Evidence

A variety of epidemiological surveys report associations between child abuse and psychopathology. Conte (1991) reviewed the literature and reported that sexual abuse has been associated with "depression, guilt, learning difficulties, sexual promiscuity, runaway behavior, somatic complaints, and sudden changes in behavior (Burgess et al. 1982); hysterical seizures (Goodwin et al. 1979); phobia, nightmares, and compulsive rituals (Weiss et al. 1955); and self-destructive or suicidal behavior (Carroll et al. 1980; de Young 1982; Yorukoglu and Kemph 1966)" (p. 292).

On the other hand, Schloredt (1993) conducted an exhaustive review of the literature and found that an estimated 3% to 30% of males (Kercher and McShane 1984; Landis 1956) and 8% to 62% of females (Fritz et al. 1981; Wyatt 1985) are sexually abused during childhood. However, few of these individuals seek mental health treatment (Divasto et al. 1984), and approximately one-third of child sex abuse victims have no symptoms at all (Kendall-Tackett et al. 1993). Schloredt (1993) concludes:

> Even though a number of investigators have examined abuse related characteristics and variables that may impact long-term psychological outcome (e.g., Finkelhor 1979), such efforts have first and foremost failed to converge on a specific set of variables that may constitute necessary experiences/conditions if abuse victims are indeed going to have long-term psychological difficulties. Secondly, they [do not contribute] to understanding possible intervening processes. (p. 3)

A Problem With Epidemiological Evidence

Clearly, sexual and physical abuse of children is associated with adult personality problems and clinical symptoms. However, it is not known why some children are vulnerable and others more hardy. It also is not clear how the effect is transmitted in vulnerable individuals. Simple counts of associations between early experience and adult psychopathology are about as informative as are simple counts of prevalence of traits or diagnoses or symptoms within groups that vary in consanguinity. Such descriptive reports of associations suggest a connection, but they do not assess relative contributions of "nature and nurture." Nor do they provide specific ideas about possible mechanisms. An organizing explanatory theory is needed. An illustrative and highly informative review of many possible theoretical and causal models for depression appears in Klein et al. (1993).

Genetic Studies that Directly Assess Environmental Factors

The research design usually used to assess the role of genetic factors is straightforward. The incidence of clinical phenomena (symptoms, diagnoses, personality traits) is compared among groups that vary in consanguinity. In the ideal study of this type, similarity is predicted to follow a hierarchy: monozygotic twins > same-sex dizygotic twins > full siblings > half siblings > unrelated individuals raised in the "same" environment (adopted).

An important newer research design adds specific continuous measures of possible environmental factors to this basic design. These studies are more likely to conclude that environmental effects are important. For example, Gatz et al. (1992) reported that the "influence of family rearing context played a substantial role in explaining twin similarity, whereas unique life experiences accounted for the greatest proportion of variance" (p. 701).

Plomin and Daniels (1987) were strong early advocates of the importance of including measures of environmental differences within groups of genetically similar individuals. They concluded, "Environmental influences make two children in the same family as different from one another as are pairs of children selected randomly from the population" (p. 1). Reiss et al. (1991) elaborated on this theme:

> . . . the genetic data suggest that the important environmental factors are those which are different for siblings in the same family. These might include differences in how they are treated by the same parent, differences in peer relationships, differences in school environment, and, when they are older, differences in their marital and occupational experiences. In current research, these influences are termed "nonshared environmental effects." (p. 284)

A related study showed that differences in perceived parental hostility within monozygotic twin pairs correlated significantly with differences in self-rated trait hostility.[1] "Thus, nongenetic variance in hostility was associated with perceived differences in early environments" (McGonigle et al. 1993, p. 23).

In sum, genetic studies that include direct assessments of environmental factors strongly suggest that developmental factors add a very important component to personality and psychopathology. These studies establish that nonshared environmental variance has a major impact on development and needs extensive study. It is likely that genetic programming can enhance or diminish the impact of developmental experiences. Hardy characters may be less vulnerable to a given experience, whereas vulnerable characters may be excessively affected by certain developmental experiences. Fascinating new possibilities have been described by Kraemer et al. (1989), who found that cerebrospinal fluid norepinephrine levels in laboratory monkeys varied depending on the type of mothering experiences and rearing conditions they had. Kraemer (1992) reached a startling conclusion: The causes of developmental psychopathology may be largely environmental, yet the effects that need to be prevented or reversed are neurobiological" (p. 22). To account for the impact of developmental experience on neurology, Kraemer (1992) has proposed a psychobiological theory of attachment that suggests the primate infant normally internalizes a neurobiological "image" of the behavioral and emotional characteristics of the caregiver that subsequently regulates core features of its brain function:

---

[1]The sample had identified monozygotic twins on the basis of complete agreement on 10 polymorphic gene markers.

The intertwined development of brain function and social attachment can sometimes go awry . . . If the attachment process fails, or
if the caregiver is incompetent as a member of the species, the developing infant will also fail to regulate its social behavior and may
be dysfunctional in the social environment. This helps to explain
how developmental psychopathology and later vulnerability to adult
psychopathology can be caused by disruption of social attachment.
(p. 539)

In a very different context (Benjamin 1993a, 1995, 1996b), I have
proposed that personality change cannot be implemented through psychotherapy until and if there is a change in the individual's relationship
with his or her important people and their internalized representations
(IPIRs). The idea that IPIRs must be changed was developed on the
basis of careful analysis of successful psychotherapies with seemingly
"intractable" cases. I believe that patients' wishes and fears in relation
to their IPIRs sustain and support maladaptive patterns. Patients must
transform their relationships with IPIRs before the maladaptive behaviors characteristic of personality disorder can be replaced with more
appropriate ones. Perhaps IPIRs are related to Kraemer's neurobiological images or "icons" (personal communication, June 1990). If IPIRs
(or icons) must change before psychotherapy with personality and
other severe mental disorders can succeed, then successful psychotherapy that truly implements personality change might have to "reverse biology." Because there are relatively rare, but clearly successful
psychotherapies with personality disordered individuals, it would follow that such psychotherapies would actually change "biology." The
possibility deserves study.

Use of Partial Correlations to Study the Relative Contributions of Nature and Nurture

Kendler et al. (1993) have presented a highly sophisticated application
of structural equation modeling (SEM) to explore the roles of nature

and nurture in the development of depression in women. They used a large sample (N = 608) of female-female twin pairs of known zygosity. Several relevant measures of environmental factors were included, such as parental warmth, childhood parental loss, lifetime traumas, social support, recent difficulties, and recent stressful life events. Reviewing the results of their SEM analysis, these investigators wrote:

> The model suggested that at least four major and interacting risk factor domains are needed to understand the etiology of major depression: traumatic experiences, genetic factors, temperament, and interpersonal relations. *Conclusions*: Major depression is a multifactorial disorder, and understanding its etiology will require the rigorous integration of genetic, temperamental, and environmental risk factors. (Kendler et al. 1993, p. 1139)

The Kendler et al. study sets a modern standard for using multivariate methods to compare and contrast nature and nurture. They carefully assessed both genetic and environmental variables, sampled longitudinally over three or more years of adulthood, and used a sophisticated statistical model for analysis. SEM is a rather complex variation on the basic statistical technique of regression analysis. In its simplest form, correlational methods use one variable (e.g., parental warmth) to predict another (e.g., degree of depression). Some versions of multiple regression analysis expand that model so that the predictions are between one set of variables (e.g., various measures related to nature and/or nurture) and another set of variables (e.g., depression, or measures of different symptoms or personality traits). Whenever more than two variables are used, the problem of covariance becomes apparent (e.g., a correlation between depression and a developmental factor like parental warmth might covary with current life stress). Many multivariate models therefore provide a means to "correct" for covariance (e.g., they assess the relation between parental warmth and depression, after correcting for current life stress). SEM (e.g., Bentler 1989) adds even more features. For example, it allows the investigator to specify which variables stand in directional causal relationships, and which variables are expected to covary. It also provides for control of other sources of variance, such as that associated with method of measurement.

Unfortunately, such complicated multivariate analyses can become conceptually overwhelming. Although they have the advantage of identifying problem cross-correlations that are not apparent with simpler models, they still are potentially vulnerable to arbitrary decision making on the part of the modeler. For example, SEM permits the investigator specifically to name covariances that are expected to be relevant. The decision about what to include and what to exclude can make major differences in results.

To consider just one example, SEM was applied in a demonstration workshop by Peter Bentler to a set of data that contained both measures of depression and of developmental factors (Benjamin 1990). The dynamic SEM model tested the hypothesis that perceived early developmental factors have a causal relation to depressive symptoms. Differences between obtained scores and scores predicted by the dynamic model were very small. The appropriate χ^2 was associated with $P < .912$, indicating an excellent fit between data and theory. The alternative medical model proposed that depression would cause patients to take a worse view of their childhood experiences. Deviation between theory and data was enormous. The χ^2 was associated with a very small P. The medical model did not fit the data at all. Then, Bentler thought of two more covariances that should be added to the medical model. With this change, the fit for the medical model improved dramatically to $P < .912$. In the end, the data were equally well described by the opposing models. One suggested that depressive state affects remembered relationships with parents. The other, that perceived childhood relationships (e.g., helplessness, isolation) cause depression. These or similar problems arise with any other SEM model, including the more frequently used linear structural relations modeling (LISREL; Byrne 1989). Such complicated multivariate analyses are always vulnerable to investigator choices of models.

Bentler advised that if causal predictions are to be made with certainty, SEM cannot come from a cross-sectional sample. Rather, there must be longitudinal data sampling. The longitudinal sampling should be made throughout childhood, the time when the developmental impact theoretically occurs. Because cause is ultimately established by observing sequences in real time (Hume 1947), data that presume to assess cause must be based on real time sequential observations.

Figure 12–1 presents an example of how simple partial correlation based on appropriate longitudinal sampling can compare nature and nurture. The purpose of the illustrative study shown in Figure 12–1 (Benjamin 1962b) was to compare the relative contributions of nurture (thumbsucking) and nature (genetic predisposition) in the appearance of dental malocclusion in baby monkeys. The measure of genetic predisposition was malocclusion at birth. The measure of the environmental factor was the baby monkeys' nonnutritive sucking (thumbsucking) observed at successive developmental periods.[2]

The basic logic of the model is as follows: 1) A genetically based predisposition to malocclusion should be relatively constant over time. The genetic plans for the shape of the teeth should not change. 2) If thumbsucking displaces teeth, the effect should be maximal if it occurs when the teeth first arrive and the mouth is still growing. Longitudinal assessments of thumbsucking made after the permanent teeth already were in place would miss vital information about cause. 3) If thumbsucking displaces teeth, maximal effects should occur in reasonable association with maximal exposure to the causal agent.

Partial correlations like those shown in Figure 12–1 can compare nature and nurture according to those three logical conditions. 1) The genetic effect should be manifest by few changes in the correlations between the dependent and the genetic variable, when the environmental variable is partialled out. The genetic effect should remain constant throughout the age range studied. 2) By contrast, the environmental effect should be manifest by a progressive increase in the magnitude of the correlations, when the genetic effect is partialled out. As more days pass during which the environmental factor is implemented, the effect should cumulate. 3) Finally, the rate of increase in the partial correlations that reflect compounding environmental effects should correspond to the rate at which the environmental events are

---

[2]The average number of 10-second periods out of 25 during which it was observed. Observations of thumbsucking were made while the monkeys were in a smooth, round Plexiglas cage. The cage was enclosed within a Masonite cubicle equipped with one-way vision glass placed so that all parts of it could be seen.

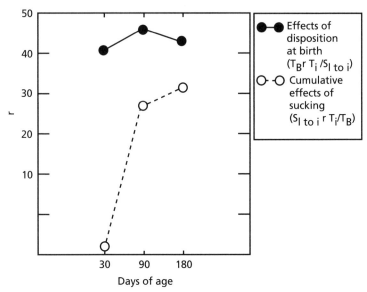

Figure 12–1. *A model for assessing the relative contributions of nature and nurture. The nature effect is represented by partial correlations between predisposition (T_B) and dental malocclusion (T_i) at successive time periods (i = 30, 90, and 180 days). Genetic effects are assessed independently of environmental input (sucking at i = 30, 90, and 180 days). The solid line shows that across this developmental period, the genetic effect remains large and constant. The nurture effect is represented by partial correlations between dental malocclusion (T_i) and thumbsucking (S_i), independently of genetic predisposition (T_B). The dashed line shows that the nurture effect becomes progressively larger with time. [Reprinted with permission from Benjamin 1962a, p. 61.]*

observed. Maximal environmental effects should be associated with maximal exposure.

The data shown in Figure 12–1 meet all three of these conditions. Results are presented at 30-day intervals from birth through 180 days. 1) The partial correlations between malocclusion and displacement[3] at birth (corrected for observed thumbsucking) remained constant throughout. 2) The partial correlations between malocclusion and observed thumbsucking (correcting for displacement at birth) increased

---

[3]A composite measure of open-bite, over-jet, and midline deviation described in Benjamin 1962a, p. 32.

over time. 3) The rate of increase in the thumbsucking effect slowed during the last period, as it should, because there was a prior decrease in the rate of thumbsucking. The figure also shows that genetic effects were consistently greater than the thumbsucking effect in the age range studied.

In applying the model shown in Figure 12–1 to the problems of personality and psychopathology, it is difficult to find equally good measures. Some promising available measures might serve. Some investigators, including Kagan (1988) and Rothbart (Rothbart and Goldsmith 1985) have developed reliable methods to assess temperament. For assessment of psychosocial experiences, the SASB model, described in this chapter, may be useful. Measures of Axis I problems are relatively advanced, for example, DSM-IV (American Psychiatric Association 1994), SCL-90-R (Derogatis 1977), and the Structured Clinical Interview for DSM-IV Axis I Disorders, Clinical Version (SCID-CV; First et al. 1996). Measures of adult personality are highly controversial but are proliferating and improving. Possibilities would include instruments that assess the DSM descriptions of personality disorder: the Personality Disorder Examination (PDE; Loranger et al. 1987), Structured Clinical Interview for DSM-IV Axis II Personality Disorders (SCID-II; First et al. 1997), or the Wisconsin Personality Inventory (WISPI; Klein et al. 1993). Finally, personality traits might be measured by the NEO Personality Inventory (NEO-PI; Costa and MacCrae 1988) or the Differential Personality Questionnaire (Tellegen 1982). The SASB methods also could measure adult interpersonal and intrapsychic patterns.

SASB Offers an Objective Method for Studying Dynamic Contributions to the Development of Personality

Since 1968, I have been working on a methodology that seeks to operationalize interpersonal and intrapsychic developmental concepts, and relate them to adult personality and psychopathology. The SASB model and methods (Benjamin 1974, 1984, 1996a) operationalize some of Sullivan's interpersonal ideas about the development of personality and symptoms, and some ideas from the Object Relations school of psychoanalysis. The SASB model is accompanied by questionnaires to assess the concepts from the perspective of the patient, family members, or clinicians. A formal coding system also permits objective analysis of videotapes of patient interactions with important others. Software is available to generate a variety of parameters that are useful in providing individual feedback or analyzing group trends. The approach can be applied to any context where there is social or intrapsychic interaction. Examples include psychotherapy process and content, group processes, parent-child interactions, and more.[4] Accumulating SASB data sets may contribute to the goal of making the concepts of dynamic psychotherapy more amenable to the standards of science.

Two illustrative data sets demonstrate how the method can contribute to assessment of developmental factors. The data show how childhood experiences can be related to adult personality and symptoms. One set demonstrates the usefulness of the SASB questionnaires, and the other illustrates the SASB observational coding system.

A Brief Description of the SASB Model

The SASB model is presented in Figure 12–2. The model has a long developmental history. Important predecessors include Sullivan's interpersonal psychiatry (Sullivan 1953), Leary's interpersonal circumplex (Leary 1957), Schaefer's circumplex model (Schaefer 1965) for parenting behavior, and more. Reviews of the history of the development of the SASB model and its relation to other circumplex models appear in Benjamin (1974, 1984, 1996a).

---

[4]The approach has been applied to a wide variety of psychotherapy approaches in addition to dynamic psychotherapy. These include client-centered, cognitive-behavioral, gestalt, family couples, group, and other forms of psychosocial intervention. The questionnaires have been translated into 10 languages, and there are more than 50 published studies using the methods. Among psychotherapy research, it has been seen as especially useful by German psychoanalysts (Tress 1993) and by Short Term Dynamic Therapy researchers (e.g., Henry et al. 1986).

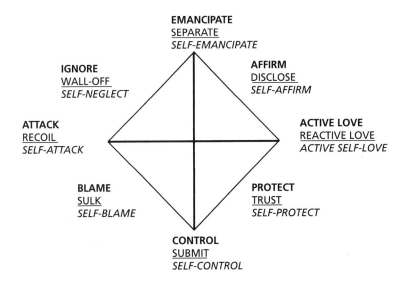

FIGURE 12–2. *The simplified SASB cluster model. The horizontal axis runs from hate to love, and the vertical axis represents a continuum from enmeshment to differentiation. The three types of focus are represented on three surfaces by different styles of print. Complementarity is shown by adjacent* **BOLD** *and* <u>UNDERLINED</u> *points. Introjection is shown by adjacent* **BOLD** *and* ITALICIZED *points. [Reprinted with permission from Benjamin 1996a, p. 55.]*

The terms shown in **boldface** describe behaviors that are prototypically parentlike and involve focus on another person. The <u>underlined</u> terms shown in Figure 12–2 are prototypically childlike and involve reactive interpersonal focus on the self. The terms shown in *italics* indicate introjections. Points that appear together on the model are closely related. Pairs of **bold** and <u>underlined</u> points are complementary and describe interpersonal positions that are likely to appear together. Pairs of **bold** and *italicized* points describe introjections. They connect specific social experiences and aspects of self-concept. The parentlike behavior, **IGNORE** is likely to be complemented by the childlike behavior, <u>WALL-OFF</u> **IGNORE**. It also is likely to lead to a self-concept that includes a strong component of *SELF-NEGLECT*.

The SASB model has additional predictive features. It specifies opposites and antitheses. Opposites are located at 180 degree positions on Figure 12–2. For example, the opposite of **IGNORE** is **PROTECT**. Antitheses are defined as the complement of the opposite. To illustrate, consider that **IGNORE** has the antithesis, TRUST. The child who has a parent who is not adequately attentive to the child's legitimate developmental needs (i.e., the parent **IGNORE**s the child) might naturally exhibit the antithetical behavior, TRUST. This provides a complementary "draw" for the parent to switch from **IGNORE** to **PROTECT**. The child's increased TRUST makes it more likely he or she receives parental behavior vital to the development of attachment, namely **PROTECT**. Still other predictive principles accompany the SASB model. One, illustrated later in Figures 12–3 and 12–4, suggests that self structure includes a reaction to an internalization of important other people (Benjamin 1994, 1996). The SASB model assesses both phenomenology and observable behaviors and provides a fine-grained analysis of interpersonal and intrapsychic interactions. These features make it appropriate to use to study nonshared environmental variance.

Application of the SASB Model to the DSM Categories of Personality

The SASB dimensional model has been applied to the DSM (American Psychiatric Association 1987, 1994) descriptions of personality disorder (Benjamin 1996a). Overlap among "categories" is diminished by requiring that symptoms of personality disorder be interpreted in interpersonal context. For example, the ubiquitous symptom of anger is exhibited in different contexts and for different reasons by individuals having the various personality disorders. Anger in individuals with borderline personality disorder is triggered by perceived abandonment or not caring. Anger in narcissistic personality disorder likely to appear in a context of failed entitlement. Other personalities use anger in still other ways. Besides reducing overlap among DSM categories, the predictive properties of the SASB model were used to generate developmental hypotheses that have specific psychosocial treatment implications. For example, passive-aggressive (negativistic) personality disorder is described interpersonally:

> There is a tendency to see any form of power as inconsiderate and neglectful, together with a belief that authorities or caregivers are incompetent, unfair, and cruel. The PAG [individual with passive-aggressive personality disorder] agrees to comply with perceived demands or suggestions, but fails to perform. He or she often complains of unfair treatment, and envies and resents others who fare better. His or her suffering indicts the allegedly negligent caregivers or authorities. The PAG fears control in any form and wishes for nurturant restitution. (Benjamin 1996a, p. 272)

The hypothetical interpersonal history includes a nurturant beginning that was abruptly terminated by unfair and cruel demands for performance. Typically this accompanied the birth of a sibling, but sometimes it was forced by a change in family fortunes. Along with requiring that the individual with passive-aggressive personality disorder (PAPD) perform beyond his or her years, there were harsh punishments for anger or for showing autonomy that interfered with serving the family needs. The person with PAPD shows the consequences of this combination of developmental events. He or she wishes for nurturance, but expects it will not be forthcoming, or that it will be flawed. Sensitivity to coercion and a characteristic position of punitive neediness also are generated by this history.

The treatment implications are that the person with PAPD must learn to distance from or transform IPIRs that have seemed so unfair. He or she has to stop resisting the imagined continued abuse and deprivation. There must be an understanding of the need to go ahead and perform "even if it is good for him or her." This analysis and treatment approach represents a testable interpersonal version of some psychoanalytic hypotheses about "oral-sadistic" characters.

Similar testable and refutable hypotheses about the developmental history for each of the respective DSM personality disorders are presented by Benjamin (1996a). The developmental understanding leads to specific psychosocial treatment suggestions for each disorder.

Models of Theoretical Parallels Among Social Behavior, Affect, and Cognition

On the assumption that behavior, affect, and cognition evolved in parallel, models for affect and cognitive style have also been drawn to parallel the SASB model for social behavior (Benjamin 1986). They are compared in Table 12–1, which illustrates how behavior, affect, and cognition might correspond. The behavior **IGNORE** is presumed to be associated with the affects of indifference and disgust, and with a diffuse irrational cognitive style. The opposite behavior, **PROTECT,** may be associated with the affect of kindliness, and a rational, clearly focused cognitive style.[5]

Most of the unpleasant affects characteristic of patients appear on the hostile side of the *childlike* surface of the SASB model. For examples, SUBMIT is associated with helplessness and apathy; SULK is accompanied by sullenness and feelings of humiliation and fear; RECOIL goes with hate and anguish; WALL OFF is characterized by pessimism, bitterness, and hopelessness.

Cognitive styles might also show orderly correspondence with characteristic behaviors. A tendency to appeal to authority and defer would be expected to go with SUBMIT. Constriction and overcautiousness would match SULK. A tendency to "shut down" or close to experience would go with RECOIL. Oppositionalism or looseness and incoherence would accompany a position described by the SASB model as WALL OFF.

Unlike the SASB model itself, these parallel cognitive and affect models have not been validated. The idea has potentially useful implications. Problems with behavior, affect, and cognition show orderly associations. The idea of parallelism opens a way to explain the vexing problems of comorbidity between personality disorders and clinical syndromes (Benjamin 1996b). Parallelism provides a potential expla-

---

[5]On the full SASB model (Benjamin 1984), items that more fully detail the interpersonal region marked by the label **PROTECT** include: "P lovingly looks after C's interests and takes steps to protect C. P gets C interested and teaches C how to understand and do things. P pays close attention to C so P can figure out all of C's needs and take care of everything."

TABLE 12–1.
Hypothetical parallels between behaviors (described by the SASB model), Affect, and Cognition.

SASB behaviors	Affective parallels	Cognitive parallels
EMANCIPATE	Indifferent	Broad scan
AFFIRM	Sympathetic	Balanced
ACTIVE LOVE	Cherishing	Expect continuity
PROTECT	Comforting	Rational
CONTROL	Energized	Sharp focus
BLAME	Arrogant	Judgmental
ATTACK	Vengeful	Terminating
IGNORE	Rejecting	Illogical
SEPARATE	Unconcerned	Immune
DISCLOSE	Confident	Honest
REACTIVE LOVE	Merry, joyful	Open
TRUST	Hopeful	Agreeable
SUBMIT	Helpless	Deferential
SULK	Humilitated	Constricted
RECOIL	Panicked	Closed
WALL OFF	Hopeless	Incoherent

Note. *From Benjamin 1996b, p. 181; Copyright 1996 by The Guilford Press. Reprinted by permission.*

nation for how developmental experience can relate to mental disorder in adulthood. It suggests that behavioral adaptations during childhood are naturally accompanied by specific affects and cognitions such as those detailed in Table 12–1. If these adaptations are maintained in adulthood and conform to patterns that are recognized as personality disordered, then their associated affects and cognitions also accompany the personality disorders. The SASB analysis of PAPD, described earlier, suggests that the behaviors represented by the model point SULK would be accompanied by certain affects (sullen, dour, anguished) and cognitive styles (constricted, overcautious). The PAPD behaviors summarized by the model point WALL OFF would be accompanied by the affects pessimistic and bitter and by the cognitive styles oppositional, loose, and incoherent. Indeed, PAPD often is accompanied by intractable depression that is reasonably well described by these forms of affect and cognition. The SASB model somewhat arbitrarily enters the system from the behavioral perspective. Whether one enters in the domain of cognition or affect or behavior, the connections hold true. The clinician can move knowledgeably among descriptions of social events, feelings, and thoughts. The researcher can understand why certain patterns of personality are regularly accompanied by specific Axis I symptoms.

Methods of Assessment Using the SASB Model of Social Behavior

SASB (Intrex) Questionnaires

SASB (Intrex) questionnaires allow patients to rate their self-concepts and relationships with important others. The standard form asks for the following ratings: introject in the best and in the worst state; a love relationship in the best and worst state; the relationship with mother when the rater was aged 5–10; the relationship with father at the same age; and finally, the observed interactions between the mother and father. In the SASB (Intrex) Long Form there are four or five items for each cluster shown in Figure 12–1. For example, footnote #5 reviewed the long form items for the cluster **PROTECT**. The items are presented to the rater in a randomly determined order and he or she uses a scale that ranges (in units of 10) from 0 (item applies never, not at all) to 100 (item applies always, perfectly). A score for each point shown in Figure 12–2 is generated by the average of endorsements for all full-model items that belong to the point or cluster (e.g., **PROTECT**).

The earliest published and the most recent reviews of the validity of the SASB were by Benjamin (1974, 1994). The present data are from a sample of psychiatric inpatients who completed self-ratings of their psychiatric symptoms on measures such as the SCL-90-R and the MMPI as well as ratings of themselves and IPIRs on the SASB (Intrex) questionnaires. Figure 12–3 shows that the remembered relationship with mother relates to self structure. Data are separated for the 102 female psychiatric inpatients (top of the figure) and the 80 males (bottom of the figure). Diagnostic groups for the female and male samples are listed in Table 12–2.[6] The sample was divided by gender to compare the impacts of attachment to mothers and fathers on the self-concept. Effects might reasonably be expected to be different for male and female children.

The top part of Figure 12–3 presents females' ratings of their introject at worst, correlated with their remembered reaction to their mothers during childhood. The introject points are represented in *italics* in the SASB model shown in Figure 12–2, while the reactions to the mother are shown by underlined points. Inspection of the correlations in Figure 12–3 shows clearly that more positive feelings about the self (*SELF-AFFIRM, ACTIVE SELF-LOVE, SELF-PROTECT*) are associated with strong reactive attachment to the mother (DISCLOSE, REACTIVE LOVE , TRUST). Conversely, negative feelings about the self (*SELF-BLAME, SELF-ATTACK,* and *SELF-NEGLECT*) are associated with disrupted attachment to the mother (SULK, RECOIL, and WALL OFF).

The orderly trends shown in Figure 12–3 are not a simple function of general factors like negative or positive affectivity. Rather than shifting abruptly from negative to positive correlations, the magnitudes of the correlations progressively change according to circumplex order (Guttman 1966). Consider the correspondence between ratings of the behavior DISCLOSE to the mother and ratings of the successive points that describe self-concept as it appears on the introject surface of Figure 12–2. Correlations become progressively larger as the point *ACTIVE SELF-LOVE* is approached, and diminish to reach a minimum at the opposite point, *SELF-ATTACK.*[7] This succession of points forms a cosine wave. The pattern defined by a cosine wave can be understood intuitively by imagining you are holding a laser beaming device as you ride on a Ferris wheel (corresponding to the circular model). Imagine the laser beam projected on a wall that is moving

---

[6]Diagnostic groups were defined by an elaborate process that began with the Diagnostic Interview Schedule (Robbins et al. 1981) and included a formal scan of the chart, use of the Physician Interview Program (Greist et al. 1976). A manual operationalized hierarchical decisions according to whether symptoms had interfered with work or love relationships. The procedure was reported by Greist et al. (1984).

[7]To correspond exactly to circumplex order, the magnitude should have been maximal at *SELF-AFFIRM* and minimal at *SELF-BLAME.*

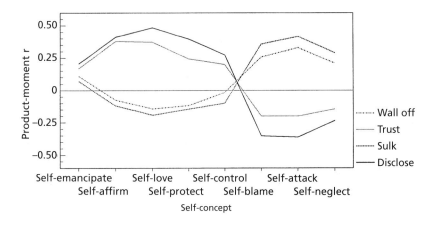

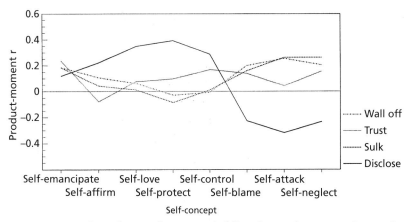

FIGURE 12–3. *Correlations between childhood attachment to the mother and self-structure in 102 female (top) and 80 male (bottom) adult psychiatric inpatients. SASB (Intrex) ratings of remembered reaction to mother were correlated with inpatients' ratings of their introjects in the worst state. Good attachment is associated with higher self-esteem; poor attachment is associated with self-attack. The progressive changes in magnitude of the correlations follow circumplex order, suggesting the effect is not due to a generalized factor like negative affectivity.*

perpendicular to the Ferris wheel. The pattern traced on the moving wall by the beam is a cosine wave.[8] The cosine pattern in Figure 12–3 suggests that the magnitude of the correlations progressively change as predicted by an underlying circular model.

---

[8]A sine wave has the same shape, displaced 90 degrees.

TABLE 12–2.
Diagnostic groups for psychiatric inpatients shown in Figure 12–3

Diagnostic group	Female (%)	Male (%)
Major depression	23.2	16.9
Psychotic depression	13.9	3.6
Borderline personality disorder	25.9	3.6
Paranoid schizophrenia	6.5	19.3
Bipolar mania	8.3	15.6
Schizoaffective disorder	7.4	12.0
Antisocial personality disorder	0.0	16.9
Bipolar depression	7.4	6.1
Chronic undifferentiated schizophrenia	1.9	3.6
Bipolar mixed	5.5	2.4

In addition to noting the circumplex order in the pattern of correlations in Figure 12–3, two other analyses suggest that the connection
between perceived attachment to the mother and self-concept is not a
simple artifact of depressive state. One is to use the technique of partial
correlations to adjust the data in Figure 12–3 for depressive state. That
operation diminishes the amplitude of the cosine wave, but does not
change its basic shape. Current depressive state magnifies the connection between reported attachment to the mother and the introject at
worst. But state does not account for the connection. The cosine pattern persists even after correcting for current depression.

Figure 12–4 presents another analysis in support of the idea that
results in Figure 12–3 are not a simple artifact of depressive state. The
circumplex pattern of Figure 12–4 appeared in a subsample of diagnostic groups that were not depressed (paranoid schizophrenic, bipolar
manic, antisocial personality, and chronic undifferentiated schizophrenia). In this smaller sample, the curves are less smooth, but the
circumplex order still was apparent.

In two analyses (male group, total sample; female group, nondepressed sample), the relations between TRUST in the mother and self-
concept did not correspond to the predicted circumplex order for the
SASB point TRUST. This interaction between gender (and/or diagnosis) and the correspondence between self-structure and TRUST in

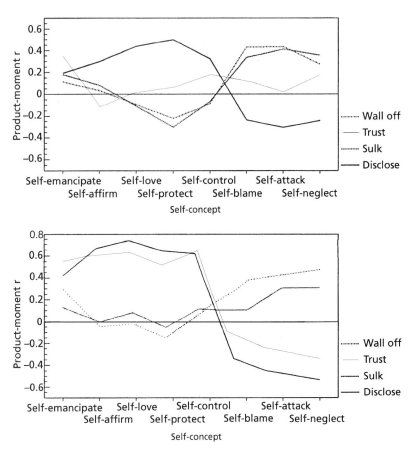

FIGURE **12–4.** *Correlations between childhood attachment to the mother and self structure in adulthood in 18 female (top) and 46 male (bottom) psychiatric inpatients who were not depressed. SASB (Intrex) ratings of remembered reaction to mother are correlated with inpatients who are not depressed rating themselves in their worst state. Similarity between Figures 12–3 and 12–4 shows that the obtained circumplex order is not accounted for by the depressed condition of the patients.*

mother may have theoretical significance. It merits further investigation.

Figures 12–3 and 12–4 drew a connection between the experienced relationship with the mother and self-structure. Figure 12–5 relates self-structure to psychiatric symptomatology as measured by the SCL-90-R and shows clear circumplex order in correlations between

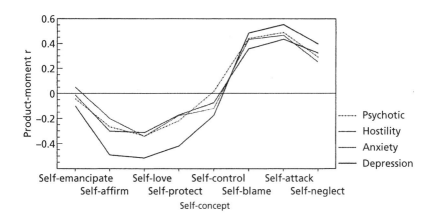

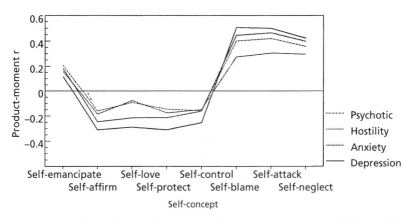

FIGURE 12–5. *Correlations between self-structure at worst and SCL-90-R symptoms in 84 female (top) and 67 male (bottom) psychiatric inpatients. For both males and females, hostile treatment of the self is associated with more Axis I symptomatology. Again, circumplex order is shown.*

self-concept at worst and four major symptom scales. The results are most sharply delineated for depression. Because there were very high correlations among the SCL-90-R scales, parallel results for all symptoms in the figure (anxiety, hostility, and psychotic thoughts) are not surprising.[9]

The trends shown in Figure 12–5 were also apparent in relation to MMPI measures of depression and anxiety. This type of circumplex order in correlations between social behavior and symptoms has been observed in still other contexts (Benjamin 1994). Schloredt (1993) found circumplex order in the correlations between introject at worst and SCL-90-R scores in a sample of undergraduate students reporting a history of sexual and/or physical abuse. The students obviously were functioning at a higher level than inpatients, but they still showed a strong association between self-concept and symptoms. University students who have a clear history of severe sexual or physical abuse may represent a hardy group. It is interesting that the control subjects[10] in Schloredt's sample did not show the same orderly associations between self-structure and symptoms on the SCL-90. Of course, they also reported significantly less symptomatology.

These orderly relations between self-structure and symptoms in patient samples, and between self-structure and perceived early parenting support the idea that developmental factors have a significant impact on adult personality and psychopathology. More specific, testable hypotheses about how this happens are presented by Benjamin (1993, 1995, 1996a, 1996b).

Observer Coding of Mother-Infant Interactions

Figure 12–6 presents preliminary results from an ongoing study of mother-infant interactions observed in the Ainsworth Strange Situation

---

[9]These samples are smaller than the ones shown in Figures 12–3 and 12–4 because not all subjects completed the SCL-90-R.

[10]Control subjects were drawn from the same population in the same manner, but they denied any history of sexual or physical abuse.

(Ainsworth et al. 1978). Fourteen of the mothers had been treated for depression; the other 19 were matched on demographics but had never been treated for depression. Mothers assigned to the depressed group had a Beck Depression Inventory score (BDI; Beck 1978) greater than 9 at the time they entered this longitudinal study. The data reported here were taken approximately 1½ years after entry into the study. Current BDI measures of depression also were available. SASB codings of videotapes of mother-infant interactions were made by raters blind to diagnosis.

Placing a toddler in a strange room, and subjecting him or her to two separations from the mother is a severe stress. Data were generated by observing the first five minutes after the second separation. The figure presents the SASB codes of the interactions during the second reunion, when the mother and baby were once again together in a room full of toys. Usually after an initial greeting, the normal mothers **EMANCIPATE**ed (top of Figure 12–6) or **AFFIRM**ed (bottom of Figure 12–6) their child by, for example, encouraging or allowing him or her to go play with toys. The child "did his or her own thing." By contrast, babies with mothers who had a history of depression were more likely continually to approach the mother for support (<u>TRUST</u>), and yet also to <u>WALL OFF</u>. Sometimes they would do both simultaneously. An example would be to come to the mother for a hug, but remain stiff and not reciprocate. The appropriate group by cluster interaction in MANOVA of the data shown in Figure 12–6 was significant at the 0.01 level. Single clusters yielding significant differences between groups were <u>DISCLOSE, REACTIVE LOVE, TRUST,</u> and <u>WALL OFF</u>. Covariance adjustments for current depression did not affect these findings. Correction with available measures of temperament also did not change the results.

Results suggest that babies with depressed mothers were ambivalent: they showed more dependency (<u>TRUST</u>) and clinging (<u>SULK</u>), and they were more autistic (<u>WALL OFF</u>). Babies with normal mothers showed better attachment (<u>REACTIVE LOVE</u> and <u>DISCLOSE</u>), and better ability to go play (<u>SEPARATE</u>) after the reunion. It appears that babies with depressed mothers are at high risk for depression because at an average age of 18 months they already showed behaviors characteristic of depression: ambivalence between submissive helplessness and social withdrawal. Normal babies showed stronger attachment and more friendly autonomy. These results are from the first half of the sample. If confirmed in the complete data set, this study will more firmly suggest that infants with depressed mothers respond differently to the stress of separation than do infants with normal mothers.[11]

Conclusions

Four lines of evidence were reviewed to suggest that childhood experience has a significant impact on adult personality and symptomatology:

1. Epidemiological surveys that associate childhood trauma with psychopathology in adulthood.
2. Genetic studies that carefully assess environmental factors.
3. Genetic studies that use longitudinal sampling and multivariate techniques that can separate nature and nurture effects. This approach has not yet been fully implemented. It might be, if the Gelfand-Teti (Teti et al. 1995) longitudinal study of depressed mothers and their children can continue through the time when the children reach adulthood.
4. Data from the SASB circumplex model that permits objective assessment of relevant interpersonal and intrapsychic factors. These data were the main focus in this chapter.

---

[11]An ideal study of this sort would add neurochemical measures.

➤

FIGURE 12–6. *Responses of infants to maternal autonomy-giving after the second separation in the Ainsworth Strange Situation. Infants with normal mothers* (n = 19) *go ahead and play with the toys in the room. Those with mothers who have a history of depression* (n = 14) *are more likely to show dependent behaviors* (TRUST, SULK). *Ambivalence about this dependency is suggested by their additional tendency to* WALL OFF.

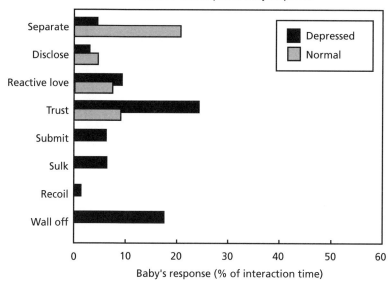

Mother emancipates, Baby responds

Baby's response (% of interaction time)

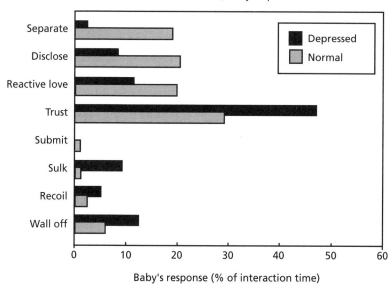

Mother affirms, Baby responds

Baby's response (% of interaction time)

SASB (Benjamin 1974, 1984, 1996a) provides a method that can quantify and help study nonshared environmental variance. The model and methods can test specific hypotheses about how childhood experiences relate to adult personality (DSM Axis II) and symptomatology (DSM Axis I). Clinical illustrations of the usefulness of the approach are offered in a monograph that analyzed the DSM descriptions of personality disorder (Benjamin 1996a). The resulting descriptions of personality disorders promise to yield less overlap among categories and provide developmental hypotheses for each of the DSM personality disorders. These testable and refutable developmental and interpersonal perspectives have specific psychosocial treatment implications.

Two data sets were presented here to illustrate research use of the SASB model: 1) A sample of psychiatric inpatients showed strong correspondence between memory of reaction to mother and self-structure. Self-structure, in turn, showed very close correspondence to symptoms measured by the SCL-90-R (and MMPI). 2) Babies of mothers with a history of depression showed disrupted attachment compared with a matched normal sample. Their ambivalent reaction to their mothers after a separation stress was similar to the ambivalent position often seen in adults with a depressive disorder. There was both helpless submission and social withdrawal. The results were independent of temperament. If babies with depressed mothers show patterns characteristic of adult depression, it may be that depressive styles are learned at a very early age. This preliminary data set will be expanded and further analyzed to more exactly assess stimulus-response contingencies between the mother and the baby.

Findings from these four research approaches suggest that interventions that directly consider developmental factors should be given increased priority in funding for research, training, and service. Examples of such interventions would include educational and social support for better childrearing and more enlightened and effective psychotherapy. Residencies would reinstate the practice of including significant training in dynamic psychotherapy.

References

Ainsworth ADF, Blehar MC, Waters E, et al: Patterns of Attachment. Hillsdale, NJ, Lawrence Erlbaum Associates, 1978

American Psychiatric Association: Diagnostic and Statistical Manual of Mental Disorders, 3rd Edition, Revised. Washington, DC, American Psychiatric Association, 1987

American Psychiatric Association: Psychosocial treatment research in psychiatry: a task force report of the American Psychiatric Association. JP Docherty (chairperson). Washington, DC, American Psychiatric Association, 1993

American Psychiatric Association: Diagnostic and Statistical Manual of Mental Disorders, 4th Edition. Washington, DC, American Psychiatric Association, 1994

Beck AT: Depression Inventory. Philadelphia, PA, Center for Cognitive Therapy, 1978

Benjamin LS: Non-nutritive sucking and the development of malocclusion in the deciduous teeth of the infant Rhesus monkey. Child Dev 33:57–64, 1962a

Benjamin LS: Non-nutritive sucking and dental malocclusion in the deciduous and permanent teeth of the Rhesus monkey. Child Dev 33:29–35, 1962b

Benjamin LS: Structural analysis of social behavior (SASB). Psychol Rev 81:392–425, 1974

Benjamin LS: Principles of prediction using Structural Analysis of Social Behavior, in Personality and the Prediction of Behavior. Edited by Zucker RA, Aronoff J, Rabin AJ. New York, Academic Press, 1984, pp 121–173

Benjamin LS: A beginner's view of Structural Equation Modeling (SEM). In a series of papers summarizing a workshop at the annual meetings of the Society for Psychotherapy Research, 1990.

Benjamin LS: Every psychopathology is a gift of love. Psychother Res 3:1–24, 1993

Benjamin LS: SASB: a bridge between personality theory and clinical psychology. Psychological Inquiry 5:273–316, 1994

Benjamin LS: Good defenses make good neighbors, in Ego Defenses: Theory and Research. Edited by Conte H, Plutchik R. New York, Wiley, 1995, pp 53–78

Benjamin LS: Interpersonal Diagnosis and Treatment of Personality Disorders, 2nd Edition. New York, Guilford, 1996a

Benjamin LS: An interpersonal theory of the personality disorders, in Major Theories of Personality Disorder. Edited by Clarkin JF, Lenzenweger M. New York, Guilford, 1996b

Bentler PM: EQS. Structural Equations Program Manual. Los Angeles, CA, BMPD Statistical Software, 1989

Byrne BM: Primer of LISREL. New York, Springer-Verlag, 1989

Carroll J, Schaffer C, Spensley J, et al: Family experiences of self mutilating patients. Am J Psychiatry 137:852–853, 1980

Conte JR: Overview of child sexual abuse, in American Psychiatric Press Review of Psychiatry, Vol 10. Edited by Tasman A, Goldfinger SM. Washington, DC, American Psychiatric Press, 1991, pp 283–307

Costa PT, McCrae RR: Personality in adulthood: a six-year longitudinal study of self-reports and spouse ratings on the NEO personality inventory. J Pers Soc Psychol 54:853–863, 1988

Derogatis LR: SCL-90 Administration, Scoring and Procedures Manuals for the Revised Version. Baltimore, Leonard R. Derogatis, 1977

Divasto PV, Kaufman A, Rosner L, et al: The presence of sexually stressful events among females in the general population. Arch Sex Behav 13:59–67, 1984

First MB, Spitzer RL, Gibbon M, et al: Structured Clinical Interview for DSM-IV Axis I Disorders, Clinical Version (SCID-CV). Washington, DC, American Psychiatric Press, 1996

First MB, Gibbon M, Spitzer RL, et al: Structured Clinical Interview for DSM-IV Axis II Personality Disorders. Washington, DC, American Psychiatric Press, 1997

Fritz GS, Stoll K, Wagner NA: A comparison of males and females who were sexually molested as children. J Sex Marital Ther 7:54–59, 1981

Gatz M, Pedersen NL, Plomin R, et al: Importance of shared genes and shared environments for symptoms of depression in older adults. J Abnorm Psychol 101:701–708, 1992

Greist JH, Klein MH, Erdman HP: Routine on-line psychiatric diagnosis by computer. Am J Psychiatry 133:1405–1407, 1976

Greist JH, Mathiesen KS, Klein MH, et al: Psychiatric diagnosis: what role for the computer? Hosp Community Psychiatry 35:1089–1090, 1984

Gunderson JG: Diagnostic controversies, in American Psychiatric Press Annual Review of Psychiatry, Vol 11. Edited by Tasman A, Riba MB. Washington, DC, American Psychiatric Press, 1992, pp 9–24

Guttman L: Order analysis of correlation matrixes, in Handbook of Multivariate Experimental Psychology. Edited by Cattell RB. Chicago, Rand McNally, 1966, pp 439–458

Henry W, Schacht T, Strupp HH: Structural analysis of social behavior: Application to a study of interpersonal process in differential psychotherapeutic outcome. J Consult Clin Psychol 54:27–31, 1986

Hume D: An enquiry concerning human understanding, reprinted in Basic Problems of Philosophy. Edited by Bronstein DJ, Krikorian YH, Wiener PP. New York, Prentice-Hall, 1947, pp 373–390

Kagan J: The meanings of personality predicates. Am Psychol 44:614–620, 1988

Kendall-Tackett K, Williams LM, Finkelhor D: Impact of sexual abuse on children: a review and synthesis of recent empirical studies. Psychol Bull 113:164–180, 1993

Kendler KS, Kessler RC, Neale MC, et al: The prediction of major depression in women: toward an integrated etiologic model. Am J Psychiatry 150:1139–1157, 1993.

Kercher G, McShane M: The prevalence of child sexual abuse victimization in an adult sample of Texas residents. Child Abuse Negl 8:495–502, 1984

Klein MK, Benjamin LS, Rosenfeld R, et al: The Wisconsin Personality Inventory (WISPI). Development, reliability, and validity. J Personal Disord 7:285–303, 1993

Klein MH, Wonderlich S, Shea MT: Models of relationships between personality and depression: toward a framework for theory and research, in Personality and Depression. A Current View. Edited by Klein MH, Kupfer DJ, Shea MT. New York, Guilford, 1993, pp 1–54

Kraemer GW: A psychobiological theory of attachment. Behav Brain Sci 14:1–28, 1992

Kraemer GW, Ebert MH, Lake CR, et al: A longitudinal study of the effects of different rearing environments on cerebrospinal fluid norepinephrine and bigenic amine metabolites in rhesus monkeys. Neuropsychopharmacology 2:175–89, 1989

Landis JT: Experiences of 500 children with adult sexual deviation. Psychiatric Quarterly Supplement 30:91–109, 1956

Leary T: Interpersonal Diagnosis of Personality: A Functional Theory and Methodology for Personality Evaluation. New York, Ronald Press, 1957

Loranger AW, Susman VL, Oldham JM, et al: The personality disorder examination: a preliminary report. J Personal Disord 1:1–13, 1987

Lowing PA, Mirsky AF, Pereira R: The inheritance of schizophrenia spectrum disorders: a reanalysis of the Danish Adoptee Study data. Am J Psychiatry 140:1167–1171, 1983

McGongile M, Smith T, Benjamin LS, et al: Hostility and nonshared family environment: a study of monozygotic twins. J Res Pers 27:23–34, 1993

National Advisory Mental Health Council: Health care reform for Americans with severe mental illnesses: report of the National Advisory Mental Health Council. Am J Psychiatry 150:1447–1463, 1993

Oldham JM, Skodol AE: Personality disorders and mood disorders, in American Psychiatric Press Review of Psychiatry, Vol 11. Edited by Tasman A, Riba MB. Washington, DC, American Psychiatric Association, 1992, pp 418–435.

Ornstein PH, Kay J: Development of psychoanalytic self psychology: a historical-conceptual overview, in American Psychiatric Press Review of Psychiatry, Vol 9. Edited by Tasman A, Goldfinger SM, Kaufmann CA. Washington, DC, American Psychiatric Press, 1990, pp 303–322

Plomin R, Daniels D: Why are children in the same family so different from one another? Behav Brain Sci 10:1–60, 1987

Reiss D, Plomin R, Hetherington EM: Genetics and psychiatry: an unheralded window on the environment. Am J Psychiatry 148:283–291, 1991

Robbins LH, Helzer JE, Croughan JL, et al: National Institute of Mental Health diagnostic interview schedule: its history, characteristics and validity. Arch Gen Psychiatry 38:381–389, 1981

Rothbart MK, Goldsmith HH: Three approaches to the study of infant temperament. Dev Rev 5:237–260, 1985

Schaefer ES: Configurational analysis of children's reports of parent behavior. J Consult Psychol 29:552–557, 1965

Schloredt K: Relations among perceived parenting, introject, and self-reported symptomatology in women abused as children. Master's thesis, Salt Lake City, University of Utah, 1993

Schulz PM, Soloff PH, Kelly T, et al: A family history study of borderline subtypes. J Personal Disord 3:217–229, 1989

Sullivan HS: The Interpersonal Theory of Psychiatry. New York, WW Norton, 1953

Teti DM, Gelfand DM, Messinger D, et al: Maternal depression and the quality of early attachment: an examination of infants, preschoolers and their mothers. Dev Psychol 31:364–376, 1995

Tellegen A: Brief Manual for the Differential Personality Questionnaire. Unpublished manuscript. Minneapolis, University of Minnesota, 1992

Tress W, (Ed.): SASB. Die Strukturale Analyse Sozial Verhaltens. Ein Arbeitsbuch fur Forschung, Praxis und Weiterbildung in der Psychotherapie. Heidelberg, Roland Asanger Verlag, 1993

Welsh GS, Dahlstrom WG (eds): Basic Readings on the MMPI in Psychology and Medicine. Minneapolis, University of Minnesota Press, 1956

Wyatt GE: The sexual abuse of Afro-American and White American women in childhood. Child Abuse Negl 9:507–519, 1985

Genetic and Environmental Structure of Personality

Andrew C. Heath, D.Phil.

Pamela A. Madden, Ph.D.

C. Robert Cloninger, M.D.

Nicholas G. Martin, Ph.D.

Behavioral genetic studies provide convincing evidence for a substantial genetic contribution to personality differences. Evidence for an important genetic influence is provided by studies of monozygotic and dizygotic twin pairs reared apart and together, conducted in the United Kingdom (Shields 1962), Finland (Langinvainio et al. 1984), Sweden (Pedersen 1993; Pedersen et al. 1988), and the United States (Tellegen et al. 1988); by studies comparing biological parent–offspring and adoptive parent–offspring correlations, conducted in the United Kingdom (Eaves and Eysenck 1980; Eaves et al. 1989) and in the United States (Loehlin 1992; Scarr et al. 1981); by large-sample studies comparing monozygotic and dizygotic twin pairs reared together, conducted in the United Kingdom (Eaves and Eysenck 1975; Eaves et al. 1989), the United States (Eaves et al. 1998; Loehlin and Nichols 1976), Sweden (Floderus-Myrhed et al. 1980), Australia (Heath et al. 1994; Martin and Jardine 1986), and Finland (Rose et al. 1988); and by

Supported by NIAAA Grants AA07535 and AA07728, and by a grant from the Australian National Health and Medical Research Council.

extended twin family studies, of twin pairs and their offspring, from Sweden (Hewitt 1984; Price et al. 1982) and the United States (Eaves et al. 1998; Loehlin 1992). Although most of these studies have used self-report measures of personality, a twin study that used informant ratings confirmed the importance of genetic influences (Heath et al. 1992). In all of these studies, the major finding has been that insofar as family members have similar personalities, it is largely because of their genetic resemblance, rather than because of any shared family environmental influences (Eaves et al. 1989; Loehlin 1992, 1993).

Various theorists have proposed competing descriptions for the structure of personality, in terms of varying numbers of personality dimensions (e.g., Cloninger 1986, 1987, 1988, 1991; Eysenck and Eysenck 1969, 1976; McCrae and Costa 1989; Tellegen 1985). The voluminous body of research that has accumulated, however, has in almost all instances involved research on samples of unrelated individuals. What has not generally been realized is that genes and environment may have very different effects on personality structure so that, in the extreme, environmental influences may generate a negative correlation but genetic influences a positive correlation between two traits (Heath and Martin 1990). Thus conventional factor analytic studies can tell us very little about the inherited structure of personality. In this chapter we examine the use of multivariate genetic factor models, combining concepts from genetic analysis and traditional factor analysis (Heath et al. 1989; Martin and Eaves 1977) to explore the genetic structure of personality. We shall focus explicitly on two personality systems that have made strong predictions for the role of personality differences in determining psychiatric disorders, namely the personality systems of Eysenck (Eysenck and Eysenck 1985) and of Cloninger (1986, 1987).

As part of a study of the inheritance of alcoholism and other psychiatric disorders in an Australian twin sample, we have obtained self-report personality data, by mailed questionnaire, using the short form of the Eysenck Personality Questionnaire: Revised (EPQ-R) (Eysenck et al. 1985), and a specially abbreviated 54-item version of the Tridimensional Personality Questionnaire (TPQ) of Cloninger et al. (1991). Results of fitting univariate genetic models to the higher-order TPQ scales and the EPQ-R scales have been presented elsewhere (Heath et al. 1994). These analyses confirmed significant genetic influences on the Eysenckian personality dimensions in this sample and provided the first demonstration of the hypothesized genetic contribution to differences in harm avoidance (HA), reward dependence (RD), and novelty seeking (NS). No significant influence of shared family environment on personality differences was found, although it should be noted that because genetic nonadditivity (e.g., genetic dominance or genetic epistasis, i.e., gene-gene interactions) may mask shared environmental effects in data on twin pairs reared together, we could not exclude the possibility of modest familial environmental influences on personality (cf., Loehlin 1992). After correcting for measurement error, estimates of broad heritability (i.e., the proportion of the reliable variation in personality attributable to additive and nonadditive genetic effects) ranged from 54% to 61% for HA, NS, and RD; 41% to 59% for the Eysenckian dimensions of extraversion (E), neuroticism (N), and toughmindedness or "psychoticism" (P), and, in women, for social conformity or "lie" (L); but only 34% for L in men. Further multivariate analyses were conducted using genetic triangular decomposition models in order to examine the extent to which the EPQ-R and TPQ were assessing the same versus different dimensions of genetic variability (Heath et al. 1994). Such models may be viewed as being more closely related to principal components analysis than to factor analysis in that they do not distinguish between common factor and specific factor genetic (or environmental) variance. Results indicated that "the personality systems of Eysenck and Cloninger are not simply alternative descriptions of the same dimensions of personality, but rather each provides incomplete descriptions of the structure of heritable personality differences" (Heath et al. 1994, p. 762). Together, the two personality questionnaires appeared to be assessing five to six dimensions of genetic variability, and at least six environmental dimensions.

In this chapter we present the results of fitting genetic models to the primary scales of the TPQ to determine whether significant genetic influences are found for each of these subscales. We then fit multivariate genetic factor models to examine the dimensions of genetic variability assessed jointly by the EPQ-R and higher-order TPQ scales. We use results of these analyses to reexamine the potential role of personality differences as mediators in the inheritance of Axis I disorders and of personality disorders.

Sample and Methods

As described elsewhere (Heath et al. 1994), completed personality assessments were obtained from both members of 2680 adult twin pairs (946 monozygotic [MZ] female pairs, 541 dizygotic [DZ] female pairs, 401 MZ male pairs, 223 DZ male pairs, 569 opposite-sex DZ pairs). We found good test-retest reliability and high internal consistency for the TPQ personality scales of HA, RD, and NS, and for three of the four Eysenckian personality scales, E, N, and L, but low internal consistency and low test-retest reliability in the oldest age cohort for the P scale. In this chapter we also present data on the primary scales of the TPQ (see Table 13–1 later in this chapter). Because, in the shortened form of the TPQ used in the present study, these primary scales consisted of only four or five items each, internal consistency and test-retest reliability must be expected to be somewhat reduced compared with the full instrument. For three primary scales, internal consistency (Cronbach's α), assessed separately by gender and for different birth cohorts (pre-1931; 1931–1945; 1946–1955; 1956–1964), was poor: disorderliness (NS4: $\alpha = 0.20$–0.44); sentimentality (RD1: $\alpha = 0.17$–0.43); and dependence (RD4: $\alpha = 0.29$–0.46). For the remaining scales, internal consistency coefficients were in the range 0.51–0.77 for HA1–HA4, 0.39–0.72 for NS1–NS3, 0.54–0.69 for RD2, and 0.70–0.82 for RD3. Short-term test-retest reliability was assessed by a 2-year follow-up mailing of 500 male and 500 female respondents, with completed questionnaires being returned by 430 males and 451 females at an average test-retest interval of 2.1 years. Estimates of test-retest reliability for the TPQ primary scales were generally in the range 0.47–0.82, with reduced reliability being observed primarily for RD1 and RD4 in young men ($r = 0.43$ and 0.38, respectively), and RD4 in middle-aged women ($r = 0.44$).

Raw scores on the abbreviated TPQ primary scales used in this study were in all cases in the range 0–4 or 0–5. Conventional methods of fitting genetic models to summary twin pair covariance matrices (e.g., Heath et al. 1989; Neale and Cardon 1992), which rely upon the assumptions of multivariate normality, would therefore be likely to give misleading results. Two-way contingency tables were therefore computed, cross-classifying scores of first twin and second twin (or female twin and male twin, in the case of opposite-sex pairs) separately for each twin group; polychoric correlations were estimated and genetic and environmental models fitted by the method of maximum likelihood (Eaves et al. 1978, 1989). The goodness-of-fit of different models was compared to that of the most general model by likelihood-ratio χ^2 test. Estimates of broad heritability uncorrected for measurement error (i.e., the proportion of the total variance attributable to additive and nonadditive genetic effects) are reported for the best-fitting model for each scale.

For the joint analysis of the EPQ-R and TPQ higher-order scales, summary covariance matrices were computed separately for each zygosity group, giving the variances and covariances of the seven personality variables measured on first and second twins (i.e., 14×14 covariance matrices). Raw personality scores were transformed and age corrected as described in Heath et al. (1994). Genetic factor models (Heath et al. 1989; Martin and Eaves 1977; Neale and Cardon 1992) were fitted to the set of five twin pair covariance matrices (including opposite-sex pairs as well as same-sex MZ and DZ pairs) by the method of maximum likelihood, using the computer package MX (Neale 1992). The goodness-of-fit of different models was compared using Akaike's information criterion (AIC) (Akaike 1987). Technical details of model-fitting are beyond the scope of this chapter, but may be found in Eaves et al. 1989, Heath et al. 1989, Neale and Cardon 1992, and similar sources.

Genetic Models

Figure 13–1 summarizes the basic univariate genetic model used for model-fitting analyses. The model distinguishes between shared family

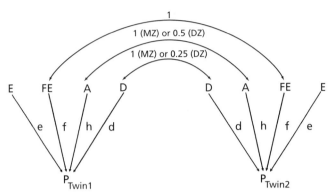

FIGURE 13–1. *Path model used for univariate genetic model-fitting. P denotes the observed phenotype (personality score); and E, FE, A, and D the underlying within-family environmental, shared family environmental, additive genetic, and dominance or epistatic (nonadditive) genetic effects on the phenotype. Genetic and environmental variance components e^2, h^2, and d^2 or f^2 were estimated (Eaves et al. 1978).*

environmental effects, assumed to be no more highly correlated in MZ than in DZ twin pairs, and within-family environmental effects that reflect those differences in environmental experience that make even an identical twin differ from his or her co-twin. Within-family environmental effects include measurement error in these univariate analyses. The model also distinguishes between additive genetic effects (i.e., the additive effects of multiple genetic loci) and also nonadditive genetic effects arising through genetic dominance or through multiplicative gene-gene interactions (genetic epistasis). In univariate data on twin pairs reared together, the effects of genetic nonadditivity will tend to mask shared environmental effects and vice versa; the former leading to DZ correlations that are less than one-half the corresponding MZ correlations, and the latter DZ correlations that are greater than one-half the corresponding MZ correlations. Thus we cannot estimate simultaneously both nonadditive genetic and shared environmental parameters. Data from separated twin and adoption studies, however, suggest that any effects of family environment on personality differences are at best extremely weak (Loehlin 1992). To test for genotype × sex interaction, the fit of a genetic model that constrained genetic and environmental parameters (h^2, e^2, and d^2 or f^2) to be the same in both genders was compared to that of a model that allowed for sex differences in these parameters, by likelihood-ratio χ^2 test. The goodness-of-fit of submodels that dropped one or more genetic parameters, or that dropped the shared environmental parameter, was likewise compared to that of the most general model by likelihood-ratio χ^2 test.

Figure 13–2 summarizes the two-factor version of the genetic factor model used for the multivariate genetic analyses. Full details of multivariate genetic factor analysis may be obtained from Martin and Eaves (1977), Heath et al. (1989), and Neale and Cardon (1992). As in conventional factor analysis (e.g., Harman 1976), we distinguish between common factor effects, which generate correlations between variables, and specific factor effects, which contribute to the variance of a variable but not to its covariance with other variables and which will therefore include measurement error effects (at least insofar as these are uncorrelated between personality variables). Our primary interest is in the number of common factors needed to account for the observed correlations between variables and in the factor loadings of those variables on the underlying common factors. Whereas a conventional factor analysis uses only the matrix of correlations within persons, and a conventional univariate genetic analysis uses only twin pair correlations within variables, multivariate genetic analysis exploits the additional information contained in the twin pair cross-variable correlations. This permits estimation of separate genetic and environmental common factor loadings, and separate genetic and environmental specific factor variances; it also permits tests of hypotheses about the number of genetic and environmental common factors needed to account for the observed twin pair covariance matrices. In contrast to the univariate case, in multivariate data it is possible to estimate simultaneously nonadditive genetic and shared environmental common factors, provided that the number of observed variables is sufficient to permit estimation of at least a two-factor model (e.g., D. Duffy, unpublished data, January 1992). One important feature of the model that we used should be noted. By assuming that additive genetic and nonadditive genetic common factor effects were mediated through the intervening genetic common factors G1 and G2, we imposed the constraint, which appears biologically plausible, that factor loadings on the first additive genetic common factor be a multiple, h_1, of factor

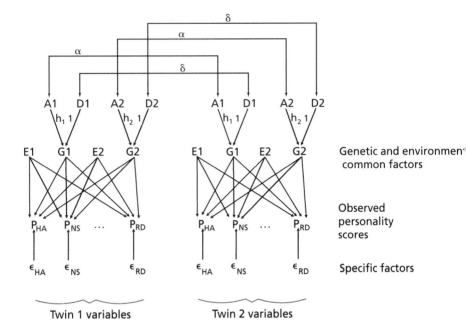

FIGURE 13–2.   *Genetic factor model used for multivariate genetic model-fitting analysis. A two-factor model, with two genetic and two within-family environmental common factors (G1 and G2, E1 and E2), is depicted. To simplify the diagram, common factor shared environmental effects, and specific factor additive and nonadditive genetic and shared environmental effects have been omitted. P_{HA}, P_{NS} . . . P_{RD} denote the observed personality scores, and ϵ_{HA}, ϵ_{NS}, ϵ_{RD} the corresponding within-family environmental specific factor effects. Path coefficients for the paths from E1, G1, E2, and G2 to the observed personality scores—which are the genetic and environmental common factor loadings of the personality measures on E1 . . . G2—have also been omitted. Genetic common factors G1 and G2 are influenced by both additive genetic effects (A1, A2) and nonadditive genetic effects (D1, D2). From genetic theory (e.g., Bulmer 1980), $\alpha = 1$ for MZ pairs; $\alpha = 0.5$ for DZ pairs; and $\delta = 1$ for MZ pairs, $\delta = 0.25$ for DZ pairs.*

loadings on the first nonadditive genetic common factor, and that factor loadings on the second additive genetic factor be a multiple, h_2, of loadings on the second nonadditive genetic common factor. Unless indicated otherwise in this chapter, in all multivariate analyses we estimated additive and nonadditive genetic and within-family environmental specific factor variances.

In conventional exploratory factor analysis, whereas a single-factor model will yield a unique solution, a model with two or more common factors will yield an infinite number of rotationally equivalent solutions; and various criteria have been proposed for factor rotation to a "simple structure" solution (Harman 1976). In multivariate genetic analysis, a single-factor model estimating one additive genetic common factor, one nonadditive genetic or shared environmental common factor, and one within-family environmental common factor will likewise yield a unique solution. Under an unconstrained two-factor solution, however, separate factor rotations of the factor loadings on the two additive genetic common factors, the two within-family environmental common factors, and so on, may be performed. In the case of the model of Figure 13–2, however, there are constraints on the additive and nonadditive genetic loadings that prevent factor rotation, (i.e., define a unique genetic factor structure), but the environmental factor loadings may be rotated in the usual fashion. Where appropriate, genetic or environmental factor loadings were rotated to an orthogonal simple structure using varimax criteria.

In some multivariate analyses, additional constraints were imposed upon the genetic and environmental factor structures. In particular, we explored the improvement in parsimony that could be obtained by 1) constraining loadings on each genetic common factor in males to differ from those in females only by a scale factor (i.e., $h_{\mathrm{m}ji} = k_i h_{\mathrm{f}ji}$, where i denotes the ith factor, j denotes the jth item, and subscripts m and f are used to distinguish factor loadings in males and females under the most general model); 2) imposing the same constraint on loadings on each environmental common factor; 3) fitting "common pathway" models (Neale and Cardon 1992) in which loadings on each genetic common factor were constrained to differ from those on the corresponding within-family environmental common factor by only a scale factor (i.e., $h_{ji} = k_i e_{\mathrm{f}ji}$). Constraints 1 and 2 allow for the possibility that the genetic structure (or environmental structure) of personality is essentially the same in men and women, except for a sex difference in the magnitudes of the genetic and environmental contributions to personality differences. Imposing constraint 3 tests whether the genetic and environmental factor structures observed for the personality variables are the same, once we allow for differences in the relative contributions of genes and environment to personality differences.

Results

Table 13–1 summarizes maximum-likelihood estimates of twin pair polychoric correlations for each of the TPQ primary scales. Correlations for the higher-order scales are also reproduced from Heath et al. (1994) for comparison. For all scales, higher MZ than same-sex DZ correlations were observed, both in women and in men, consistent with a genetic contribution to personality differences. There were only two scales in women (fear of uncertainty [HA2] and sentimentality [RD1]) and one in men (disorderliness [NS4]) where the same-sex dizygotic twin pair correlation was apparently more than one-half the corresponding monozygotic correlation, the pattern that would be predicted if there were shared environmental as well as genetic contributions to personality differences. Formal results of model-fitting are not presented here. However, in every case it was possible to reject the hypothesis of no genetic effects at the 5% significance level, by likelihood-ratio χ^2 test; and in no case was the effect of shared environment found to be significant. For three of the four HA primary scales (HA1–HA3), and for NS4, significant genotype $\times$ sex interaction (i.e., significant heterogeneity of genetic and environmental parameters as a function of gender) was observed. Significant nonadditive genetic as well as additive genetic effects were found for the four HA primary scales as well as for NS4 and RD2, but for the remaining scales the data were consistent with a simple additive genetic mode of inheritance.

Estimates of broad heritability for each of the TPQ primary scales (and, for comparison, the higher-order scales) are summarized in Table 13–2. Estimates ranged from a high of 47% (for HA3 in men) to a low of 27% (HA1 in men). These estimates were not corrected for measurement error and thus will underestimate "true score" heritabilities by 25%–50%, depending upon the reliability of the scale, at least under the assumption that response inconsistency is not itself heritable. A

TABLE 13-1.

Univariate twin correlations for TPQ higher-order scales (from Heath et al. 1994) and primary scales

N pairs	MZ female 924–937	DZ female 526–537	MZ male 394–399	DZ male 220–223	DZ opposite-sex 560–567
Harm avoidance (HA)	0.44	0.20	0.42	−0.03	0.09
Anticipatory worry (HA1)	0.42	0.17	0.27	−0.03	0.08
Fear of uncertainty (HA2)	0.37	0.26	0.36	−0.04	0.02
Shyness with strangers (HA3)	0.39	0.14	0.47	0.15	0.10
Fatigability (HA4)	0.34	0.10	0.27	0.09	0.12
Novelty seeking (NS)	0.42	0.14	0.35	0.06	0.07
Excitability (NS1)	0.35	0.15	0.31	0.11	0.09
Impulsiveness (NS2)	0.33	0.13	0.28	0.10	0.05
Extravagance (NS3)	0.38	0.19	0.32	0.10	0.14
Disorderliness (NS4)	0.29	0.04	0.37	0.25	0.04
Reward dependence (RD)	0.38	0.11	0.39	0.18	0.06
Sentimentality (RD1)	0.39	0.27	0.35	0.18	0.11
Persistence (RD2)	0.39	0.12	0.41	0.12	0.12
Attachment (RD3)	0.39	0.16	0.35	0.10	0.11
Dependence (RD4)	0.30	0.20	0.33	0.17	0.05

Note. Polychoric correlations are tabulated for primary scales; product-moment correlations for higher-order scales.

TABLE 13–2.

Estimates of broad heritability, uncorrected for measurement error, for TPQ higher-order scales (from Heath et al. 1994) and primary scales

	Men	Women		Men	Women		Men	Women
Harm avoidance	42	44	Novelty seeking	41	(41)	Reward dependence	39	37
HA1	27	42	NS1	32	(32)	RD1	38	(38)
HA2	36	37	NS2	29	(29)	RD2	40	(40)
HA3	47	38	NS3	35	(35)	RD3	36	(36)
HA4	33	(33)	NS4	29	(29)	RD4	30	(30)

Note. _Estimates given in parentheses for women do not differ significantly from those for men._

striking finding was that for three of the four RD scales, the heritability estimates obtained were comparable in magnitude to the broad heritability of the higher-order RD dimension.

Table 13–3 reports the results of fitting genetic factor models to twin pair covariance matrices for the EPQ-R and higher-order TPQ personality scales. No model gave an adequate fit to the data by χ^2 test of goodness-of-fit, a common finding in multivariate problems (e.g., Bollen 1989), so the fit of different models was compared by AIC (Akaike 1987). The most parsimonious model will be the one with the lowest AIC value. Models 1–3, which allowed for common factor shared environmental effects, and which assumed no common factor genetic effects, but did allow for trait-specific genetic effects, gave a very poor fit to the data. Models 4–6, which allowed for common factor genetic effects, but not shared environmental effects, gave a substantially better fit. A model with three genetic and three within-family environmental common factors (model 6)—the largest number that could be estimated with only seven observed variables—gave a substantially better fit than models with only one or two genetic and within-family environmental common factors (models 4 and 5). Allowing for nonadditive as well as additive genetic effects for the first genetic common factor led to a substantial further improvement in fit, comparing model 7 with model 6; but a model that allowed for nonadditive genetic effects on the second genetic factor as well (model 8) gave a slightly worse fit by AIC. Adding a single shared environmental common factor to model 7 did yield a substantial improvement in fit (model 9), but the addition of a second shared environmental factor (model 10) once again led to a less parsimonious fit. Although not shown in Table 13–3, dropping either one additive genetic common factor from model 9 ($\chi^2_{397} = 590.09$, AIC $= -203.91$) or one within-family environmental common factor ($\chi^2_{397} = 647.36$, AIC $= -146.64$) in each case led to a substantial deterioration in fit. Thus our best-fitting model included three genetic factors (with one of these allowing for nonadditive as well as additive effects), one shared environmental common factor, and three within-family environmental common factors. This model also estimated additive and nonadditive genetic and within-family environmental-specific factor variances for each personality scale.

TABLE 13-3.

Results of fitting multivariate genetic factor models: EPQ-R and TPQ scales

	Number of common factors				Goodness-of-fit		
Model	Additive genetic	Nonadditive genetic	Shared environment	Within-family environment	df	χ^2	AIC
1	0[a]	0	1[a]	1	455	2,658.04	1,748.04
2	0[a]	0	2[a]	2	427	1,317.72	463.72
3	0[a]	0	3[a]	3	399	770.84	−27.16
4	1	0[b]	0	1	455	2,193.50	1,283.50
5	2	0[b]	0	2	427	996.97	142.97
6	3	0[b]	0	3	399	600.72	−197.28
7	3	1[c]	0	3	397	568.70	−225.30
8	3	2[c]	0	3	395	566.94	−233.06
9	3	1[c]	1	3	383	511.37	−254.63
10	3	1[c]	2	3	369	488.03	−249.97

[a]Specific-factor additive genetic and shared and within-family environmental variances were estimated.
[b]Specific-factor nonadditive genetic variances were estimated.
[c]Nonadditive genetic common factor loadings were constrained to be a multiple of additive genetic loadings on the corresponding factor.

356

Environmental Structure of Personality

Table 13–4 summarizes varimax-rotated environmental factor loadings under the best-fitting model. Because the factors are orthogonal, a factor loading is equivalent to the correlation between a personality scale and the underlying environmental (or genetic) factor. In women, within-family environmental factors I–III clearly represented environmental influences on HA, RD, and NS, respectively. Factor I was also modestly associated with increasing N and decreasing E; factor II had a modest positive loading of E; and factor III had modest positive loadings of E and P, and a negative loading of L. In men, a somewhat different pattern of loadings was observed. Factor I had substantial loadings of both N and HA, with a modest negative loading of L; factor II had a substantial positive loading of E, with modest positive loadings of NS and RD, and a negative loading of HA; factor III had a substantial loading only of NS, with all other loadings less than 0.2 in absolute magnitude. Thus whereas factor rotation in women clearly identified HA, RD, and NS environmental factors, the rotated factor solution in men was more readily interpretable in terms of N/HA, E, and NS environmental factors.

Also given in Table 13–4 are the item-specific within-family environmental variances. These include error variance and so were quite substantial in magnitude. Estimates for L and P were large in both sexes, implying that there was substantial nonerror variance for these variables that was not explained by the within-family environmental common factors. Very low estimates were obtained for specific environmental variances for HA and RD in women, and E and NS in men. This was most probably an artifact of attempting to estimate a three-factor model when we had only seven observed variables; ideally we would require three variables per factor.

The single shared environmental common factor estimated in both sexes had a substantial negative loading of L in both sexes, as well as a modest negative loading of P in men. All other shared environmental common factor loadings were less than 0.2 in absolute magnitude. Even with the increased power of multivariate genetic analysis to detect shared environmental effects, we found only modest shared

TABLE 13-4.

Environmental factor loadings under best-fitting model

	Women					Men				
	Within-family environment				Shared environment common factor loadings	Within-family environment				Shared environment common factor loadings
	Common factor loadings			Specific variance		Common factor loadings			Specific variance	
	I	II	III			I	II	III		
E	-0.33	0.26	0.23	0.31	0.10	-0.03	0.71	0.10	0.00	-0.01
N	0.41	0.02	0.04	0.39	-0.05	0.59	-0.14	-0.16	0.26	0.12
L	-0.07	0.03	-0.21	0.49	-0.44	-0.30	-0.06	-0.11	0.64	-0.35
P	-0.10	-0.15	0.24	0.58	-0.13	-0.05	0.02	0.17	0.69	-0.24
HA	0.75	-0.08	-0.05	0.02	-0.11	0.47	-0.31	-0.17	0.22	0.19
NS	-0.08	0.13	0.46	0.33	0.17	0.16	0.24	0.78	0.01	0.01
RD	-0.05	0.64	-0.03	0.17	0.11	-0.05	0.28	0.06	0.58	0.19

environmental contributions to personality differences, accounting for less than 4% of the variance in the case of the TPQ scales.

Genetic Structure of Personality

Table 13–5 summarizes genetic common factor loadings and specific factor variances. We consider first the genetic factor structure in women. The first genetic factor allowed for both additive and nonadditive genetic effects, although additive genetic effects predominated, accounting for approximately 73% of the total genetic variance associated with the first factor. Similar to the first within-family environmental factor in women, the first genetic factor had a high positive loading of HA, a more modest loading of N, and a negative loading of E. The second genetic factor had positive loadings of RD and E, a small positive loading of N, and a negative loading of P. With the exception of the N loading, this pattern was also very similar to that observed for the second within-family environmental common factor in women. The third genetic factor had positive loadings of NS, N, and also P, a negative loading of L, and a small positive loading of HA. The low E loading and higher positive loadings of HA and N presented a different pattern from that observed for the corresponding within-family environmental factor. Specific-factor genetic variances, summing additive plus nonadditive variances, were largest for RD (accounting for 19% of the total phenotypic variance) and for NS (12%), with all other specific factor genetic variances accounting for no more than 10% of the total phenotypic variance.

Despite genetic factor loadings in men and women that were estimated jointly in a five-group analysis that included opposite-sex pairs, a procedure that was expected to maximize our chances of obtaining consistent results across sexes, we did find some pronounced gender differences in the genetic structure of personality. In men, additive genetic loadings on the first genetic factor were estimated at zero, so that effectively all of the genetic variance in that factor was nonadditive. The pattern of loadings on that first factor was also somewhat different in men compared with women: loadings of NS and E were smaller, but there were also positive loadings of L and RD in males,

TABLE 13-5.
Genetic factor loadings under best-fitting model

	Women						Men					
	Additive genetic				Nonadditive genetic		Additive genetic				Nonadditive genetic	
	Common factor loadings			Specific variance	Common factor loadings	Specific variance	Common factor loadings			Specific variance	Common factor loadings	Specific variance
	I	II	III		I		I	II	III		I	
E	-0.44	0.36	0.10	0.03	-0.27	0.05	0.00	0.57	0.05	0.03	-0.13	0.15
N	0.34	0.23	0.39	0.05	0.21	0.05	0.00	-0.05	0.33	0.05	0.43	0.00
L	-0.02	0.14	-0.33	0.00	-0.01	0.10	0.00	0.04	-0.29	0.00	0.31	0.00
P	-0.23	-0.30	0.33	0.10	-0.14	0.00	0.00	0.00	0.52	0.10	-0.29	0.00
HA	0.53	0.05	0.22	0.00	0.33	0.00	0.00	-0.43	0.08	0.00	0.36	0.02
NS	-0.29	0.10	0.36	0.12	-0.18	0.00	0.00	0.34	0.36	0.12	-0.14	0.16
RD	-0.13	0.35	0.02	0.13	-0.08	0.06	0.00	0.46	-0.07	0.13	0.27	0.01

in addition to the positive loadings of HA and N observed in both sexes. Loadings on the third genetic factor in men were more consistent with those observed in women, with moderate positive loadings observed for NS and N, a negative loading for L, but also a positive loading for P that was quite substantial in men (0.52). The pattern of loadings on the second genetic factor, in contrast, exhibited a marked sex difference. Although there were positive loadings of RD and E in both sexes, these loadings were much higher in men than in women. In men, but not in women, this second factor had a strong negative loading of HA and positive loading of NS. The negative loading of P on this second factor in women was not found in men. The pattern of common factor genetic loadings observed in men, at least in the case of genetic factor I, was also rather different from the within-family environmental common factor loadings. In contrast to the moderately large loadings of RD and P on the first genetic factor, these variables had negligible loadings on the corresponding within-family environmental factor. The sign of the loading of L was actually reversed between the first genetic and first within-family environmental factors. As for genetic-specific factor variances, substantial residual genetic variance was observed for RD and for NS for men, as for women, accounting for 28% and 14% of the total phenotypic variance in these traits; but substantial residual genetic variance for E was also observed (18%).

Factor Structure Differences

How could these apparently disparate findings for the genetic and environmental structure of personality in men and women be reconciled? The first question that had to be addressed was whether the apparent gender differences that we observed were nonsignificant, or alternatively whether we had obtained rotationally equivalent solutions such that genetic factor loadings in women could be rotated to reproduce the pattern of loadings for men. To address this issue, we fitted a modified version of model 9 that constrained genetic common factor loadings in men to be a multiple of corresponding loadings in women, thereby testing the hypothesis that the genetic structure of personality in men and women was identical but for a scaling factor for each genetic factor. Whether we constrained loadings on only the first genetic factor ($\chi^2_{390} = 536.60$, AIC $= -243.40$) or on all three genetic factors ($\chi^2_{402} = 556.38$, AIC $= -247.62$), these models gave less parsimonious fits than the model that allowed for sex differences in genetic factor loadings. In similar fashion, we fitted a modified version of model 9 that allowed the environmental structure of personality to differ by only four scaling factors (for the three within-family environmental and one shared environmental common factors). This gave a much worse fit to the data ($\chi^2_{407} = 669.97$, AIC $= -126.22$). Thus the observed gender differences in the genetic and environmental structure of personality cannot be dismissed as merely due to chance differences in factor rotation. In similar fashion, it was necessary to confirm whether the apparent differences within genders between genetic and environmental factor structures were merely rotational differences, by fitting a multivariate genetic common pathway model. Once again, this model gave a poor fit to the data ($\chi^2_{431} = 654.11$, AIC $= -207.89$), confirming the importance of the observed differences between the genetic and environmental factor structure.

Discussion

We have presented results of univariate genetic analyses of the primary subscales of the TPQ. We were able to confirm for each of the subscales the genetic influence reported previously for the higher-order personality dimensions of HA, RD, and NS (Heath et al. 1994). We have also presented results of fitting genetic factor models to the higher-order scales of the TPQ and the EPQ-R, an instrument that has been used extensively in behavioral genetic research (e.g., Eaves et al. 1989; Loehlin 1992). Several findings that are consistent with analyses of other behavioral genetic data sets emerge from these analyses: 1) shared family environment makes only a modest contribution to personality differences, its major influence being on the SC or L scale of the EPQ-R; 2) within-family environmental influences are substantial; 3) additive and nonadditive genetic influences on personality are also of major importance. As others have noted from conventional univariate genetic analyses (Eaves et al. 1989; Loehlin 1992), we have found that twin pair resemblance for personality cannot be explained by simple additive genetic inheritance: substantial effects of genetic dominance or gene-gene interactions are observed for HA, NS, N, and E. Thus although estimates of broad heritability for these traits are high, predicted correlations between first-degree relatives are modest. Our ability to demonstrate a mediating role of these personality variables in the inheritance of Axis I or Axis II disorders is likely to be poor if we are using only a conventional family study approach, but will be substantially improved if we use a twin design.

In multivariate genetic model-fitting analyses, we observed important gender differences in the genetic structure of personality. Non-additive genetic influences on personality were more important in men than in women, confirming a difference noted in the univariate genetic analysis of the higher-order scale scores (Heath et al. 1994). Gender differences were observed in the pattern of loadings for genetic common factors I and II, in particular. It seems implausible that there should be important gender differences in the mode of inheritance of personality, at least when considered at the level of the dimensions of biological variability that underlie personality differences. It is much more plausible that there is only a very imperfect relationship between the paper and pencil measures of personality used in this research and the underlying dimensions of biological variability, and that this relationship differs as a function of gender. Alternatively, it is possible that fitting genetic factor models, as we have done here, when the number of personality variables will permit estimation of no more than three additive genetic common factors, but we suspect at least five to six underlying dimensions of genetic variability, may account for the observed gender differences. This explanation might apply also to the observed differences between genetic and environmental factor structures, though we have noted elsewhere (Heath and Martin 1990) that there is no reason in principle why genes and environment need play the same role in shaping the structure of personality. An important implication of this problem is that we are much more likely to gain an understanding of the mediating role of personality differences in the inheritance of psychiatric disorders by fitting genetic Cholesky decomposition models (e.g., Madden et al. 1993a, 1993b), in effect estimating genetic and environmental correlations between the personality variables and psychiatric disorders, than by exploratory genetic factor analysis. It remains to be seen how well extensions of Cloninger's theory for the genetic structure of personality to assess dimensions of character as well as temperament (e.g., Cloninger et al. 1993; Svrakic et al. 1993) will clarify this picture.

References

Akaike H: Factor analysis and AIC. Psychometrika 52:317–332, 1987

Bollen KA: Structural Equations With Latent Variables. New York, Wiley, 1989

Bulmer MG: The Mathematical Theory of Quantitative Genetics. Oxford, Clarendon Press, 1980

Cloninger CR: A unified biosocial theory of personality and its role in the development of anxiety states. Psychiatr Dev 3:167–226, 1986

Cloninger CR: A systematic method for clinical description and classification of personality variants: a proposal. Arch Gen Psychiatry 44:573–588, 1987

Cloninger CR: Anxiety and theories of emotions, in Handbook of Anxiety, 2nd Edition. Edited by Noyes R, Roth M, Burrows GD. Amsterdam, Elsevier, 1988, pp 1–29

Cloninger CR: Brain networks underlying personality development, in Psychopathology and the Brain. Edited by Carroll BJ, Barrett JE. New York, Raven, 1991, pp 183–208

Cloninger CR, Przybeck TR, Svrakic DM: The tridimensional personality questionnaire: U.S. normative data. Psychol Rep 69:1047–1057, 1991

Cloninger CR, Svrakic DM, Przybeck TR: A psychobiological model of temperament and character. Arch Gen Psychiatry 50:975–990, 1993

Eaves LJ, Eysenck HJ: The nature of extraversion: a genetical analysis. J Pers Soc Psychol 32:102–112, 1975

Eaves LJ, Eysenck HJ: The genetics of smoking, in The Causes and Effects of Smoking. Edited by Eysenck HJ. London, Maurice Temple Smith, 1980, pp 140–314

Eaves LJ, Last K, Young PA, et al: Model-fitting approaches to the analysis of human behavior. Heredity 41:249–320, 1978

Eaves LJ, Eysenck HJ, Martin NG: Genes, Culture, and Personality: An Empirical Approach. London, Academic Press, 1989

Eaves LJ, Heath AC, Neale MC, et al: Sex differences and non-additivity in the effects of genes on personality. Twin Research 1:131–137, 1998

Eysenck HJ, Eysenck SBG: Personality Structure and Measurement. London, Routledge & Kegan Paul, 1969

Eysenck HJ, Eysenck SBG: Psychoticism as a Dimension of Personality. London, Hodder & Stoughton, 1976

Eysenck HJ, Eysenck MW: Personality and Individual Differences. New York, Plenum, 1985

Eysenck SBG, Eysenck HJ, Barrett P: A revised version of the psychoticism scale. Personality and Individual Differences 6:21–29, 1985

Floderus-Myrhed B, Pedersen N, Rasmuson I: Assessment of heritability for personality, based on a short-form of the Eysenck Personality Inventory. Behav Genet 10:153–162, 1980

Harman H: Modern Factor Analysis. Chicago, University of Chicago Press, 1976

Heath AC, Martin NG: Psychoticism as a dimension of personality: a multivariate genetic test of Eysenck and Eysenck's psychoticism construct. J Pers Soc Psychol 58:1–11, 1990

Heath AC, Neale MC, Hewitt JK, et al: Testing structural equation models for twin data using LISREL. Behav Genet 19:9–35, 1989

Heath AC, Neale MC, Kessler RC, et al: Evidence for genetic influences on personality from self-reports and informant ratings. J Pers Soc Psychol 63:85–96, 1992

Heath AC, Cloninger CR, Martin NG: Testing a model for the genetic structure of personality. J Pers Soc Psychol 66:762–765, 1994

Hewitt JK: Normal components of personality variation. J Pers Soc Psychol 47:671–675, 1984

Langinvainio H, Kaprio J, Koskenvuo M, et al: Finnish twins reared apart. III: Personality factors. Acta Genet Med Gemellol 33:259–264, 1984

Loehlin JC: Genes and Environment in Personality Development. Individual Differences and Development Series, Vol. 2. Newbury Park, CA, Sage, 1992

Loehlin JC: What has behavioral genetics told us about the nature of personality, in Twins as a Tool of Behavioral Genetics. Edited by Bouchard TJ, Propping P. Chichester, England, Wiley, 1993, pp 109–120

Loehlin JC, Nichols RC: Heredity, Environment, and Personality: A Study of 850 Sets of Twins. Austin, University of Texas Press, 1976

Madden PA, Heath AC, Bucholz KK, et al: The genetic relationship between problems related to alcohol use, smoking initiation and personality. Paper presented at the meeting of the Research Society on Alcoholism, San Antonio, TX, June 19–24, 1993a

Madden PA, Heath AC, Bucholz KK, et al: Novelty seeking and the genetic determinants of smoking initiation and problems related to alcohol use in female twins. Paper presented at the 23rd annual meeting of the Behavior Genetics Association, Sydney, Australia, July 13–16, 1993b

Martin NG, Eaves LJ: The genetical analysis of covariance structure. Heredity 28:79–95, 1977

Martin NG, Jardine R: Eysenck's contributions to behavior genetics, in Hans Eysenck: Consensus and Controversy. Edited by Modgil S, Modgil C. Lewes, Sussex, Falmer, 1986, pp 13–62

McCrae RR, Costa PT: The structure of interpersonal traits: Wiggins's circumplex and the five-factor model. J Pers Soc Psychol 56:586–595, 1989

Neale MC: Mx Statistical Modeling. Richmond, Department of Psychiatry, Medical College of Virginia, 1992

Neale MC, Cardon LR: Methodology for Genetic Studies of Twins and Families, NATO ASI Series. Dordrecht, The Netherlands, Kluwer Academic, 1992

Pedersen NL: Genetic and environmental continuity and change in personality, in Twins as a Tool of Behavioral Genetics. Edited by Bouchard TJ, Propping P. Chichester, England, Wiley, 1993, pp 147–164

Pedersen NL, Plomin R, McClearn GE, et al: Neuroticism, extraversion, and related traits in adult twins reared apart and reared together. J Pers Soc Psychol 55:950–957, 1988

Price RA, Vandenberg SG, Iyer H, et al: Components of variation in normal personality. J Pers Soc Psychol 43:328–340, 1982

Rose RJ, Koskenvuo M, Kaprio J, et al: Shared genes, shared experiences, and similarity of personality: data from 14,288 adult Finnish co-twins. J Pers Soc Psychol 54:161–171, 1988

Scarr S, Webber PL, Weinberg RA, et al: Personality resemblance among adolescents and their parents in biologically related and adoptive families. J Pers Soc Psychol 40:885–898, 1981

Shields J: Monozygotic Twins: Brought Up Apart and Brought Up Together. Oxford, Oxford University Press, 1962

Svrakic D, Whitehead C, Przybeck TR, et al: Differential diagnosis of personality disorders by the seven factor model of temperament and character. Arch Gen Psychiatry 50:991–999, 1993

Tellegen A: Structure of mood and personality and their relevance to assessing anxiety, with an emphasis on self-report, in Anxiety and the Anxiety Disorders. Edited by Tuma AH, Maser JD. Hillsdale, NJ, Lawrence Erlbaum Associates, 1985, pp 681–706

Tellegen A, Lykken DT, Bouchard TJ, et al: Personality similarity in twins reared apart and together. J Pers Soc Psychol 54:1031–1039, 1988

Emerging Neuroscience Approaches to Understanding Cognition and Psychopathology: Positron-Emission Tomography Imaging

Wayne C. Drevets, M.D.

The development of functional brain imaging technologies such as positron-emission tomography (PET) has vastly improved our capabilities for noninvasively studying the distributed neural networks that support the specific mental operations related to cognitive processes. Compared with techniques involving lesion effects, electrical stimulation and recording, postmortem neuroreceptor assessment, neurochemical measures from body fluids, or neuropsychological test performance, functional imaging affords superior spatial resolution and the ability to image multiple structures functioning simultaneously in vivo. Currently, PET measurements of regional cerebral blood flow (BF) permit spatial resolution of ≈ 5 mm and temporal resolution of 40 sec (Raichle 1987). However, methods for dynamically measuring BF and metabolism with magnetic resonance imaging (MRI) are being developed that may permit measurements with spatial resolution < 5 mm and temporal resolution of a few hundred milliseconds (Ogawa et al. 1992).

The application of PET and other modern imaging technologies such as MRI and magnetic resonance spectroscopy to investigations of psychopathology holds the potential to transport psychiatry into a new era in which pathophysiology, rather than signs and symptoms, guides the nosology of psychiatric disorders. These emerging neuroscience approaches may also identify "normal" variations in the neural networks employed in cognitive processing that underlie some differences in personality and temperament.

This chapter discusses some of the principles relevant to the design and interpretation of functional imaging studies. Experimental series performed in our laboratory to delineate the functional anatomical correlates of language and major depression are specifically described to illustrate the application of these principles in investigations of cognitive processing and psychopathology, respectively. Although the image data reviewed here were acquired using PET technology, the principles of experimental design and data interpretation discussed below generally apply to measurements of BF and metabolism obtained using other functional imaging modalities as well.

PET Imaging of Brain Function

The PET camera tomographically images the annihilation radiation generated as positrons are absorbed in matter, recording highly accurate spatial representations of the distribution of a radionuclide that has previously been inhaled or infused (Figure 14–1; for reviews see Phelps et al. 1986; Raichle 1987). The PET image is effectively equivalent to a quantitative tissue radiogram in laboratory animals but affords the advantage that it is noninvasive and can be performed in a living human. A variety of positron-emitting radionuclides are available for administration during PET scanning, permitting three-dimensional imaging of BF, blood volume, glucose or oxygen metabolism, water extraction (across the blood-brain barrier), or neuroreceptor binding.

The Relationship Between Brain Function, BF, and Metabolism

In 1890 Roy and Sherrington published their pioneering observations that an "automatic mechanism" exists in the brain such that local var-

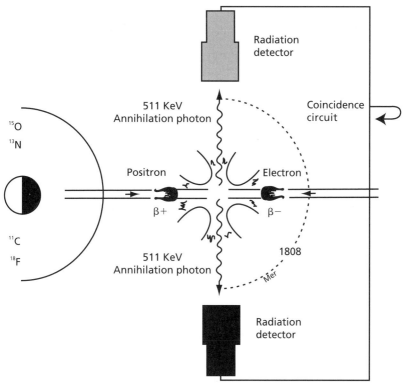

FIGURE **14-1.** *Detection scheme for PET. Radionuclides employed in PET decay by emission of positrons from a nucleus unstable because of a deficiency in neutrons. Positrons lose their kinetic energy after traveling a finite distance (~1–6 mm) and, when brought to rest, interact with electrons. The 2 particles annihilate, and their mass is converted to 2 annihilation photons traveling at ~180 degrees from each other with an energy of 511 KeV. Annihilation photons are detected by the PET camera, using opposing radiation detectors connected by electronic coincidence circuits that record an event when 2 photons arrive simultaneously. A major factor determining the ultimate resolution of PET is the distance traveled by the positron before its annihilation. [Reprinted with permission from Raichle 1983.]*

iations in functional activity are accompanied by local variations in blood supply (Roy and Sherrington 1890). This hypothesis has been corroborated by numerous experiments both before and since the development of modern tracer methodology (for review see Raichle 1987). These experiments have specifically demonstrated that local alterations in neuronal activity are associated with rises in regional BF and metabolism that follow the cortical electrical activity by ≈0.5 sec (Figure 14–2). Therefore, by acquiring measurements of regional BF or metabolism, functional imaging techniques provide detailed pictures of local neuronal work.

The ability to noninvasively image regional neuronal work in terms of BF and metabolism affords unprecedented opportunities to map the cortical regions involved in cognitive processing. Functional imaging techniques have identified the neuroanatomical correlates of motor, somatosensory, visual, auditory, linguistic, and purely cognitive tasks

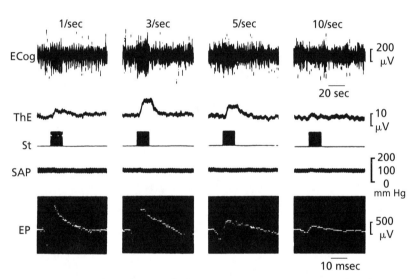

FIGURE 14–2. *Recordings of electrocorticogram (ECoG), local BF recorded with a thermoelement (ThE) in the cortical projection field of left forepaw in right sensorimotor cortex, systemic arterial blood pressure (SAP), and sensory evoked potential (EP) in a cat during stimulation of left forepaw with 15-V rectangular pulses of 0.3 msec duration. Output of stimulator (St) records stimulation time. Changes in ThE do not appear until stimulus frequency reaches 3 Hz, as the average ThE during period of measurement is not appreciably affected at stimulation frequencies as low as 1 Hz. At stimulation frequencies >3 Hz the amplitude of EP and ThE decline in parallel. [K.-A. Hossman, personal communication, as reported by Raichle (1987), reproduced with permission from Raichle 1987, p. 659.]*

using strategies that compare dynamic images obtained during an experimental task with images acquired during a control task (Figures 14–3 and 14–4). Such experimental paradigms may eventually prove fruitful in elucidating and distinguishing the functional anatomy of the experience, evaluation, and expression of human emotion, and variations in cognitive processing that are related to personality and temperament.

Brain mapping studies using PET are generally limited to measurements of regional BF using oxygen-15 labeled water or butanol. This is because the short half-life ($t_{1/2}$) of ^{15}O (about 2 min) permits image acquisition over a sufficiently short time period (40 sec) to capture functional changes related to neuronal activity before the BF signal decays (Mintun et al. 1989). In addition, the short $t_{1/2}$ of ^{15}O permits BF measurements to be repeated at 10 min intervals, so that BF scans can be acquired in different cognitive-behavioral states during the same scanning session (see Figure 14–3).

In contrast to measurements of BF, PET measurements of metabolism are less suitable for activation paradigms. Although the increases

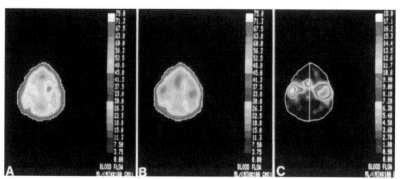

FIGURE 14–3. *PET images of a single subject. A. Image showing the cerebral BF in the resting control state. B. Image showing BF during bilateral vibrotactile stimulation of the fingers. Images A and B were obtained 10 minutes apart and pass through the same plane. C. Image showing the difference between Images A and B to demonstrate the increase in cerebral BF induced by finger stimulation. The lateral response areas are in the first somatosensory cortex. The single medial response area is in the supplementary motor area. [Reprinted from Fox et al. 1987 with permission.]*

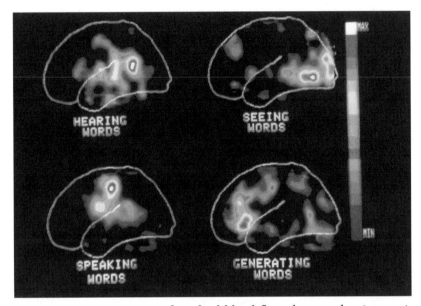

FIGURE 14–4. *PET images of cerebral blood flow changes showing cortical areas in the left hemisphere activated by single word processing (Petersen et al. 1988, 1989). The sagittal image sections shown are from composite images of mean blood flow changes generated by superimposing and subtracting images acquired during the experimental and control tasks and then averaging the resulting blood flow difference images across subjects. The Seeing Words image demonstrates areas where flow increases as subjects passively view nouns presented on a video screen, as compared with when they view a cross-hair on the same screen. The Hearing Words image reveals areas where flow increases as nouns are presented auditorily, rather than visually. The Speaking Words comparison shows areas where flow increases as subjects repeat aloud the nouns (presented either visually or auditorily) as compared with when they "passively" view or hear the noun. Finally, the Generating Words image shows flow increases as subjects view or hear nouns and then generate aloud a verb related to each noun, relative to when they simply repeat the noun aloud. See text for description of the anatomical areas shown and interpretation of the results. Anterior is to the left, dorsal to the page top. [Reprinted with permission from Raichle 1991.]*

in regional BF and glucose metabolism during cortical activity are correlated with each other, rising, for example, 51% and 50%, respectively, in the striate cortex during visual stimulation (Fox et al. 1988), the long $t_{1/2}$ of the radionuclide involved in measurements of ^{18}F-deoxyglucose metabolism (about 2 hours) mandates a longer image acquisition period (generally 45 min). This limits the ability to repeat measurements during the same scan session and is generally too long a period to sustain a cognitive task because of subject fatigue, signal decay, and rehearsal effects over time (see the end of the next section).

In contrast to the tight coupling between BF and glucose metabolism, focal uncoupling of BF and oxidative metabolism occurs during the first ≈ 2 min of sensory stimulation (Fox and Raichle 1986, 1987), making PET measurements of oxygen metabolism less satisfactory for functional mapping studies. For example, during neural activation induced by somatosensory stimulation, the mean BF elevation (29%) far exceeds the concomitant local increase in oxygen utilization (5%) (Fox and Raichle 1986). However, in spite of the limitations of PET measurements of oxygen utilization, signal changes related to oxygen uptake can be very sensitively measured during sensory stimulation with functional MRI (Ogawa et al. 1992). These and other functional MRI techniques may eventually replace PET measurements of BF for brain mapping endeavors because of their superior spatial resolution, freedom from radiation exposure, and lesser expense.

The experimental strategies employed in brain mapping studies using PET typically rely upon paired comparisons involving BF scans acquired in two different cognitive-behavioral states. These BF images are superimposed and subtracted from one another to highlight regional BF changes that presumably reflect the mental events distinguishing the two states (see Figures 14–3 and 14–4). Because each subject serves as his or her own control, nonspecific BF variations related to differences in anatomy and head positioning are avoided, and the sensitivity and specificity of measured BF changes are enhanced. The superior sensitivity of the paired image subtraction technique is especially critical in studies of higher cognitive functions such as memory, language, or attention, because the BF changes associated with these activities are relatively subtle.

The number of possible interpretations for each BF change observed in a brain mapping paradigm increases with the number of mental operations that differ between the experimental and control tasks. Thus complex cognitive processes such as memory, language, or attention must be dissected into a series of simple, component mental operations. These elemental steps are imaged in successive control-activation subtraction pairs so that the distributed neural networks involved in each aspect of a more complex task can be isolated from one another.

Investigating the Cortical Anatomy of Language With PET

A series of experiments performed in our laboratory to investigate the cortical anatomy of single-word processing demonstrates the application of these principles in a PET study of language (Petersen et al. 1988, 1989, 1990). Extant knowledge in cognitive psychology, linguistics, and clinical neurology was used to parse single-word processing into three component steps that were isolated from one another by scanning subjects in each of four behavioral conditions (Coltheart 1985; Damasio 1984; LaBerge and Samuels 1974). The four behavioral tasks were used to form a three-level subtractive hierarchy such that each task state added a small number of mental operations to the previous task state.

The first level of comparison involved the subtraction between a BF image acquired as the subject passively viewed nouns presented on a video screen (at 1 Hz) and a BF image acquired while the subject viewed a crosshair on the same screen (see Figure 14–4). This comparison demonstrated the neuroanatomical correlates of visual input and involuntary word processing. The BF responses were interpreted as indicating two levels of computation: passive sensory processing, which was associated with BF increases in the primary visual (striate) cortex,[1] and modality-specific word-form processing, which was associated with BF increases in the extrastriate cortex.[2]

---

[1]Other simple visual stimuli also produce BF increases in this area (Fox et al. 1986).

[2]Subsequent experiments demonstrated that this area is also activated by words and pronounceable non-words, but not by consonant letter strings or false fonts (Petersen et al. 1990).

In a separate but parallel comparison, the nouns were presented auditorily instead of visually (see Figure 14–4). This resulted in BF increases in areas of the temporal cortex, where BF had not changed when the nouns were presented visually (Petersen et al. 1988, 1989). However, BF increases could be elicited in these temporal cortical regions if a pair of words were presented visually and the subjects were required to judge in silence whether the two words rhymed (Raichle 1990). This exemplifies the functionally flexible nature of the distributed, modular organization of the brain.

In the second level of comparison in the investigation of single-word processing, the subjects were again presented a series of nouns, but this time they repeated the words aloud during the PET scan. The previous task in which the subjects passively viewed nouns served as the control task for comparison with the higher level "repeat words" task. Flow increased in the brain areas related to motor output and articulatory coding: the mouth area of the primary sensorimotor cortex, the supplemental motor area, and a portion of the insular cortex (it was later demonstrated that BF increased in this insular area if subjects moved their mouth and tongue in the absence of visual word presentation or verbal output). These same brain areas were activated if the nouns were presented auditorily rather than visually (see Figure 14–4).

In the third and final level of comparison, subjects were asked to view the nouns but to generate and state aloud a verb related to each noun. Whether the words were presented visually or auditorily, BF increased in the inferior prefrontal cortex (PFC: see Figure 14–4) and the anterior cingulate gyrus. The cingulate area was thought to participate in an anterior attention system engaged in selection for action, while the prefrontal area was thought to be involved in the process of semantic association.

It is noteworthy that the BF responses in the anterior cingulate and inferior prefrontal cortices during the verb generation task were most evident while the task was still novel and required active attention. If the subjects were permitted to repeatedly practice generating verbs for the same noun list before the PET scan was acquired, significantly smaller BF increases occurred in these areas during the verb generation task, and a reciprocal BF increase appeared in the sylvian-insular cortex (Raichle et al. 1991). The practice-related decrement in prefrontal and cingulate BF correlated with the practice-related decrease in reaction times associated with performing the task. This demonstration that the neurophysiology associated with a task changes as the performance of the task becomes more automatic with rehearsal introduces another level of complexity in the selection of behavioral tasks.

Potential Applications of Functional Imaging in Studies of Personality and Temperament

The data presented in the previous section, along with other evidence, indicate that the human brain is characterized by a functionally flexible modular organization consisting of multiple routes that may be used depending upon factors related to stimulus characteristics, task demands, habit formation, or behavioral output. It is conceivable that variations in cognitive processing contribute to the interpersonal differences in patterns of behavior, thinking, and emotion that underlie differences in personality and temperament. Toward this end dynamic imaging during cognitive and emotional activation paradigms may provide important insights into the neurophysiologic concomitants of personality and temperament.

For example, in contrast to the relatively stable constellation of neural structures that participate in single word processing (in right-handed subjects), diverse patterns of BF change have been observed in our laboratory during an activation paradigm that involves a short-term memory task (Fiez et al. 1986). These data have suggested that during short-term memory processing different individuals employ distinct cognitive strategies that are supported by different functional anatomical correlates. It is conceivable that such interindividual differences in "normal brain function" may relate to differences in personality and temperament. Perhaps individuals who consistently behave, think, or feel differently from one another do so because of differences in information acquisition or retrieval. It may thus be possible to associate personality or temperament traits with distinct patterns of

BF change during the performance of attentional, memory, or language tasks.

Activation paradigms involving emotional induction tasks could also prove fruitful in understanding personality and temperament. Because emotional responsiveness appears important in governing personality factors such as reward dependence or harm avoidance (Cloninger 1987), activation paradigms that examine emotional processing could be used to investigate the neurophysiologic basis of differences in these traits. For example, our laboratory previously employed a paradigm involving the anticipation of a painful electrical stimulus to induce anxiety. Perhaps this paradigm could be used to identify differences in the regional BF changes during anticipatory fear in subjects who are low as opposed to high in harm avoidance.

Another type of functional imaging paradigm that may yield valuable data regarding personality and temperament involves pharmacologic activation. Besides the utility of PET in quantitating neuroreceptor binding using radiolabeled receptor ligands (for review see Wong and Young 1991), PET can also provide information about the functional sensitivity of receptor systems by measuring changes in BF or metabolism during pharmacologic challenges (Rowe and Perlmutter 1991; Roy-Byrne et al. 1993). Pharmacologic activation paradigms could be employed to explore whether differences in personality or temperament correlate with differences in the responsiveness of various receptor systems. For example, the hypothesis that dopamine receptor sensitivity varies with novelty seeking (Cloninger 1987) could be approached by comparing neurophysiologic responses to the administration of dopamine agonists in subjects who are low as opposed to high in novelty seeking.

In the experiments proposed here, specific structures would be targeted based upon a priori hypotheses. Where less information exists, however, omnibus techniques for image analysis have been developed to guide hypotheses regarding the regions involved in cognition or psychopathology (Drevets et al. 1992a; Friston et al. 1992). For example, correlational images (created by computing correlation coefficients of the relationship between regional physiology and clinical ratings for each image voxel) have been used to identify brain regions involved in auditory hallucinations (Friston et al. 1992). Statistical maps that correlate regional BF or metabolism with dimensional ratings of personality traits could similarly be used to investigate the neurophysiologic correlates of personality and temperament.[3]

In contrast to measurements obtained during cognitive, emotional, or pharmacologic challenges, measures of BF or metabolism in the resting condition are less likely to be sensitive to differences related to personality or temperament. The magnitudes of the resting abnormalities reported in subject samples with affective, psychotic, or anxiety disorders have typically been small, with differences ranging from about 5% to 15% relative to control subjects. Resting physiologic differences associated with personality traits are expected to be even more subtle and may fail to rise above the background level of statistical noise in a PET image. Thus, the superior sensitivity of the activation paradigm makes it the more promising experimental design for functional imaging studies of personality and temperament.

PET Imaging in the Investigation of Psychopathology

Functional imaging technologies are also capable of identifying the pathophysiologic concomitants of disease states. PET has been used to study neurologic disorders such as Parkinson's disease, Huntington's disease, dementia, and epilepsy, and psychiatric disorders such as schizophrenia, affective illness, anxiety disorders, and substance abuse (Andreason 1989; Drevets 1992a; Phelps et al. 1986). Imaging holds particular promise in studies of psychiatric disorders because the absence of gross neuropathological changes in these disorders has previously obscured their pathophysiologic concomitants. Moreover, the absence of gross anatomical changes in most psychiatric disorders makes them well suited for functional imaging studies, because differ-

---

[3] However, the large number of computations required to create statistical images mandates that such analyses be used only for generating hypotheses regarding the regions that contain intergroup differences or intragroup correlations. These hypotheses should be rigorously tested in separate subject samples using measurements confined to the regions-of-interest indicated by the original statistical map (Drevets et al. 1992a).

ences in BF or metabolism can only be expected to reflect functional activity in the brain if the underlying neuroanatomy remains intact.[4]

Nevertheless, comparisons between ill and normal subjects are more complicated to interpret than activation paradigms involving normal subjects. This is because differences in BF or metabolism between patients and control subjects have many possible interpretations. They may represent 1) the pathophysiologic abnormalities associated with the genetic and/or environmental predisposition to a disorder; 2) the state dependent changes that reflect the cognitive, emotional, or behavioral manifestations of the illness; or 3) the potential structural changes resulting from the illness or past treatment (for review see Drevets 1993). Because functional image data are affected by so many variables, a thoughtful strategy is required so that successive experiments systematically isolate each possible cause of physiologic difference.

Ultimately, information from disciplines capable of exploration on more basic levels (e.g., in vivo or postmortem neuroreceptor imaging, histopathologic investigations, and electrophysiologic recording) may be required to answer some of the questions raised by functional imaging data. Toward this end PET data should prove useful in directing basic scientists to the specific brain regions where such analyses are likely to prove fruitful. Even if the molecular nature of the abnormalities identified by PET remains obscure, by elucidating the neurophysiologic correlates of psychiatric disorders imaging may provide the ability to subclassify broad diagnostic categories such as major depression (see next section) or schizophrenia. The definition of subtypes based upon pathophysiology rather than upon symptoms could prove invaluable to studies investigating prognosis, treatment outcome, biochemical markers, and genetic linkage. For example, if trait markers for a particular disorder can be identified using PET, image data could guide genetic linkage analyses by identifying genotypic carriers who have not yet manifested phenotypic changes within a family lineage.

---

[4]In contrast, the presence of atrophy in neurodegenerative disorders such as dementia confounds the interpretation of PET image data, because tomographic image data are affected by the inclusion of metabolically inactive cerebrospinal fluid spaces resulting from atrophy (known as the "partial volume effect") (Mazziotta et al. 1981). In patient samples in whom atrophy exists it becomes difficult to determine whether measured decreases in BF or metabolism reflect changes in physiology, loss of tissue, or combinations of the two.

Finally, imaging may eventually prove clinically useful in guiding diagnostic and treatment decisions.

PET Imaging in Major Depression

A series of studies performed in our laboratory to investigate the regional BF abnormalities in unipolar depression illustrates some of the methodologic considerations relevant to PET studies of psychopathology. Primary major depression is an illness well suited for functional imaging studies, because neurochemical, neuroendocrine, and neuropsychological assessments have indicated that dysfunction may exist within several parts of the central nervous system in major depression (Goodwin and Jamison 1990), yet gross pathological changes are generally absent.[5]

Moreover, the episodic nature of major depression and its excellent response to treatment permit the application of a number of strategies to differentiate the physiologic correlates of symptoms from the pathophysiologic changes that may underlie the tendency to become depressed. For example, state-related differences (present only when symptomatic) may be distinguished from trait differences (present whether symptomatic or asymptomatic). In addition, because many of the symptoms of major depression represent exaggerations or extensions of cognitive and emotional states that can be experienced by subjects who are not depressed, the nature of BF changes related to the depressed state can be explored by imaging normal subjects during experimentally induced sadness, anxiety, self-depreciation, or sleep deprivation.

One of the challenges facing imaging studies of major depression stems from the likelihood that this disorder actually encompasses a heterogeneous group of disorders (Winokur 1982). Besides the obvious

---

[5]An important exception to this are the arteriosclerotic/ischemic lesions that have been identified in subjects with the onset of depression after age 60 (Chimowitz et al. 1992; Deicken et al. 1989; Fiegel et al. 1991). The presence of such lesions would render PET images uninterpretable since measured decreases in BF and metabolism could no longer be presumed to reflect neuronal activity. This problem probably confounds the PET studies that have included such elderly subjects with depression in their sample.

clinical heterogeneity extant within affective disease, biological heterogeneity also exists. For example, neuroendocrine and neurochemical abnormalities are typically present in subgroups, but not in entire samples of subjects with depression (Goodwin and Jamison 1990). The diversity of responses to distinct antidepressant therapies also suggests biological heterogeneity. If major depression is associated with multiple pathophysiologic states, it is presumably be associated with an assortment of different PET images (discussed later in this chapter). Thus the results of imaging studies may vary depending on the composition of their subject sample.

For example, subjects with unipolar and bipolar depression appear to be neurochemically, pharmacologically, and genetically distinct (Goodwin and Jamison 1990; Moldin et al. 1991; Rice et al. 1987; Schatzberg et al. 1989). Consistent with these differences, several imaging studies have reported that they substantially differ in their respective circulatory and metabolic correlates (Baxter et al. 1985; Buchsbaum et al. 1986; Delvenne et al. 1990; Drevets et al. 1992b; O'Connell et al. 1989; Schwartz et al. 1987). Consequently, studies combining unipolar and bipolar subjects (which constitute the majority of imaging studies of affective disorders) are difficult to interpret. In fact, many of the discrepancies across studies may simply be due to differences in their subject composition.

In our initial investigation of major depression we attempted to select a homogeneous sample of subjects with primary, unipolar depression using criteria for familial pure depressive disease (FPDD; Winokur 1982), defined as primary major depression in an individual who has a first degree relative with primary depression but no family history of alcoholism, antisocial personality, or mania. Because this classification identifies three subtypes of primary, unipolar depression based upon a trait variable, namely family history, as well as upon clinical criteria, it may pertain to pathophysiology, given the heritability of affective disorders (Moldin et al. 1991; Rice et al. 1987). In addition, FPDD was associated with a much higher rate of abnormal cortisol suppression following dexamethasone administration than the other two subtypes of primary unipolar depression included in this classification (depression spectrum disease and sporadic depressive disease), suggesting that FPDD may be the more likely subtype to be associated with biologic markers (Winokur 1982). Finally, by excluding subjects with a family history of mania, the criteria for FPDD enhance the likelihood of obtaining subjects with genetic purity for unipolar depression (Moldin et al. 1991; Rice et al. 1987), a critical concern for PET imaging studies because, as described later, subjects with unipolar and bipolar depression differ in their respective circulatory and metabolic correlates.

The Functional Anatomy of FPDD

We have been investigating the functional neuroanatomy of FPDD using PET measurements of regional BF. In our initial study we obtained evidence that flow is increased in the left PFC and the left amygdala in the depressed phase of FPDD (Drevets et al. 1992a; Figures 14–5 and 14–6). In a group of subjects with FPDD who were scanned in remission, regional BF was normal in the left PFC but remained elevated in the left amygdala (Figure 14–7). These data suggested that FPDD is associated with an abnormality related to the state of being depressed in the left PFC and possibly with an abnormality related to the trait of being susceptible to depression in the amygdala.

Increased BF in the amygdala and the PFC in the depressed phase of FPDD may represent either physiologic concomitants of their roles in mediating the cognitive, emotional, or behavioral symptoms of depression, or disrupted physiology associated with the primary pathophysiologic defect causing such symptoms. Although one cannot yet decide which interpretation is correct, determining the state versus trait nature of these abnormalities begins to address this question. Because the abnormality in the left PFC appeared to be a state marker in FPDD, it presumably reflected the physiology underlying the expression of at least part of the depressive syndrome. In contrast, if the abnormality in the amygdala is a trait marker, it may represent a more fundamental aspect of the disease process and the vulnerability to major depression. The following discussion demonstrates our attempt to integrate these PET findings in the PFC and amygdala with other PET imaging, electrophysiology, lesion analysis, and neuroanatomy data in order to generate hypotheses regarding these structures' involvement in depression.

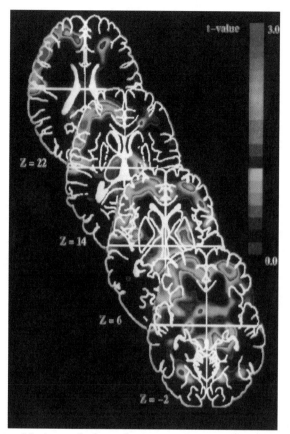

FIGURE 14–5. *Horizontal slices from an image consisting of unpaired t-values that compared stereotaxically standardized BF scans from 13 subjects with unipolar depression with FPDD and 35 control subjects (Drevets et al. 1992a; Winokur 1982). The areas of positive t-values illustrated correspond to areas where BF in the subjects with depression exceeded that of the control subjects. The area of increased flow in the left PFC involved much of the ventrolateral PFC and extended through the tissue immediately caudal to the frontal pole to include part of the left medial PFC (which includes the pregenual portion of the anterior cingulate gyrus). The t-image is used to generate hypotheses regarding regions-of-interest that may contain intergroup differences. The existence of a significant BF elevation in this PFC region in unipolar depression has been confirmed in two additional samples of subjects who also met criteria for FPDD. The t-image planes are overlaid on corresponding atlas section outlines, and located by their distance in mm from the bicommissural line by the Z-axis coordinate listed beneath each slice (Talairach et al. 1967). The x and y axes locate the midpoint of the bicommissural line. Left is toward the reader's left, anterior is toward the page-top.*

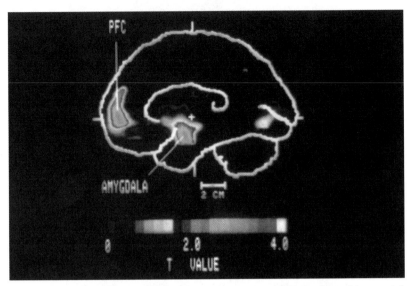

FIGURE 14–6. *t-Image corresponding to increased BF in the subjects with depression at the sagittal plane through the center of the amygdala (x = 21 mm left of midline). Anterior is toward the reader's left. The z and y axes locate the midpoint of the bicommissural line. The most rostral part of the left PFC region is also demonstrated (see Figure 14–5 for the full extent of this region). [Reprinted with permission from Drevets et al. 1992a.]*

The PFC. The abnormality in the left PFC appeared to include lateral, anterior, and medial components (see Figure 14–5). The lateral component contained much of the left ventrolateral PFC (VLPFC), and the medial component involved the medial orbital cortex and the pregenual portion of the anterior cingulate gyrus. All of these regions are heavily interconnected with the ipsilateral amygdala (Amaral and Price 1984).

The PFC contains relatively high proportions of cells that undergo sustained change in their rate of discharge during the delay period between a reward-linked sensory cue and the subsequent response to it (Fuster 1989). It has been suggested that the PFC in general is concerned with the use of short-term, representational memory, such that behavior is guided by representations of a stimulus instead of the stimulus itself (Goldman-Rakic 1987). This allows behavior to be gov-

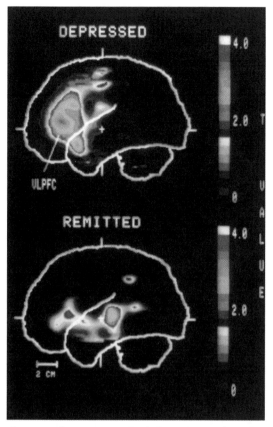

FIGURE 14–7. *Increased activity in the left PFC was found in the subjects with depression but not the subjects in remission. Each t-image indicates areas where subjects in the depressed (top) and remitted (bottom) phases of FPDD have increased flow relative to the control subjects. Mean voxel t-values for the sagittal planes from 47–57 mm left of the bicommissural line are demonstrated. Legend: VLPFC, ventrolateral PFC. [Reprinted with permission from Drevets et al. 1992a.]*

erned by concepts or memories in the absence of informative external cues (Fuster 1989; Goldman-Rakic 1987).

In the area of the left VLPFC where BF was elevated in depression, BF also increased in normal subjects during the performance of two tasks that involved making associations with information being held in representational memory. In the first, subjects were presented nouns (for 150 msec) and asked to generate related verbs (Petersen et al. 1989), while in the second, subjects were asked to contemplate sad thoughts or memories to self-induce a sad mood (Pardo et al. 1993). A common feature of both tasks was the process of associating thoughts or emotions with a previous thought. The subjects with depression were also engaged in a similar associative operation, as they reported experiencing incessant negative thoughts during the PET scan.

The three experimental conditions that resulted in increased BF in the left VLPFC (generating verbs, contemplating sad thoughts, and depressive ruminations) all involved making associations with information being held in representational memory: semantic associations in the case of the language task and emotional associations in the case of depressive ruminations and the sad thoughts task. Thus, increased flow in the left VLPFC in depression may reflect a physiologic correlate of the associative computations that accompany depressive ruminations. Possibly consistent with this hypothesis, Perris and Monakhov (1979) found that left frontal electroencephalogram (EEG) activity in subjects with depression correlated with ruminative ideation, but not with depressed mood.

Although PET is incapable of distinguishing whether the same neuronal populations within the VLPFC are involved in each of the three conditions (major depression, induced sadness, and verb generation), it would appear that rather than serving as an emotion specific area, the left VLPFC may serve a more general function in mediating associative computations. The specificity for cognitive versus emotional states may arise via the distributed networks that involve other neural structures. For example, flow increased in the left dorsolateral PFC during verb generation (Petersen et al. 1989), but not during induced sadness or major depression. In contrast, BF was increased in the medial orbital cortex in both the depressed phase of FPDD and the sadness induction task, but not in the verb generation task.

Flow changes in the anterior cingulate cortex also differed between the emotion-related conditions and the verb generation task. During verb generation, flow increased in the portion of the anterior cingulate cortex that was dorsocaudal to the genu of the corpus callosum, an area which has been implicated in attention and selection for action by a variety of PET data (Petersen et al. 1989). Flow was unchanged in this portion of the anterior cingulate in major depression. In contrast, BF was increased in the pregenual portion of the anterior cingulate gyrus (which is heavily connected with the amygdala) in depression and induced sadness, but not in the verb generation task (Drevets et al. 1992a; Drevets and Raichle 1995).

The medial orbital and pregenual cingulate regions that distinguished the emotion-related conditions have previously been implicated in emotional processing (LeDoux 1987; Papez 1937). In the orbital cortex nearly one-half of all cells demonstrate altered firing rates during the delay period between stimulus and response, and posttrial activity is related to the presence or absence of reward (Rosenkilde et al. 1981). One type of cells appears to encode the availability of reward, and a second type encodes deviations from expectancy of reward (Rosenkilde et al. 1981). Damasio et al. (1990) has reported that humans with destruction of the medial orbital cortex lose the experience and expression of emotion related to concepts that would ordinarily evoke emotion, yet they have no difficulty forming plans or working intellectually through problems. It has been suggested that the association of concept with emotion may be mediated by the ventral PFC (Collins 1988; Damasio et al. 1990).

In the medial PFC, the anterior cingulate cortex appears to participate in the motivational aspects of stimulus coding, as has been suggested by reinforcement associated with appetitive rewards, affective responses to noxious stimuli, and significance coding (Vogt 1993). Vogt (1991) has hypothesized that in the cingulate cortex perceptual events are constructed from distributed representations of sensory space and integrated with affective features. Bilateral cingulate ablation has been associated with akinetic mutism, characterized by the absence of motivation to behave or speak (Damasio and Van Hoesen 1983). In contrast, more limited surgical lesions within the anterior cingulate ameliorate severe depressive and anxiety syndromes (Ballantine et al. 1987).

The functions of the cingulate gyrus differ across its ≈ 15 cm length. For example, electrical stimulation produces arousal and heightened attention, simple motor movements, or affective changes such as euphoria, anguish, sadness, or fear (Damasio 1983) depending upon which portion of the cingulate is stimulated (Laitinen 1979; Talairach et al. 1973). In PET studies of language and attention, sites of increased activity in the anterior cingulate have been identified in the portion of the cingulate caudal and dorsal to the genu of the corpus callosum (Corbetta et al. 1991; Pardo et al. 1990; Petersen et al. 1989; Posner and Petersen 1990). The role of this cingulate area has been interpreted to be related to attention and selection for action (Corbetta et al. 1991; Posner and Petersen 1990). In contrast, the pregenual portion of the anterior cingulate cortex (area 32) may be more specifically involved in emotion, as BF increases there in major depression and induced sadness but not in the language or attentional tasks (Drevets et al. 1992a; Drevets and Raichle 1997).

The amygdala.   There is considerable evidence that the amygdala plays a role in assigning affective significance to experiential stimuli (Gloor et al. 1982; LeDoux 1987; Neill 1988; Nishijo et al. 1988). The amygdala receives highly processed exteroceptive input from all sensory modalities, and it has outputs both to areas of the hypothalamus and brainstem that are involved in organizing the autonomic and behavioral responses associated with emotion and to the PFC and other limbic forebrain structures (LeDoux 1987; Price et al. 1987; Ricardo and Koh 1978; Sarter and Markowitsch 1985; Turner et al. 1980). Individual cells within the amygdala respond to a variety of sensory and visceral stimuli, and some of these show differential responses to aversive and rewarding stimuli (Nishijo et al. 1988). Bilateral destruction of the amygdala results in the "psychic blindness" of the Klüver-Bucy syndrome, such that the significance of stimuli cannot be recognized (Aggleton and Passingham 1981; Weiskrantz 1956). In addition, bursts of EEG activity have been recorded in the amygdala during recollection of specific emotional events (Halgren 1981), and electrical stimulation of the amygdala can evoke emotional experiences (Gloor et al. 1982).

It is conceivable that dysfunction of the amygdala in evaluating affective significance could yield a state where negative affective labels are inappropriately assigned to all stimuli—resulting in depressed mood, or where positive affective labels are not assigned to any stimuli—resulting in anhedonia. Our data suggested that increased BF in the amygdala reflects a trait abnormality in FPDD, and that the magnitude of this abnormality correlates with the severity of the depressive symptoms (Drevets et al. 1992a). As discussed later, we have hypothesized that abnormal activity in the amygdala could potentially drive both the severity of depression and the propensity to relapse following remission.

Exploring the Neural Circuitry of Depression With PET

Local changes in BF and metabolism generally reflect the energy utilization associated with synaptic activity, rather than the electrophysiologic activity of cell bodies (Raichle 1987; Schwartz et al. 1979). Because synaptic activity may originate from cell bodies distantly located from observed changes as well as from local intercellular communication, consideration of the neural circuitry involving the site of a BF difference becomes imperative in interpreting PET image data. For example, in our study of FPDD, we explored the neural circuitry that may involve the PFC and the amygdala and obtained additional evidence that BF is abnormal in the left medial thalamus and the caudate (Figure 14–8; Drevets et al. 1992a). These data along with other evidence suggested that circuits involving the PFC, amygdala and related parts of the striatum, pallidum, and medial thalamus participate in the functional neuroanatomy of FPDD (Folstein et al. 1991; McHugh 1989; Swerdlow and Koob 1987).

Our findings of increased BF in the amygdala and the PFC coupled with indications of increased flow in the medial thalamus and reduced flow in the medial caudate specifically suggest that two interconnected circuits are involved in the pathophysiology of unipolar depression: a limbic-thalamo-cortical circuit involving the amygdala, the mediodorsal nucleus of the thalamus (MD; located in the medial thalamus) and the ventrolateral and medial PFC; and a limbic-striatal-pallidal-thalamic (LSPT) circuit involving related parts of the striatum and the ventral pallidum as well as the components of the other circuit (Figure 14–9). The first of these circuits can be conceptualized as an excitatory triangular circuit whereby the amygdala and the PFC are interconnected by excitatory projections with each other and with MD

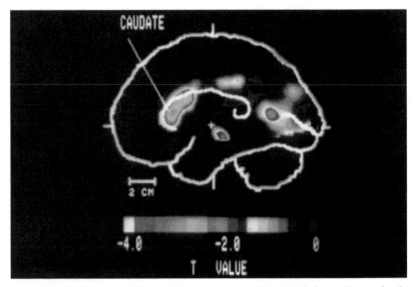

FIGURE **14–8.** *Decreased activity was observed in the left caudate of subjects with unipolar depression . The t-image demonstrates areas of decreased activity in the subjects with depression relative to the control subjects in a sagittal projection of the greatest voxel t-values in all planes between the midline and 10 mm left of midline. Anterior is to the reader's left. The coordinates for the affected area include the head of the caudate nucleus and an arc passing posteriorly, dorsally, and laterally, suggesting that the caudate body may also be involved. The color bar is reversed to indicate negative t-values. [Reprinted with permission from Drevets et al. 1992a.]*

(Amaral and Price 1984; Carnes and Price, 1988; Kuroda and Price 1991; Russchen et al. 1987). Through these connections the amygdala is in a position both to directly activate the PFC and to modulate the reciprocal interaction between the PFC and MD.

The LSPT circuit constitutes a disinhibitory sideloop between the amygdala or the PFC and MD. The amygdala and the PFC send excitatory projections to overlapping parts of the ventromedial caudate and nucleus accumbens (Fuller et al. 1987; Russchen et al. 1985). As with the more extensively studied dorsal striatal-pallidal pathway, this part of the striatum sends an inhibitory projection to the ventral pallidum (Graybiel 1990), which in turn sends GABA-ergic, inhibitory fibers to MD (Kuroda and Price 1991). Because the pallidal neurons

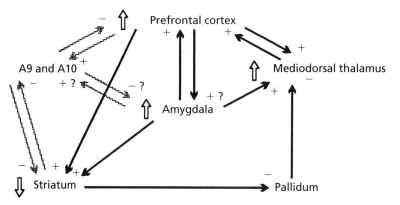

FIGURE **14–9.** *Neuroanatomical circuits hypothesized to participate in the functional anatomy of unipolar major depression. Regions containing BF differences have adjacent open arrows that indicate the direction of change in flow in the subjects with depression relative to control subjects. The regions' monosynaptic connections with each other are illustrated (closed arrows) with (+) indicating excitatory and (−) inhibitory projections, and with (?) indicating where experimental evidence is limited. The portions of the PFC referred to involve primarily the ventrolateral and medial PFC (see text). The parts of the striatum under consideration are the ventral medial caudate and nucleus accumbens, which particularly project to the ventral pallidum (Nauta and Domesick 1984). The major dopaminergic projections from the substantia nigra (A9) and the ventral tegmental area (A10) to these structures are illustrated with the shaded tone. [Reprinted with permission from Drevets et al. 1992a.]*

have relatively high spontaneous firing rates (DeLong 1972), activity in the PFC or amygdala that activates the striatum and in turn inhibits the ventral pallidum would release MD from an inhibitory pallidal influence. Thus, if the amygdala is abnormally active in major depression it can potentially produce an episode of abnormal activity in the PFC and MD both directly and through the striatum and pallidum.

One of the major theories regarding the pathogenesis of major depression holds that a process analogous to kindling or behavioral sensitization occurs in limbic structures such as the amygdala in subjects who are susceptible to major depressive episodes and drives abnormal limbic activity (Post et al. 1984). Relevant to this hypothesis, the amygdala has been implicated as a primary target of both the acute and chronic pharmacologic actions of antidepressant drugs (Broek-kamp and Lloyd 1981; Drevets and Raichle 1992; Duncan et al. 1986; Gorka et al. 1979; Horovitz 1966; Ordway et al. 1991). Compatible with the latter data, we found that chronic antidepressant drug treatment decreased regional BF in the amygdala of subjects with unipolar depression (Drevets et al. 1993). Our additional finding that BF in the amygdala may again be increased in the subjects in remission with FPDD who are no longer taking antidepressant drugs is particularly intriguing in this regard. Because kindling-related phenomena appear to represent permanent changes in neuronal sensitivity, according to Post's hypothesis this abnormal amygdala activity would reemerge in subjects with depression who are not being treated, leading to relapse and the recurrent episodes that characterize major depression.

In a potentially related hypothesis regarding the pathophysiology of major depression, Swerdlow and Koob (1987) proposed a neural model for depression involving the LSPT circuit that is compatible with our data, and may additionally explain the observation of decreased BF in the caudate. Based in part upon evidence of decreased dopaminergic activity in depression (Jimerson 1987), they hypothesized that decreased dopaminergic transmission into the ventromedial caudate and nucleus accumbens (Nauta and Domesick 1984) enhances reverberatory activity between the PFC, amygdala, and MD. They proposed that this leads to perseveration of a fixed set of cortical activity manifested by the emotional, cognitive, and motor processes of depression. Dopaminergic projections from the substantia nigra and ventral tegmental area to the striatum, amygdala, and PFC comprise an important inhibitory or modulatory input into these structures (see Figure 14–9; Graybiel 1990; Rowlands and Robert 1980; Smith and Bolam 1990; Thierry et al. 1988). Thus, the effect of mesostriatal dopamine deficiency would be to increase striatal output, thereby inhibiting the pallidum and disinhibiting MD (Wooten and Collins 1981). This, together with the decrease in direct dopaminergic effects in the amygdala and PFC, would increase activity in the limbic-thalamo-cortical circuit, potentially yielding the BF increases found here (see Figure 14–9). Moreover, if mesostriatal dopaminergic transmission is reduced, decreased synaptic activity at striatal dopamine receptors would likely appear as decreased BF in the caudate (Brown and Wolfson 1978; McCulloch et al. 1982), also consistent with our observations (see Figure 14–8).

The hypothesis that disinhibition and consequent reverberation of the limbic-thalamo-cortical circuit is important in the pathophysiology of FPDD provides an intriguing model for investigations of antidepressant treatment mechanisms. Effective antidepressant treatments may correct or compensate for the pathophysiology of FPDD through modulation of limbic-thalamo-cortical activity. We previously reviewed evidence from electrophysiology, receptor pharmacology, and imaging studies suggesting that somatic antidepressant treatments inhibit activity within the limbic-thalamo-cortical circuit, possibly by enhancing the sensitivity of dopaminergic and serotonergic ($5HT_{1A}$) receptors within this circuit (Drevets and Raichle 1992). Compatible with these data, we found that BF decreases in the VLPFC, the medial orbital cortex, and the amygdala in subjects with FPDD during chronic antidepressant drug treatment (Drevets et al. 1993).

The Limbic-Cortico-Striatal-Pallidal-Thalamic Circuit and Induced Depression

In humans, lesions that involve the parts of the PFC that participate in these circuits and diseases of the basal ganglia (e.g., Parkinson's disease) are associated with higher rates of major depression than other similarly debilitating conditions (Folstein et al. 1991; Jeste et al. 1988; Mayeux 1983; Starkstein and Robinson 1989). For example, Starkstein and Robinson (1989) reported that the two cerebral sites where cerebrovascular accident lesions were most consistently associated with the development of unipolar major depressive syndromes were the left frontal cortex and the left caudate. Thus dysfunction at multiple points within the LSPT circuit may give rise to the major depressive syndrome.

Because these conditions affect this circuit in different ways, we hypothesized that imbalances within these circuits, rather than overall increased or decreased synaptic activity within a particular structure, may produce the major depressive syndrome. For example, in Parkinson's disease increased striatal-pallidal transmission results from the loss of the inhibitory effects of nigrostriatal dopaminergic neurons, whereas in Huntington's disease, decreased striatal-pallidal transmission results from the degeneration of striatal neurons (Rougemont et al. 1984; Young et al. 1986). Both diseases are associated with risks for developing major depression that are up to fourfold higher than those associated with other similarly disabling illnesses. If imbalances within these circuits, rather than overall increased or decreased synaptic activity in a single structure, produce mood disorders, this would resemble the case in the motor circuit, where disrupted modulation at various points results in movement disorders (the motor circuit involves the primary and supplementary motor cortices, the dorsolateral striatum, the dorsal pallidum, and the motor thalamus) (DeLong 1972).

The LSPT Circuit and Other Depressive Subtypes

If different types of modulatory dysfunction within the LSPT circuit can result in mood disturbances, then diverse patterns of BF or metabolism within this circuit may distinguish depressive subtypes. For example, in contrast to the PET findings in subjects with primary unipolar depression, subjects with bipolar depression generally display decreased BF and metabolism in the PFC[6] and normal caudate metabolism (Baxter et al. 1985; Buchsbaum et al. 1986; Delvenne et al. 1990; O'Connell et al. 1989). In our own investigation of bipolar depression, the *decreases* in prefrontal flow were located in the portion of the anterior cingulate gyrus ventral to the corpus callosum (i.e., the subgenal prefrontal cortex), an area where flow was also abnormally *decreased* in the subjects with unipolar depression with FPDD (Drevets et al. 1997). Nevertheless, discriminant analysis of the covariance of BF in the left PFC, amygdala, caudate, and medial thalamus sensitively distinguished FPDD subjects from bipolar subjects (see Drevets et al.

---

[6]These prefrontal decreases, however, could be accounted for by partial volume effects, since frontal lobe volume has been reported to be decreased in depression, and PET studies of bipolar depression have not corrected their image data for regional atrophy (Coffey et al. 1993; Nasrallah et al. 1989; Videen et al. 1988).

1992b). The differences in the patterns of BF abnormalities within the LSPT circuit in unipolar versus bipolar depression could conceivably reflect neuromodulatory disturbances affecting the LSPT circuit that differ between unipolar and bipolar affective disorder.

The few careful imaging studies performed in other major depressive subtypes have also emphasized metabolic abnormalities in limbic-cortical regions. In subjects with depression with seasonal affective disorder, Cohen et al. (1992) reported increased medial orbital metabolism and left greater than right asymmetry in the mid-PFC, similar to our findings in FPDD (Drevets et al. 1992a). In contrast, PET image data in induced depressive syndromes associated with partial-complex seizure disorder, Parkinson's disease, or Huntington's disease demonstrate decreased BF in the ventral PFC compared with nondepressed control subjects with the same disorders (Bromfield et al. 1992; Mayberg et al. 1990, 1992).

Discriminative Ability of PET Measurements of Regional BF in FPDD

To date none of the abnormalities identified in individual brain regions in depression have had sufficient separation from normative values to be useful diagnostically. However, the implication of a neural circuit in which functional activity covaries among component structures suggests that multivariate statistics may provide greater power to distinguish depressed from normal subjects (Drevets et al. 1992b). To test the discriminative power of the covariance matrix involving the LSPT circuit, we obtained regional BF measurements for the left PFC, amygdala, medial thalamus, and medial caudate in additional subjects with FPDD and in subjects in the depressed phase of bipolar affective disorder. In the subjects from our original study, the FPDD subjects were correctly classified into the FPDD group in 89% of cases, and the control subjects into the control group in 92% of cases (Wilks' lambda = 0.42, $F = 9.5$, $P < .0001$). In the new subjects with FPDD, 75% were classified by this covariance matrix as FPDD. In the subjects with bipolar disorder depression, only 11% were classified into the FPDD group and 89% into the normal group. However, 50% of the normal subjects scanned while thinking sad thoughts (described earlier) were incorrectly classified in the FPDD category.

In spite of this misclassification of "sad normal subjects" into the FPDD category, the FPDD category may be distinguishable from normal subjects scanned while thinking sad thoughts if the limbic-thalamocortical circuit is considered alone. This is because while flow increased in the left PFC and medial thalamus in the sad thoughts versus the resting condition (flow was increased in these same areas in the subjects with depression and FPDD relative to resting control subjects), it decreased in the amygdala (Wilks' lambda $= 0.000012; F = 35; P < .00001$; Drevets et al. 1992b). This contrasted with FPDD, where BF in the amygdala was abnormally elevated relative to the normative condition.

Functional Activation in a Disease State

While the image data described earlier were obtained with subjects at rest, a potentially more powerful strategy for investigating psychopathology using PET involves dynamic imaging during activated states. For example, differences in the regional BF responses during cognitive or emotional tasks that are known to activate a specific neural circuit could potentially identify the point within that circuit which is dysfunctional. Moreover, scans acquired during an activated state may identify functional abnormalities in brain areas where BF or metabolism appears normal in the resting state. Finally, if subjects with a disease employ aberrant neural circuits in the cognitive processing associated with a particular task, this could be identified in dynamic images acquired as subjects perform the task. The demonstration of such an aberrant functional anatomical pathway in a psychiatric disorder could provide the most sensitive means available for separating normal individuals from patients with the disorder.

However, the selection of appropriate experimental tasks for dynamic imaging paradigms that compare normal subjects with patients is exceedingly complicated. The patient and control groups must be matched for stimulus and behavioral performance variables in order to conclude that observed physiologic differences are related to differences in cognitive processing. For example, elementary stimulus variables such as repetition rate have profound effects on the BF responses to stimulation (for review see Raichle 1987). Somatosensory stimulation does not produce a measurable BF response in the cat somatosensory cortex until the stimulus frequency reaches 3 Hz.[7] Thereafter, the measured BF declines until the frequency reaches 10 Hz where it is again no longer measurable (see Figure 14–2). A different relationship exists between BF and stimulus frequency in the human visual cortex, where photic stimulation produces a significant rise in striate cortex BF at <1 Hz, peaks at 7.8 Hz, and is still evident at 61 Hz (Fox and Raichle 1985). Thus, unless stimulus variables such as rate and response variables such as speed and accuracy can be controlled between experimental groups, ambiguity remains as to whether BF response differences between subjects are due to regional dysfunction or simply to alterations in stimulus or behavioral performance variables.

An important implication of the relationship between BF and stimulus variables is that if behavioral performance differs between two groups, one cannot be certain that stimulus rates involving the structure in question were identical. For example, Weinberger et al. (1986) reported that the BF response in the dorsolateral PFC differs between schizophrenic and control subjects scanned while performing the Wisconsin Card Sorting Test (WCST; Heaton 1985). However, the schizophrenic subjects successfully completed an average of 1.5 categories during the scan, while the control subjects completed an average of 7.5 categories. Because the dorsolateral PFC was presumed to be involved in the performance of the WCST, it could not be determined whether the BF response differed between groups because the rate at which the stimulus reached the dorsolateral PFC differed, the behavioral output differed (which likely involved structures efferent to the dorsolateral PFC), or cognitive processing within the dorsolateral PFC differed.

Thus far little insight into the dysfunctional neural processing re-

---

[7]Because of the limited spatial and temporal resolution of measurements of BF and metabolism, neuronally induced changes in BF or metabolism must occupy a sufficient portion of the measurement time and be present in a large enough area within the region-of-interest to produce measurable changes in BF (Raichle 1987).

lated to psychopathology has been gained from PET imaging in activated states. Nevertheless, dynamic imaging during the performance
of cognitive or emotional tasks remains a potentially powerful applications of functional brain imaging. As experimental tasks are developed that can be meaningfully applied in comparisons between patients and control subjects, activation paradigms involving cognitive,
emotional, or pharmacologic challenges should eventually prove fruitful in elucidating the pathophysiology of psychiatric disorders.

References

Aggleton JP, Passingham RE: Syndrome produced by lesions of the amygdala
in monkeys (Macaca mulatta). J Comp Physiol Psychol 95:961–977, 1981

Amaral DG, Price JL: Amygdalocortical projections in the monkey. J Comp
Neurol 230:465–496, 1984

Andreasen NC (ed): Brain Imaging: Applications in Psychiatry. Washington,
DC, American Psychiatric Press, 1989

Ballantine HT Jr, Bouckoms AJ, Thomas EK, et al: Treatment of psychiatric
illness by stereotactic cingulotomy. Biol Psychiatry 22:807–819, 1987

Baxter LR, Phelps ME, Mazziotta JC, et al: Cerebral metabolic rates for glucose in mood disorders. Arch Gen Psychiatry 42:441–447, 1985

Broekkamp CL, Lloyd KG: The role of the amygdala on the action of psychotropic drugs, in The Amygdaloid Complex. Edited by Ben-Ari Y. Amsterdam, Elsevier-North Holland Biomedical, 1981, pp 219–225

Bromfield EB, Altshuler L, Leiderman DB, et al: Cerebral metabolism and
depression in patients with complex partial seizures. Arch Neurol 49:617–
623, 1992

Brown LL, Wolfson LI: Apomorphine increases glucose utilization in the
substantia nigra, subthalamic and corpus striatum of the rat. Brain Res
140:188–193, 1978

Buchsbaum MS, Wu J, DeLisi LE, et al: Frontal cortex and basal ganglia
metabolic rates assessed by positron emission tomography with [^{18}F]2-
deoxyglucose in affective illness. J Affective Disord 10:137–152, 1986

Carnes KM, Price JL: Sources of presumptive glutaminergic/aspartergic afferents to the rat mesial prefrontal cortex. Soc Neurosci Abstr 14:480,
1988

Chimowitz MI, Estes ML, Furlan AJ, et al: Further observations on the pathology of sub-cortical lesions identified on magnetic resonance imaging. Arch Neurol 49:747–752, 1992

Cloninger CR: A systematic method for clinical description and classification of personality variants. Arch Gen Psychiatry 44:573–588, 1987

Coffey CE, Wilkinson WE, Weiner RD, et al: Quantitative cerebral anatomy in depression—a controlled magnetic resonance imaging study. Arch Gen Psychiatry 50:7–16, 1993

Cohen RM, Gross M, Nordahl TE, et al: Preliminary data on the metabolic brain pattern of patients with winter seasonal affective disorder. Arch Gen Psychiatry 49:545–552, 1992

Collins RC: Prefrontal-limbic systems: evolving clinical concepts, in Advances in Contemporary Neurology. Edited by Plum F. Philadelphia, FA Davis, 1988, pp 185–204

Coltheart M: Cognitive neuropsychology and the study of reading, in Attention and Performance XI. Edited by Posner MI, Marin OSM. Hillsdale, NJ, Lawrence Erlbaum Associates, 1985, pp 3–37

Corbetta M, Miezin FM, Dobmeyer S, et al: Selective and divided attention during visual discriminations of shape, color, and speed: functional anatomy by positron emission tomography. J Neurosci 11:2383–2402, 1991

Damasio AR: The neural basis of language. Annu Rev Neurosci 7:127–147, 1984

Damasio AR, Van Hoesen GW: Emotional disturbance associated with focal lesions of the limbic frontal lobe, in Neuropsychology of Human Emotion. Edited by Heilman K, Satz P. New York, Guilford, 1983, pp 85–110

Damasio AR, Tranel D, Damasio H: Individuals with sociopathic behavior caused by frontal damage fail to respond autonomically to social stimuli. Behav Brain Res 41:81–94, 1990

Deicken RF, Van Dyke C, Fein G, et al: Phosphorous magnetic resonance spectroscopy of deep white matter lesions in human brain (abstract). Am Col Neuropsychopharmacology Annual Meeting 1989;149.

DeLong MR: Activity of basal ganglia neurons during movement. Brain Res 40:127–135, 1972

Delvenne V, Delecluse F, Hubain PP, et al: Regional cerebral blood flow in patients with affective disorders. Br J Psychiatry 157:359–365, 1990

Drevets WC: Brain imaging in psychiatry, in Behavioral Science for Medical Students. Edited by Sierles FS. Baltimore, Williams & Wilkins, 1993, pp 212–235

Drevets WC, Raichle ME: Neuroanatomical circuits in depression: Implications for treatment mechanisms. Psychopharmacol Bull 28:261–274, 1992

Drevets WC, Raichle ME: PET imaging studies of human emotional disorders, in The Cognitive Neurosciences. Edited by Gazzaniga MS. Cambridge, MA, MIT Press, 1995, pp 1153–1164

Drevets WC, Raichle ME: Reciprocal suppression of regional cerebral blood flow during emotional versus higher cognitive process: implications for interactions between emotion and cognition. Cognition and Emotion 12:353–385, 1998

Drevets WC, Videen TO, Price JL, et al: A functional anatomical study of unipolar depression. J Neurosci 12:3628–3641, 1992a

Drevets WC, Spitznagel EL, MacLeod AK, et al: Discriminatory capability of PET measurements of regional blood flow in familial pure depressive disease. Soc Neurosci Abstr 18:1596, 1992b

Drevets WC, Videen TO, MacLeod AK, et al: Regional blood flow changes during antidepressant treatment. Soc Neurosci Abstr 19:7, 1993

Duncan GE, Breese GR, Criswell H, et al: Effects of antidepressant drugs injected into the amygdala on behavioral responses of rats in the forced swim test. J Pharmacol Exp Ther 238:758–762, 1986

Drevets WC, Price JL, Simpson JR, et al: Subgenual prefrontal cortex abnormalities in mood disorders. Nature 386:824–827, 1997

Fiegel GS, Krishnan KRR, Doraiswamy PM, et al: Subcortical hyperintensities on brain magnetic resonance imaging: A comparison between late onset and early onset elderly depressed subjects. Neurobiol Aging 26:245–247, 1991

Fiez J, Raife E, Balota D, et al: A positron emission tomography study of the short term maintenance of verbal information. J Neurosci 16:808–822, 1996

Folstein SE, Peyser CE, Starkstein SE, et al: Subcortical triad of Huntington's disease—a model for a neuropathology of depression, dementia, and dyskinesia, in Psychopathology and the Brain. Edited by Carrol BJ, Barrett JE. New York, Raven, 1991, pp 65–75

Fox PT, Raichle ME: Stimulus rate determines regional blood flow in striate cortex. Ann Neurol 17:303–305, 1985

Fox PT, Raichle ME: Focal physiological uncoupling of cerebral blood flow and oxidative metabolism during somatosensory stimulation in human subjects. Proc Natl Acad Sci U S A 83:1140–1144, 1986

Fox PT, Raichle ME: Cerebral blood flow and oxidative metabolism are focally uncoupled in physiological activation: a positron-emission tomographic study, in Cerebrovascular Diseases. Edited by Raichle ME, Powers WJ. New York, Raven, 1987, pp 129–140.

Fox PT, Mintun MA, Raichle ME, et al: Mapping human visual cortex with positron emission tomography. Nature Lond 323:806–809, 1986

Fox PT, Raichle ME, Mintun MA, et al: Nonoxidative glucose consumption during focal physiologic neural activity. Science 241:462–464, 1988

Friston KJ, Liddle PF, Frith CD, et al: The left medial temporal region and schizophrenia. Brain 115:367–382, 1992.

Fuller TA, Russchen FT, Price JL: Sources of presumptive glutaminergic/aspartergic afferents to the rat ventral striatopallidal region. J Comp Neurol 258:317–338, 1987

Fuster JM: The Prefrontal Cortex—Anatomy, Physiology, and Neuropsychology of the Frontal Lobe. New York, Raven, 1989

Gloor P, Olivier A, Quesney LF, et al: The role of the limbic system in experiential phenomena of temporal lobe epilepsy. Ann Neurol 12:129–144, 1982

Goldman-Rakic PS: Circuitry of primate prefrontal cortex and regulation of behavior by representational memory, in Handbook of Physiology—The Nervous System V. Edited by Mills J, Mountcastle VB. Baltimore, Williams & Wilkins, 1987, pp 373–417

Goodwin FK, Jamison KR (eds): Manic-Depressive Illness. New York, Oxford University Press, 1990

Gorka Z, Ossowska K, Stach R: The effect of unilateral amygdala lesion on the imipramine action in behavioral despair in rats. J Pharm Pharmacol 31:647–648, 1979

Graybiel AM: Neurotransmitters and neuromodulators in the basal ganglia. Trends Neurosci 13:244–254, 1990

Halgren E: The amygdala contribution to emotion and memory: current studies in humans, in The Amygdaloid Complex. Edited by Ben-Ari Y. Amsterdam, Elsevier-North Holland Biomedical, 1981, pp 395–408

Heaton R: Wisconsin Card Sorting Test. Odessa, TX, Psychological Assessment Resources, 1985

Horovitz ZP: The amygdala and depression, in Antidepressant Drugs. Edited by Garattini S, Dukes M. Amsterdam, Excerpta Medica, 1966, pp 121–129

Jeste DV, Lohr JB, Goodwin FK: Neuroanatomical studies of major affective disorders—a review and suggestions for further research. Br J Psychiatry 153:444–459, 1988

Jimerson DC: Role of dopamine mechanisms in the affective disorders, in Psychopharmacology: The Third Generation of Progress. Edited by Meltzer HY. New York, Raven, pp 505–511, 1987

Kuroda M, Price JL: Synaptic organization of projections from basal forebrain structures to the mediodorsal nucleus of the rat. J Comp Neurol 303:513–533, 1991

LaBerge D, Samuels SJ: Toward a theory of automatic information processing in reading. Cognitive Psychol 6:293–323, 1974

Laitinen LV: Emotional responses to subcortical electrical stimulation in psychiatric patients. Clin Neurol Neurosurg 81:148–157, 1979

LeDoux: Emotion, in Handbook of Physiology—the Nervous System V. Edited by Mills J, Mountcastle VB, Plum F, Geiger SR. Baltimore, Williams & Wilkins, 1987, pp 373–417

Mayberg HS, Starkstein SE, Sadzot B, et al: Selective hypometabolism in the inferior frontal lobe in depressed patients with Parkinson's disease. Ann Neurol 28:57–64, 1990

Mayberg HS, Starkstein SE, Peyser CE, et al: Paralimbic frontal lobe hypometabolism in depression associated with Huntington's disease. Neurology 42:1791–1797, 1992

Mayeux R: Emotional changes associated with basal ganglia disorders, in Neuropsychology of Human Emotion. Edited by Heilman KM, Satz P. New York, Guilford, 1983, pp 141–164.

Mazziotta JC, Phelps ME, Plummer D, et al: Quantitation in positron emission computed tomography. 5. Physical-anatomical effects. J Comput Assist Tomogr 5:734–743, 1981

McCulloch J, Savaki HE, McCulloch MC, et al: The distribution of alterations in energy metabolism in the rat brain produced by apomorphine. Brain Res 243:67–80, 1982

McHugh PR: the neuropsychiatry of basal ganglia disorders. Neuropsychiatry Neuropsychol Behav Neurol 2:239–247, 1989

Mintun MA, Raichle ME, Quarles RP: Length of PET data acquisition inversely affects ability to detect focal areas of brain activation. J Cereb Blood Flow Metab 9(S1):S349, 1989

Moldin SO, Reich T, Rice JP: Current perspectives on the genetics of unipolar depression. Behav Genet 21:211–242, 1991

Nasrallah HA, Coffman JA, Olson SC: Structural brain-imaging findings in affective disorders: an overview. J Neuropsychiatry Clin Neurosci 1:21–26, 1989

Nauta WJH, Domesick V: Afferent and efferent relationships of the basal ganglia. CIBA Found Symp 107:3–29, 1984

Neill D: Distinct dopamine terminal areas controlling behavioral activation and reward value of hypothalamic stimulation, in The Mesocorticolimbic Dopamine System. Edited by Kalivas PW, Nemeroff CB. New York, New York Academy of Sciences, 1988, pp 520–522

Nishijo H, Ono T, Nishino H: Single neuron responses in amygdala of alert monkey during complex sensory stimulation with affective significance. J Neurosci 8:3570–3583, 1988

O'Connell RA, Van Heertum RL, Billick SB, et al: Single photon emission computed tomography (SPECT) with [^{123}]IMP in the differential diagnosis of psychiatric disorders. J Neuropsychiatry Clin Neurosci 1:145–153, 1989

Ogawa S, Tank DW, Menon R, et al: Intrinsic signal changes accompanying sensory stimulation: functional brain mapping with magnetic resonance imaging. Proc Natl Acad Sci U S A 89:5951–5955, 1992

Ordway GA, Gambarana C, Tejani-Butt SM, et al: Preferential reduction of binding of 125(super)I-iodopindolol to beta-1 adrenoceptors in the amygdala of rats after antidepressant treatments. J Pharmacol Exp Ther 257:681–690, 1991

Papez JW: A proposed mechanism of emotion. Arch Neural Psychiatry 79:217–224, 1937

Pardo JV, Pardo PJ, Janer KW, et al: The anterior cingulate cortex mediates processing selection in the Stroop attentional conflict paradigm. Proc Natl Acad Sci U S A 87:256–259, 1990

Pardo JV, Pardo PJ, Raichle ME: Neural correlates of self-induced dysphoria. Am J Psychiatry 150:713–719, 1993

Perris C, Monaknov K: Depressive symptomatology and systemic structural analysis of the EEG, in Hemisphere Asymmetries of Function in Psychopathology. Edited by Gruzelier J, Flor-Henry P. Amsterdam, North Holland-Elsevier, 1979, pp 223–236

Petersen SE, Fox PT, Posner MI, et al: Positron emission tomographic studies of the cortical anatomy of single word processing. Nature 331:585–589, 1988

Petersen SE, Fox PT, Posner MI, et al: Positron emission tomographic studies of the processing of single words. J Cogn Neurosci 1:153–170, 1989

Petersen SE, Fox PT, Snyder AZ, et al: Activation of extrastriate and frontal cortical areas by visual words and word-like stimuli. Science 249:1041–1044, 1990

Phelps ME, Mazziotta JC, Schelbert HR (eds): Positron Emission Tomography and Autoradiography—Principles and Applications for the Brain and Heart. New York, Raven, 1986

Posner MI, Petersen SE: The attention system of the human brain. Annu Rev Neurosci 13:25–42, 1990

Post RM, Putnam F, Contel NR, et al: Electroconvulsive seizures inhibit amygdala kindling: implications for mechanisms of action in affective illness. Epilepsia 25:234–239, 1984

Price JL, Russchen FT, Amaral DG: The limbic region. II: the amygdaloid complex, in Handbook of Chemical Neuroanatomy, Vol. 5. Edited by Bjorklund A, Hokfelt T, Swanson LW. New York, Elsevier, 1987, pp 279–388

Raichle ME: Positron Emission Tomography. Ann Rev Neurosci 6:249–267, 1983

Raichle ME: Circulatory and metabolic correlates of brain function in normal humans, in Handbook of Physiology, Vol 5, The Nervous System, pt 2. Edited by Mountcastle VB, Plum F, Geiger SR. Baltimore, Williams & Wilkins, 1987, pp 643–674.

Raichle ME: Exploring the mind with dynamic imaging. Semin Neurosci 2:307–315, 1990

Raichle ME: [Book Cover], in Mapping the Brain and its Functions. Edited by Pechura CM, Martin JB. Washington, DC, National Academy Press, 1991

Raichle ME, Fiez J, Videen TO, et al: Practice-related changes in human brain functional anatomy. Soc Neurosci Abstr 17:21, 1991

Rice J, Reich T, Andreasen N, et al: The familial transmission of bipolar illness. Arch Gen Psychiatry 44:441–447, 1987

Richardo JA, Koh ET: Anatomical evidence of direct projections from the nucleus of the solitary tract to the hypothalamus, amygdala, and other forebrain structures in the rat. Brain Res 153:1–26, 1978

Rosenkilde CE, Bauer RH, Fuster JM: Single cell activities in ventral prefrontal cortex of behaving monkeys. Brain Res 209:375–394, 1981

Rougement D, Baron JC, Collard P, et al: Local cerebral glucose utilization in treated and untreated patients with Parkinson's disease. J Neurol Neurosurg Psychiatry 47:824–830, 1984

Rowe CC, Perlmutter JS: Pharmacological activation of dopaminergic pathways in the baboon studied with PET. Soc Neurosci Abstr 17:1300, 1991

Rowlands GJ, Robert PJ: Specific calcium-dependent release of endogenous glutamate from rat striatum is reduced by destruction of the corticostriatal tract. Exp Brain Res 39:239–240, 1980

Roy CS, Sherrington CS: On the regulation of the blood supply of the brain. J Physiol Lond 11:85–108, 1890.

Roy-Byrne P, Fleishaker J, Arnett C, et al: Effects of acute and chronic alprazolam treatment on cerebral blood flow, memory, sedation, and plasma catecholamines. Neuropsychopharmacology 8:161–169, 1993

Russchen FT, Bakst I, Amaral DG, et al: The amygdalostriatal projections in the monkey—an anterograde tracing study. Brain Res 329:241–257, 1985

Russchen FT, Amaral DG, Price JL: The afferent input to the magnocellular division of the mediodorsal nucleus of the thalamus in the monkey, Macaca fascicularis. J Comp Neurol 256:175–210, 1987

Sarter M, Markowitsch HJ: Involvement of the amygdala in learning and memory: a critical review, with emphasis on anatomical relations. Behav Neurosci 99:342–380, 1985

Schatzberg AF, Samson JA, Bloomingdale KL, et al: Toward a biochemical classification of depressive disorders. Arch Gen Psychiatry 46:260–268, 1989

Schwartz JM, Baxter LR, Mazziotta JC, et al: The differential diagnosis of depression: relevance of positron mission tomography studies of cerebral glucose metabolism to the bipolar-unipolar dichotomy. J Am Med Assoc 258:1368–1374, 1987

Schwartz WJ, Smith CB, Davidsen L, et al: Metabolic mapping of functional activity in the hypothalamo-neurohypophysial system of the rat. Science 205:723–725, 1979

Smith AD, Bolam JP: The neural network of the basal ganglia as revealed by the study of synaptic connections of identified neurons. Trends Neurosci 13:259–265, 1990

Starkstein SE, Robinson RG: Affective disorders and cerebral vascular disease. Br J Psychiatry 154:170–182, 1989

Swerdlow NR, Koob GF: Dopamine, schizophrenia, mania and depression: toward a unified hypothesis of cortico-striato-pallido-thalamic function. Behav Brain Sci 10:197–245, 1987

Talairach J, Zilka G, Tournoux P, et al: Atlas d'Anatomie Stéréotaxique du Télencéphale. Paris, Masson, 1967

Talairach J, Bancaud J, Geier S, et al: The cingulate gyrus and human behavior. Electroencephalogr Clin Neurophysiol 34:45–52, 1973

Thierry AM, Mantz J, Milla C, et al: Influence of the mesocortical/prefrontal dopamine neurons on their target cells, in The Mesocorticolimbic Dopamine System. Edited by Kalivas PW, Nemeroff CB. New York, New York Academy of Sciences, 1988, pp 101–111

Turner BH, Mishkin M, Knapp M: Organization of the amygdalopetal projections from modality—specific cortical association areas in the monkey. J Comp Neurol 191:515–543, 1980

Videen TO, Perlmutter JS, Mintun MA, et al: Regional correction of positron emission tomography data for the effects of cerebral atrophy. J Cereb Blood Flow Metab 8:662–670, 1988

Vogt BA: The role of layer I in cortical function, in Cerebral Cortex, Vol 9. Edited by Peters A, Jones EG. New York, Plenum, 1991, pp 49–80

Vogt BA: The structural organization of cingulate cortex, in The Neurobiology of Cingulate Cortex and Limbic Thalamus. Edited by Vogt BA, Gabriel M. Boston, MA, Birkhäuser, 1993, pp 19–70

Weinberger DR, Berman KF, Zec RF: Physiologic dysfunction of dorsolateral prefrontal cortex in schizophrenia. Arch Gen Psychiatry 43:114–124, 1986

Weiskrantz L: Behavioral changes associated with ablation of the amygdaloid complex in monkeys. J Comp Physiol Psychol 49:381–391, 1956

Winokur G: The development and validity of familial subtypes in primary unipolar depression. Pharmacopsychiatry 15:142–146, 1982

Wong DF, Young LT: Quantification of human neuroreceptors in neuropsychiatric disorders with positron-emission tomography, in Positron-Emission Tomography in Schizophrenia Research. Edited by Volkow ND, Wolf AP. Washington, DC, American Psychiatric Press, 1991, pp 101–124

Wooten GF, Collins RC: Metabolic effects of unilateral lesion of the substantia nigra. J Neurosci 1:285–291, 1981

Young AB, Penney JB, Starosta-Rubinstein S, et al: PET scan investigations of Huntington's disease: cerebral metabolic correlates of neurological features and functional decline. Ann Neurol 20:296–303, 1986

PART V

Treatment and Outcome of Personality Disorders

15

Cognitive Aspects of Personality Disorders and Their Relation to Syndromal Disorders: A Psychoevolutionary Approach

Aaron T. Beck, M.D.

When I first started seeing patients in the 1950s, I believed—in line with the psychodynamic dogma of the day—that the syndromal disorders (or what we now call Axis I disorders), such as depression, anxiety disorders, and phobias, were only the surface manifestation of an underlying personality disorder. Within the symptomatic adult was a "frightened, angry, needy child." This immaturity was reflected in a personality disorder that was regarded as "the cause" of the depression or anxiety disorder or phobia. I believed that if you cured the personality disorder, the neurosis would go away.

Later, under the influence of the behavior therapy movement I came to believe that the problem was on the surface and not in some deep unconscious recesses of the mind: The symptomatology produced a secondary reaction that appeared to be the personality disorder; that is, the Axis I symptoms so disabled the person that he or she only appeared to have a personality disorder. If you cured the symptom disorder, the personality disorder would go away.

This formulation seemed satisfactory in the early years while I was conducting cognitive therapy of depression. When patients were over their depression, the problematic characteristics such as overdependency, demandingness, and negativism were no longer apparent. I eventually found, however, that even though they were no longer clinically depressed or anxious, a significant proportion of these patients still showed sufficient persistent, unremitting, enduring dysfunctional behaviors and cognitive distortions as well as subjective distress to justify the attribution of an underlying personality disorder. Further, these characteristics appeared to have been present for the most part since childhood. The emergence of this subgroup of patients among our symptomatically improved depressed and anxious patients prompted me to accept the notion that at least some had an underlying personality disorder and to formulate a cognitive theory and therapy of the personality disorders (Beck et al. 1990).

Evolution of Syndromal Disorders

At the same time, I was beginning to see psychiatric disorders in the broader perspective of our prehistoric (phylogenetic) heritage. It appeared plausible that the selective pressures of our evolutionary history made us susceptible to syndromal (Axis I) and personality (Axis II) disorders. Natural selection was relentless in molding the durable predispositions of humans as well as their reactions to acute situations.

It became clear to me that although the basic evolutionary goals—survival and reproduction—and the basic strategies (competition, cooperation, nurturance-eliciting, sexuality, etc.) for achieving these goals had not changed, our specific environmental niche, specifically, the social milieu, had changed substantially from the conditions of the wild to a technologically advanced society, resulting in a poor fit—what I call the "evolutionary friction rub."

Evolution of Dysfunctional Anxiety and Depression

According to this evolutionary perspective, the forerunner of anxiety disorders was a set of strategies that were activated to deal with an acute challenge to the individual's ordinary adjustment by sudden aversive happenings. These noxious events either actually threatened the individual's resources, including personal safety, or were erroneously perceived to reduce these resources. In response to the perception of acute threat, for example, the strategies of fight, flight, freeze, or faint became mobilized (Beck and Emery 1985). When the system was unable to return to a normal state, an anxiety disorder or paranoid state was produced.

Acute anxiety and continuous vigilance, the expression of our hypersensitive alarm system, became the tribute we had to pay in order to stay alive and make a contribution to the gene pool. The "better safe than sorry principle" reflected the fact that false positives (false alarms) could be tolerated whereas a false negative could cancel us out and snap the line of transmission of our genes. Thus, the price for maintaining our lineage was a susceptibility to a life of hypervigilance.

Evolution of Depression

The predisposition to depression followed a different path. The expected negative consequences of an interpersonal loss or a loss of status laid the groundwork for depression. In the wild, the loss of a crucial relationship or the loss of status could remove critical resources and impede access to other resources. A defeat, for example, would lead to loss of status and consequently reduced opportunities for mating or access to food. A loss of a close relation would deprive the individual of support and nurturance. Loss of health or competence would also handicap the individual in fulfilling evolutionary demands of survival and reproduction. Consequently, an innate program consisting of giving up and withdrawal (in other words, depression) would serve to reduce the individual's "needs" until new resources were developed. Because people can survive and continue to procreate in contemporary society despite loss of status or loss of a close relationship, it is apparent that these threats or losses leading to anxiety or depression are largely anachronistic symbols inherited from the past.

Conservation of energy and resources. Because humans operate to a large extent according to symbols, a symbolic loss can have the same degree of impact as an actual loss. A reduction of status (e.g., receiving a lower than expected rating in a popularity contest or being passed over for promotion to a tenured position) may have a powerful impact because they represent symbolically a defeat in the evolutionary race. The loss of status may represent a selective decline of power and influence, diminished opportunities for successful competition for limited resources, and the reduction of peer support in attaining phylogenetic goals. Similarly, separation from or loss of a nurturant person may represent a significant loss of external resources (Beck 1983).

These circumstances of perceived defeat or deprivation can trigger the phylogenetic program, namely a depression. The apparent reduction of resources or loss of access to resources is manifested clinically as either a "defeat depression" or "deprivation depression" (Beck 1983). The psychobiological organization shuts down until such time as resources are perceived to be available. Because people can survive and continue to procreate in contemporary society despite loss of status or loss of a close relationship, it is apparent that these threats or losses leading to anxiety or depression are largely anachronistic symbols inherited from the past. The mechanism can be analogized to the shutdown of industries in economic depression. When evidence indicates that further expenditure of energy would yield little or no return, the automatic response is to reduce productive activity until such time that there is a likelihood of a payoff from further expenditure of energy. Until that time, further expenditure of energy is counterproductive because the scarcity of external resources would lead to a dangerous reversal of the intake-output ratio and consequently a total depletion of energy. In terms of behavior in the wild, exploratory activity, foraging, sex, group participation would constitute a drain and thus would be automatically limited by a biological program of anorexia, loss of interest, fatigability, and loss of libido; in other words, the classic picture of depression.

Evolution of Personality Disorders

To get a complete picture of the distal antecedent of personality disorders, one has to reflect on the role of evolutionary processes. Whereas psychoanalysis has proposed that adults react according to patterns inculcated by their personal past history, the evolutionary approach suggests that we react according to patterns shaped by our evolutionary history—a more remote determinant. This notion brings us to a consideration of the Axis II—the personality disorders. In essence, personality and its disorders may be conceptualized in terms of the persistence of phylogenetic patterns designed to accommodate to the vicissitudes of prehistoric life.[1]

If Axis I disorders represent a way of coping with a destabilization of normal conditions, the personality and its Axis II disorders represent an enduring adjustment (or maladjustment) to the more stable set of circumstances, including the normal demands and stressors of everyday life. The adjustment strategies are manifested in many of the characteristics that constitute personality as we understand it. *These strategies represent each individual's unique solutions to the problem of reconciling internal pressures for survival and bonding and external obstacles, threats, and demands. These solutions, although unique for each individual, are drawn from a common substrate of evolved strategies shaped by the evolutionary history of the species.* The specific strategic repertoire of the individual is determined by the interaction of his or her specific heritage with relevant developmental experiences. In keeping with the ethological literature, I have applied the label *strategy* to denote the specific behavioral patterns.

The Environmental Niche

For many individuals these stable characteristics are not well designed to promote satisfaction and adaptation to the present-day social environment. In fact, these evolutionary-derived strategies are likely to produce excessive and useless distress in many individuals and may inflict suffering on their intimates or other people.

This state of affairs is due in part to a mismatch between an individual's inherited strategies and the changed environmental niche—

---

[1]It is also conceivable that a psychological mechanism analogous to morphological neotomy or juvenilization may be operative. In this sense, we never completely "grow up" or mature. Despite our overall maturation, we retain the playfulness (Gould 1977) and some dysfunctional cognitive-affective patterns of childhood.

the circumstances of contemporary life. Developmental experiences also play a critical role in the formation of dysfunctional strategies. The genetic material we inherited is not plastic enough to deal easily with the subtleties and complexities of our social environment and at the same time to satisfy the tacit goals of preserving our lineage. The strategies derived from genetic endowment and personal experience that evolved to solve evolutionary problems (survival and procreation) thus create other problems for the individual and for other people and may be manifested in personality disorders.

Let us look at some of the traits that presumably make up normal personality. These specific traits can be thought of as interpersonal strategies derived from our archaic heritage. Among the specific strategies we use in dealing with other people are dominant-submissive, competitive-cooperative, dependent-nurturant, and assertive-avoidant patterns of behavior.

If we are able to adapt these strategies to meet our innate phylogenetic goals, to mold our environment, to harmonize our disparate strategies, to satisfy our "needs," and to solve external problems, we have a functional personality. If particular strategies are excessive, compulsive, and inappropriate, they interfere with our adjustment and our behavior is categorized by clinicians as a "personality disorder." Sometimes, a particular strategy that is dysfunctional in ordinary circumstances may be well suited to an unusual environment (for example, in wartime), in which case this label, dysfunctional, is no longer applicable. On the other hand, when a satisfying environment (for example, a supportive network) is suddenly changed (for example, by the death of a nurturant relative or friend), the individual may experience not only depression but the resurgence of a latent personality disorder.

Personality and its disorders are defined in the psychiatric nomenclature in terms of observable *behaviors*, which may be translated into *strategies*. As we shall see, however, the strategies are driven, in part, by beliefs, attitudes, and assumptions, which are the fundamental targets of therapy.

As shown in Table 15–1, certain strategies were developed in the wild to advance the evolutionary goals. *Predation* served the purpose of acquisition of essential supplies through aggressive behavior. *Help-eliciting* behavior, particularly in the young and weak, was essential for survival. Successful *competition* for acquisitions and status provided

TABLE 15–1.

The primeval strategies and their representation in specific personality disorders

Strategy	Personality disorder
Predatory	Antisocial
Help-eliciting	Dependent
Competitive	Narcissistic
Exhibitionistic	Histrionic
Autonomous	Schizoid
Defensive	Paranoid
Withdrawal	Avoidant
Ritualistic	Compulsive

Source. *Reprinted with permission from Pretzer and Beck 1993, p. 61.*

access to essential resources. *Exhibitionism* was important for mating through attracting partners, but also provided a method for attaining status. An *autonomous* pattern was the basis for physical and psychological independence—important for survival. *Defensive* strategies were crucial for self-protection. *Withdrawal* or avoidance also served as protection against physical or psychological harm. Finally, *ritualistic* behaviors were important for control over self and others and implementing of goals. These rituals involved routines used in diverse activities such as communication, courtship, and organization of resources.

Table 15–1 lists those personality disorders whose dominant features correspond to a particular primal strategy. For example, the antisocial personality manifests actions reminiscent of predatory behavior (for instance, attacking others for personal gain), whereas the dependent personality manifests the overattachment and clinging behavior associated with help-eliciting behavior in other primates.

Why do some people develop personality disorders and others do not? First, the "genetic shuffle" plays an important role: There are huge individual differences in the inheritance of the predispositions to these strategies. Some individuals seem to be extroverted and confident, whereas others are shy and retiring from early childhood. Some seem to have the deck stacked against them. They are dealt an unbalanced "hand": strong in some suits (traits) but weak in others. Thus, chance plays a role in determining whether the inherited patterns will facilitate or interfere with mature development in a given environment.

Secondly, life experience can lead to the expression and full development of certain genetic patterns whereas other adaptive patterns do not receive the appropriate environmental stimulation in order to develop. Consequently, those individuals who are deficient in certain strategies may have difficulties in coping with problems that require using these strategies. These individuals may draw on more adequate strategies to compensate for their more deficient strategies. These compensatory patterns, however, may not fully protect the individuals' vulnerabilities. Further, the compensatory patterns tend to be compulsive, inflexible, and maladaptive and, consequently, present the classic picture of a personality disorder.

The uneven distribution of the innate factors at a genotypic or ideographic level may then be aggravated by life experience, especially during the formative period. The net result is that for certain individuals some strategies are overdeveloped and others are underdeveloped. This may result in their being overprepared to deal with certain stressors and underprepared to deal with others. This imbalance may be manifested in chronic anxiety disorders and phobias as one example, a hyperactive alarm system. Conversely, a hypoactive alarm system is manifested in excessive risk-taking. Similarly, some people may be depression-prone because of an excessive weighting of the systems relevant to curbing energy output.

The overdeveloped and underdeveloped strategies in the Axis II disorders (i.e., personality disorders) are illustrated in Table 15–2. It may be noted that when a personality disorder is overweighted with one set of strategies it is likely to be underrepresented in the complementary set. The compulsive personality disorder, for example, is characterized by an excessive emphasis on control strategies but is deficient in other strategies such as spontaneity.

Structural Aspects of Syndromal and Personality Disorders

Strategies are observable in overt behavior and form the basis for the Axis II (personality disorder) diagnoses. Strategies, however, are only

TABLE 15–2.

Typical overdeveloped and underdeveloped strategies

	Overdeveloped	Underdeveloped
Compulsive	Control Responsibility Systematization	Spontaneity Impulsivity
Dependent	Help-seeking Clinging	Self-sufficiency Mobility
Passive-aggressive	Autonomy Resistance Passivity Sabotage	Intimacy Assertiveness Activity Cooperativeness
Paranoid	Vigilance Mistrust Suspiciousness	Serenity Trust Acceptance
Narcissistic	Self-aggrandizement Competitiveness	Sharing Group Identification
Antisocial	Fight Deprive others Exploit	Empathy Reciprocity Social sensitivity
Schizoid	Autonomy Withdrawal	Intimacy Reciprocity
Avoidant	Social vulnerability Avoid Inhibit	Self-assertion Gregariousness
Histrionic	Exhibitionism Expressiveness Impressionistic	Reciprocity Control Systematization

the observable manifestation of adaptive or maladaptive processes. They are functional components of a structural complex consisting of cognitive, affective, and behavioral patterns (Beck and Emery 1985; Beck et al. 1990). These patterns—or systems—make up the personality organization. The cognitive component is crucial because it is

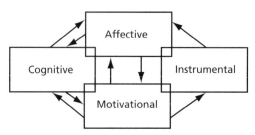

FIGURE 15–1. *Components of information processing.*

the medium for integrating data from our various senses into useful information. By its transactions, as it were, with our internal and external worlds, information processing plays a key role in survival.

The way that the cognitive component processes information influences behavior. The basic information processes have been labeled "schemas" (Beck 1964). The functions of the schemas include attending to, selecting, interpreting, storing, and retrieving information. Schemas include a specific content and structural characteristics such as density, breadth, permeability, and salience (Beck et al. 1990). Their specific content includes concepts, beliefs, assumptions, formulas, and rules (Beck 1964).

The relation of the cognitive schemas to the other components is illustrated in Figure 15–1.[2] The contiguity of the various components provides for the smooth operation of the personality.

Because information processing is crucial to the evocation of appropriate affect and the initiation of the relevant behavior, the activation of cognitive schemas generally precedes the activation of the other components. Cognitive and the affective structures interact, however, so that the individual not only experiences the affective state as a *result* of information processing but also uses the affective state as a source of information. For example, the processing of an external threat leads to anxiety and associated increase in heart rate. The increase in heart rate may be "read" as a sign that there is a danger and may also constitute a new "threat" in itself (for example, a possible sign of an impending heart attack, as in patients with panic disorder).

The sequence from external event through cognition and affect to

---

[2]For a more comprehensive illustration of the operation of schemas see Beck 1997.

motivation and instrumental behavior may be formulated in linear terms (although there is a degree of reciprocal interaction) as follows: SITUATION → INTERPRETATION → AFFECT → BEHAVIOR. For example, an individual sees a dark yellowish animal with black stripes, determines that it is a tiger, that it is loose, and that it is approaching him. (These are all components of primary appraisal.) The individual simultaneously determines he has no available defense (secondary appraisal) and that the best strategy is to escape from the situation. This rapid information processing leads to a physiological mobilization for flight. In addition, the individual feels anxious—nature's back-up system for assuring that the individual attaches top priority to attending to and responding to the danger. This subjective anxiety continues until the individual perceives that he is no longer in danger.

The sequence described here is incomplete. Individuals cannot survive if they have to puzzle out each time whether a danger exists and improvise an appropriate strategy. In a sense, the rapid adaptive response is like a program. What is missing from our description of the "program" is the inclusion of the cognitive entity that determines what is truly dangerous—in other words, the belief or rules that are applicable to a given configuration. These rules are embodied in schemas. Thus, the appropriate sequence would be SITUATION → [SCHEMA] → INTERPRETATION → AFFECT → BEHAVIOR.

Information processing in anxiety depends on the activation of certain enduring cognitive schemas relevant to the perception and assessment of physical danger. The content of the schemas thus contains certain themes such as "A large striped yellowish animal is a tiger" and "Tigers on the loose are dangerous." There is a logical sequence from "The tiger is dangerous" to the coping strategy of flight. The content of the schema determines the interpretation of the event.

If certain schemas are highly activated, they will play a preferential role in information processing and will lead to excessive mobilization (as in anxiety disorders or pathological hostility) or demobilization (depression). Thus, an individual with the belief "I am weak" is likely to interpret a multitude of relatively innocuous situations as signs of his vulnerability and will experience anxiety. A person who has a core schema "I am a failure" will be prone to depression if this schema is activated for a prolonged period.

Strategies

The salient beliefs, incorporated into schemas, not only influence the content of interpretations and conclusions but also form the basis for the characteristic strategies used by individuals and, particularly, the kind of social environment they will try to create for themselves. For example, an individual with a dominant belief such as "I am helpless" may seek nurturant individuals for help whenever challenged, threatened, or thwarted. Such an individual, often diagnosed with dependent personality disorder, is likely to gravitate toward an environment relatively free of problems. Similarly, an individual with a dominant motif of "I may get hurt" in interpersonal relations may be likely to show a disproportional number of avoidant behaviors and will (unsuccessfully) seek a relatively risk-free environment.

When stereotyped attitudes and behaviors interfere significantly with the individual's conscious goals and adjustments, the person is likely to be diagnosed as having a personality disorder. These disorders are also manifested in symptoms such as overreacting to situations, chronic dysphoria, and increased susceptibility to full-blown clinical disorders (Axis I) such as mood disorders or generalized anxiety disorder.

Table 15–3 shows the relationship between some of the characteristic beliefs and the corresponding strategies for the personality disorders.[3] Note the consistency from basic belief to strategy. The strategy can be seen as a logical derivative from the basic belief. For example, the notion "I am helpless" would logically lead to a strategy that would compensate for the presumed helplessness; namely, seeking a stronger person for help. Similarly, the narcissistic belief "I am special" would lead to self-aggrandizing behavior.

Once we start focusing on the conglomerate of beliefs, affects, and behavioral patterns, we are well on our way to understanding personality disorders as we observe them in our patients. As shown in Table 15–3, each of the personality disorders has its own set of unique basic

---

[3]Borderline personality disorders have been omitted from this formulation because 1) they may manifest a wide variety of core beliefs and behaviors representative of the other disorders and 2) they are uniquely characterized by "ego defects" in impulse control, affect stability, and reality testing rather than by a specific content.

TABLE 15–3.

Idiosyncratic beliefs for each personality disorder

Personality disorder	Basic beliefs and attitudes	Strategy (overt behavior)
Dependent	I am helpless.	Attachment
Avoidant	I may get hurt.	Avoidance
Passive-aggressive	I could be stepped on.	Resistance
Paranoid	People are potential adversaries.	Wariness
Narcissistic	I am special.	Self-aggrandizement
Histrionic	I need to impress.	Dramatics
Compulsive	Errors are bad.	Perfectionism
Antisocial	People are there to be taken.	Attack
Schizoid	I need plenty of space.	Isolation

beliefs. Yet, in working with these patients, we have found that those patients with a full-fledged personality *disorder*, in contrast to those who have simply a personality type, seemed to be struggling with a more general—and more basic—set of beliefs—what I call the *core beliefs*.

Role of the Self-Concept

Aside from some people having a greater inherited predisposition, are there "learned psychological factors"? In working with the personality disorders, I have tried to discern that they share some common denominator. Influenced perhaps by theorists in self psychology and object relations, I have narrowed my focus to the self-concept.

I have finally arrived at the notion that two forms or aspects of the self-concept are prepotent: the beliefs "I am helpless" and "I am unlovable." One should note that these two beliefs belong, respectively, to a class relevant to survival (helpless) and bonding (unloved). These notions are also relevant to the two personality types I have described previously, viz. the autonomous and the sociotropic (Beck 1983).

Autonomous: schizoid, narcissistic, antisocial, paranoid, compulsive
Sociotropic: dependent, histrionic, avoidant, passive-aggressive, borderline

The core belief "I am helpless" may be manifested in a number of permutations. Each of the descriptors listed under *Helpless* incorporates in some way the bipolar constructs of helpless and effective. The *Effective* list represents the positive concepts that individuals acquire as they mature, develop a myriad of skills, and prove their efficacy. These concepts may serve to neutralize the negative self-concepts but may become attenuated after stress and allow the negative core belief to emerge.

Helpless: passive, weak, defective, inadequate, inferior, incompetent, trapped, exposed, defenseless, stupid, powerless
Effective: assertive, strong, (perfect?), adequate, superior, competent, free, protected, defended, smart, powerful

The core belief may be inferred by trying to extract the meaning of a number of events that produce a dysphoric reaction. For example, a patient felt weak and sad in the context of several apparently unconnected events: not being able to think of the answer to a question; being inhibited in making a request; not being able to find the keys to his car. These experiences' common denominator was, "There's something wrong with me." Underlying this theme of presumed disability was the belief "I am helpless," which influenced his reactions to everyday demands and problems. Patients are not generally conscious of these core beliefs, although they can become aware of them as a consequence of explorative therapy. If the patients become depressed, however, these beliefs become very salient, dominating their thinking: "I am helpless (weak, inept, inadequate)."

The core structure "I am helpless" radiates out into a number of other cognitive facets that largely influence an individual's susceptibilities, reactions, and behavior. One set of beliefs that produce dysfunctional reactions and are oriented to specific life situations are called "specific cognitive vulnerability" (Beck 1984). The cognitive content of the cognitive vulnerability tends to be dichotomous and absolutistic. The vulnerability is formed as a cluster of conditional beliefs such as "If I am left alone, I will be unable to cope" or "If I don't have complete freedom of action, I am helpless." If a negative event impinges on the specific vulnerability, it activates the core belief, which is expressed in absolutistic terms: *"Because* I am controlled (dominated, manipulated, defeated, blocked), *I am helpless."*

If this core belief is subjected to an additional negative evaluation relevant to worth, then the helpless notion may be paired with the self-concept "I am worthless," or it may reflect the abysmally low self-regard embedded in the term, "I am nothing." Again, it should be noted that when the patient is depressed, these beliefs pervade his or her consciousness.

The same kind of sequence may be observed in light of the other core belief: "I am unloved." If this is regarded as a permanent state, the individual is likely to attribute it to an irreversible defect, "I am unlovable." The rock bottom belief may be "If I am unlovable, I am nothing."

As shown here, the "I am unloved" or ". . . unlovable" may be expressed in a variety of ways:

Unloved: unattractive, undesirable, rejected, alone, unwanted, uncared for, bad, dirty.

Examples of the type of vulnerability relevant to a person's efficacy and functioning are 1) "If I make a mistake, it means I'm stupid," 2) "If I am thwarted in an activity, it means I'm incompetent." When the individual does make a mistake or is thwarted, the belief, which was latent up until this point, becomes activated. Once the conditional part of the formula is satisfied, ("If . . ."), then the negative conclusion becomes salient. The full expression of this formula would then be "(Because I failed), *I am a failure."* It should be noted that the conditional phrase (*if* or *because*) is generally silent and the individual is aware only of the conclusion ("I am a failure" or "I am unlovable"). Clinical observations have indicated that when there is a congruence between the conditional belief and particular adverse circumstances, the individual will be prone to develop a syndromal disorder.

As individuals mature, they develop strategies and skills for dealing with the problems of living. These strategies are also used to compensate for the negative core beliefs. If the core beliefs are hyperactive, however, the strategies may become hypertrophied — as a form of *overcompensation.* Overcompensating strategies are rigid, overgeneralized, and, consequently, dysfunctional. An individual with a core belief "I am weak and inferior," for example, may compensate for this by over-developing a narcissistic strategy of demonstrating his power and competence. This strategy may be directed not only to excelling but also to proving his superiority to other people. He trades on the belief that he is entitled to special attention, to waiving rules and regulations, and to getting greater recognition. However, this strategy obviously does not prevent the occurrence of setbacks and letdowns. When his narcissistic beliefs are discredited by inevitable disregard by other people or failure to reach his perfectionistic goals, he is likely to experience self-doubts about his superiority and feel psychic pain.

To forestall such reverses and to implement the strategies, individuals build up a series of rules. For the narcissistic individual, the rules constitute a "bill of rights"; for example, "I am entitled to special privileges, attention, respect, recognition, deference, etc." Built into the bill of rights are sanctions for violations of the rules: "If people don't show me consideration (respect) they are wrong (bad, disrespectful) and should be punished (criticized, demeaned, reproached)." The rules are generally framed in imperatives such as "People should show me respect at all times," "My friends must always be kind and considerate (to me)." When these rules are violated, the individual considers himself wronged and wants to punish the offender.

Other rules are directed against the self: "I should do my best all the time" or "I must never make a mistake." When these rules are broken, the individual is prone to criticize himself. According to Ellis (1962), the demandingness, whether directed against the self or others, constitutes the basic mechanism in psychological disturbance. The function of the "musts" and "shoulds" can best be understood, however, in terms of their relation to the core beliefs and the conditional beliefs. The imperatives follow from the underlying conditional beliefs. The imperatives (the shoulds and musts) provide the driving force for the individual to attain his goals and to avert presumed undesirable happenings.

Figure 15–2 represents the sequence extending layer by layer from the underlying core belief to its representation in the conditional belief to the consequent compensatory belief and the strategy responsible for implementing the goal of the compensatory belief. In conducting cognitive therapy it is essential to formulate the case according to this diagram.

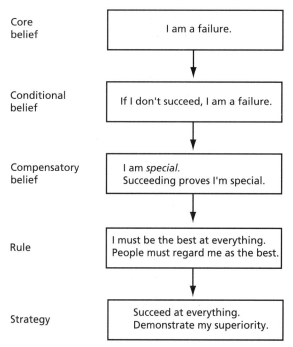

FIGURE 15–2. *Layers of beliefs in narcissistic personality disorder.*

In many cases, the core belief will become apparent after exploration of the individual's automatic thoughts. There is one condition, however, in which the core belief is fully conscious and, indeed, is salient and perseverative: depression. The thought content of depression frequently contains repetitive thoughts such as "I am a failure," "I am unlovable," and "There's something totally wrong with me." When the clinician hears patients who are depressed express these thoughts, he or she has direct access to the rock-bottom core beliefs that drive the personality disorders as well as the mood disorders.

Summary

The personality disorders (Axis II) and the syndromal disorders (Axis I) may be considered from two standpoints. First, in terms of their distal, phylogenetic origins: What were the ancestral precursors of these disorders? Second, in terms of their structures and functions: What role do they play in everyday life?

From an evolutionary standpoint, the syndromal disorders such as anxiety and depression may be viewed as preprogrammed reactions: a perceived threat (anxiety) to or a perceived depletion (depression) of the individual's resources. Thus, the perception of a danger to oneself or to one's significant others produces a mobilization of available resources to reduce the danger (fight, flight, freeze). In contrast, the perception of a substantial depletion of resources by virtue of loss of status and influence through defeat or loss of a significant interpersonal relationship leads to a demobilization, a "shutdown of power," to conserve energy (depression).

The stable components of personality draw on the inherited phylogenetic strategies to meet the demands and problems of everyday life. These strategies are designed ultimately to fulfill the evolutionary goals of adaptation or "inclusive fitness"; specifically, survival and procreation. Disorders of the personality may arise from a skewed distribution of the adaptive strategies in the genetic endowment or from adverse experiences that impinge on the individual in such a way as to produce hypertrophy of some strategies and atrophy of others. The end result is that the individual's coping strategies are excessive in some ways, deficient in others.

For clarification of the dysfunctionality of the strategies in the personality disorder, it is important to examine the role of cognitive, affective, and motivational structures (schemas). It is proposed that the interaction of the genetic endowment with the environmental influences leads to the formation of two sets of core beliefs: the self-concept of "I am helpless" or the self-concept "I am unlovable" (or both). The two self-concepts working independently or collectively lead to hypersensitivity to certain problems and to the formation or reinforcement of a variety of strategies designed to compensate for the depreciated self-concept. Although these strategies may have been adaptive in the wild, they do not fit well into our highly complex psychosocial environment and, hence, are ultimately dysfunctional. They tend to be compulsive, inflexible, and brittle. Further, the failure of the strategies can lead to the evocation of the syndromal disorders.

References

Beck AT: Thinking and depression: 2. Theory and therapy. Arch Gen Psychiatry 10:561–571, 1964

Beck AT: Cognitive therapy of depression: new perspectives, in Treatment of Depression: Old Controversies and New Approaches. Edited by Clayton P. New York, Raven, 1983, pp 265–290

Beck AT: Cognitive approaches to stress, in Clinical Guide to Stress Management. Edited by Lehrer C, Woolfolk RL. New York, Guilford, 1984, pp 255–305

Beck AT, Emery G (with Greenberg RL): Anxiety Disorders and Phobias: A Cognitive Perspective. New York, Basic Books, 1985

Beck AT, Freeman A, and associates: Cognitive Therapy of Personality Disorders. New York, Guilford, 1990

Beck JS: Cognitive Therapy: Basics and Beyond. New York, Guilford, 1997.

Ellis A: Reason and Emotion in Psychotherapy. New York, Lyle Stuart, 1962

Gould SJ: Ontogeny and Phylogeny. Cambridge, MA, Belknap Press, 1977

Pretzer J, Beck AT: A cognitive therapy of personality disorders, in Major Theories of Personality Disorder. Edited by Clarkin J. New York, Guilford, 1993, pp 36–105.

16

Pharmacotherapy of Impulsive-Aggressive Behavior

Magda Campbell, M.D.

Jeanette E. Cueva, M.D.

Phillip B. Adams, Ph.D.

Aggressive behavior has been defined as physical attacks on other persons, or property, or on one's self, with destructive intent (Campbell et al. 1982; Eichelman 1987, 1992). Aggressive behavior is relatively common in a variety of psychiatric disorders. Aggression is seen in conduct disorder, in attention-deficit hyperactivity disorder (ADHD), in autistic disorder, mania, and schizophrenia, and in some individuals with mental retardation.

Aggression characterizes a subgroup of children diagnosed as conduct disorder. This subgroup of conduct disorder children represent the majority of children 6 to 12 years of age hospitalized in an inpatient psychiatric service. These children have a poor prognosis (Keller et al. 1992) and outcome includes antisocial behavior, substance abuse as well as criminal behaviors (for review see Kazdin 1987a; Loeber 1990).

This work was supported in part by U.S. Public Health Service Grant MH-40177 (Dr. Campbell) and MH-18915 (Drs. Campbell and Cueva) from the National Institute of Mental Health; the Hirschell E. and Deanna E. Levine Foundation; the Marion O. and Maximillian E. Hoffman Foundation, Inc.; and the Beatrice and Samuel A. Seaver Foundation (Dr. Campbell).

Understanding the psychosocial environmental influences (Quay 1986; Robins 1978), the underlying pathophysiology and neurochemistry of aggressive behaviors (Kruesi et al. 1992; for review see Eichelman 1987, 1992), and their effective treatment are important areas of research, but they have been neglected in children. Several investigators have made important contributions to the biological aspects of this maladaptive behavior (Kruesi et al. 1992; Rogeness et al. 1982, 1987; Stoff et al. 1989). Of the currently available treatments, perhaps behavioral interventions have been studied most, though the results are not impressive and are of limited value (for review see Barrnett et al. 1991; Kazdin 1987a, 1987b; Werry and Wollersheim 1989).

This chapter does not exhaustively review the literature on pharmacotherapy of impulsive-aggressive behavior. It will focus on methodological and clinical issues as related to pharmacotherapy in children and adolescents, diagnosed as conduct disorder, with a profile of chronic and severe aggressive behavior accompanied by explosive affect.

Conduct Disorder and Antisocial Personality Disorder

Almost 50% of the most severely afflicted children with conduct disorder will become adults with antisocial personality disorder (Robins 1978). In children the validity of personality disorders has not been well established. A few reports suggest that traits or personality disorders can be reliably diagnosed in adolescents (Brent et al. 1990), though most are based on small sample sizes (Brent et al. 1990; Kutscher et al. 1990), and even the study by Brent et al. (1990) has a modest reliability. Baron et al. (1983), whose objective was to determine the age of onset of schizotypal personality disorder, reported a mean age of onset of 17.5 years for males and 19.1 for females.

It has been shown that conduct disorder with childhood onset associated with multiple and severe symptoms often has a chronic and persistent course (Robins 1981). Furthermore, early onset predicts a worse outcome (Loeber 1990; Robins 1981) than onset in adolescence. Conduct disorder with onset in childhood is a strong predictor of antisocial personality disorder in adulthood as well as of substance abuse disorder. The parents of these children frequently have antisocial personality disorder, substance abuse disorder, or alcohol dependence (Campbell et al. 1984; Sanchez et al. 1994; for review see Kazdin 1987a; Robins 1981). The prevalence of antisocial and delinquent behavior, including aggressive conduct disorder, has increased in the past decades (Loeber 1990).

Types of Conduct Disorder and of Aggression

Conduct disorder is the most common disorder in childhood. It is behaviorally heterogeneous, and it encompasses a variety of chronic and repetitive antisocial behaviors including aggressiveness, fighting, temper outbursts, truancy, stealing, lying, fire setting, destroying property, and cruelty to people and to animals. Conduct disorder is also etiologically heterogeneous and a variety of biologic, genetic, temperamental, and psychosocial influences are known to be contributing factors (for review see Kazdin 1987a; Quay 1986). Patterson (1982) classifies this population into aggressive and delinquent types (stealers) and recommends different treatments for these two subtypes. Antisocial behaviors were classified into overt and covert types. The overt type is characterized by arguing, fighting, bullying, defiance, and temper tantrums, whereas the salient symptoms in the covert type consist of concealed acts, such as stealing, truancy, lying, and fire setting (Loeber and Schmaling 1985a, 1985b). The overt aggressive subtype has been further subdivided into reactive/retaliatory and proactive in children (Dodge and Coie 1987; Price and Dodge 1989) and in animals into predatory aggression and affective aggression (Reis 1971, 1974).

In a sample of 73 children, ages 10 to 18 years, characterized by recurrent aggressive behavior, cluster analysis identified two clusters: planned and self-controlled aggressive behavior (predatory aggression in animals) and a second pattern, impulsive and unplanned (affective aggression) (Vitiello et al. 1990). Research is needed in order to identify subgroups responsive to different treatment modalities and outcome (Malone et al. 1998). In regard to response to treatment, Dostal (1972) found that in a group of 17 institutionalized adolescents with mental retardation severe aggressiveness was reduced by lithium only when accompanied by excitability and emotional lability, but not in those lacking the affective component. In a pilot study involving 10 children with autism, administration of lithium had a dramatic reduction of severe self-injurious behavior, temper tantrums, irritability, and explosiveness in 1 subject, a six-year-old boy who had a lifelong history of these symptoms (Campbell et al. 1972). Concerning outcome, antisocial/hostile aggression and not eruptive/impulsive aggression predicted development of conduct disorder in children with ADHD (Klein and Manuzza 1989).

Problems of Rating Aggression

All types of aggressive behaviors (both overt and covert) are low frequency behaviors and therefore difficult to capture and assess (Hinshaw et al. 1989; Kafantaris et al. 1991; Pelham and Hoza 1987) and measure reliably (for review see Campbell 1982; Hinshaw 1991). Furthermore, the conditions under which the raters assess the subjects also influence the occurrence of disruptive behavior (Romanczyk et al. 1973; for review see O'Leary and Johnson 1979). Environmental factors and ecological variables clearly affect the occurrence, rate, and severity of aggression. Multiple assessment methods are needed to capture this low frequency behavior and to reduce measurement bias.

Both diagnosis and assessment of aggressive behaviors can be carried out by clinically derived diagnosis (categorical or typological systems) or by multivariate approaches: factor analysis (symptoms) or cluster analysis (typology or subtyping). By cluster analysis, aggressive behavior can be subtyped into aggression and delinquent behavior (for review, see Kazdin 1987a). There are only a small number of rating instruments for aggressive behaviors (Table 16–1) and standardized instruments are even fewer in number (for review see Eichelman 1992; Kafantaris et al. 1991). Some of these instruments are general measures

TABLE 16–1.
Aggression rating scales

Rating scale	Author(s)
Direct observation	Campbell et al. 1984
Ratings of videotapes	Campbell and Palij 1985
Children's Psychiatric Rating Scale (CPRS)	Psychopharmacology Bulletin 1985
Conners Teacher Questionnaire (CTQ)	Psychopharmacology Bulletin 1985 Conners 1969
Peer nomination of aggression	Lefkowitz et al. 1977
Parent daily report	Patterson et al. 1982
ABC scale (antecedents, aggressive behavior, and consequences)	Cohen, unpublished data Employed in Campbell et al. 1984
Modified Profile of Mood Scale (POMS)	Walker 1982 Adapted from McNair et al. 1971
Aggression questionnaire	Vitiello et al. 1990
Overt Aggression Scale (OAS)	Yudofsky et al. 1986 Employed in Kafantaris et al. 1991, 1992; Cueva et al. 1996; Malone et al. 1994
Behavior Problem Checklist	Quay 1977
Child Behavior Checklist (CBCL)	Achenbach 1983

of psychopathology or are measures of antisocial behaviors and contain a few aggression items; however, tools developed specifically for the assessment of aggression are also available as shown in Table 16–1. Some of the methodological problems of measuring aggressiveness were addressed by the Overt Aggression Scale (OAS) developed by Yudofsky et al. (1986) (for review see Kafantaris et al. 1991). The OAS is suitable for inpatients and yields ratings of 24-hour observation; it has been found useful in hospitalized children ages 5 to 16.9 years with severe symptoms of aggressiveness. The OAS was shown to be sensitive to reflect changes associated with administration of psychoactive agents in two pilot studies (Kafantaris et al. 1992; Malone et al. 1994) and in a major double-blind and placebo-controlled clinical trial (Cueva et al. 1996).

Psychoactive Agents

There appears to be a consensus that the overt type of aggressive behavior, specifically the affective type, requires drug treatment as part
of a comprehensive treatment program. Psychosocial interventions are
indicated for the treatment of the covert type (Barrnett et al. 1991;
Kazdin 1987a, 1987b; Werry and Wollersheim 1989). The clinical decision for the type of treatment to be employed will be influenced by
the severity of aggressiveness.

Stimulants

In laboratory animals the effect of amphetamines on aggression is influenced by the type of animal, conditions, and dosages (for review see
Miczek 1987). In human subjects, too, the effects may also vary (for
review see Miczek 1987). Administration of benzedrine to a diagnostically heterogeneous group of children in a residential treatment center was associated with a decrease of aggressiveness (Bradley 1937). In
a double-blind parallel groups design, methylphenidate failed to reach
superiority over placebo in a sample of institutionalized delinquent
boys ages 9 to 14 years (Conners et al. 1971). The children were rated
on the Cottage Parent Symptom List and on the School Report list
(Conners et al. 1971); both instruments included the items fighting,
destructiveness, temper outbursts, and "quarrelsome, disturbs other
children." It is interesting that stereotypic self-biting (fingers) associated
with administration of dextroamphetamine and with methylphenidate
was reported in four children diagnosed with ADHD (Sokol et al.
1987), a side effect analogous to findings in nonhuman primates
(Goldstein et al. 1986a, 1986b).

Several studies, some based on small samples of subjects, indicate
that stimulants are effective in decreasing aggressiveness in patients
with ADHD with or without conduct disorder (Gadow et al. 1990;
Hinshaw 1991; Kaplan et al. 1990; Murphy et al. 1992). Both dextroamphetamine and levoamphetamine reduced aggressiveness sig-

nificantly in hyperkinetic children who participated in a placebo-controlled study employing a crossover design (Arnold et al. 1973).

Hinshaw (1991) presents a detailed analysis of the literature on the effects of stimulant drugs on aggression in children with ADHD. Data based on research suggest that low doses of stimulants have only weak effect on overt aggression in laboratory or playroom settings (Hinshaw 1991; Hinshaw et al. 1984; Murphy et al. 1992). In contrast, under the conditions of naturalistic observations, outdoors or in classroom, drug effects on aggression are significant (Gadow et al. 1990; Murphy et al. 1992). In addition, two reports concur that the effects on aggressiveness seem to be specific (Gadow et al. 1990; Hinshaw et al. 1989).

However, it should be noted that hyperactivity is a more prominent feature in children and adolescents with ADHD than is aggressiveness (Kaplan et al. 1990), and it is conceivable that severe aggressiveness may not be reduced to a clinically meaningful degree by a stimulant drug. Furthermore, the findings cited here are based on outpatients. Clinical experience shows that severe aggressiveness that is prominent in children diagnosed as conduct disorder leading to hospitalization is not reduced by methylphenidate and requires more potent psychoactive agents (for review see Campbell et al. 1992).

Antidepressants (Tricyclics)

There is some suggestion that tricyclics may increase aggressiveness in certain laboratory animals and in human subjects, although not all reports are in agreement (for review see Miczek 1987). While Winsberg et al. (1972) and Waizer et al. (1974) reported reduction of aggressiveness with imipramine and Yepes et al. (1977) with amitriptyline, Rapoport et al. (1974) found no effect of imipramine on conduct problem factors as rated by teachers and parents in hyperactive children. Pallmeyer and Petti (1979) reported on clear-cut emergence and increase in aggressiveness (requiring locked seclusion) associated with administration of imipramine (3.5 and 5.0 mg/kg/day) in two boys, ages 11 and 6 years, treated for depression. Administration of clomipramine was associated with decrease of aggressiveness in a 13-year-old boy and reduction in self-injurious behavior in a 29-year-old woman, both outpatients diagnosed with autistic disorder (McDougle et al. 1992), whereas an increase and/or emergence of these symptoms were observed in three hospitalized autistic children, ages 5.2–7.6 years (Sanchez et al. 1994).

Neuroleptics

Neuroleptics are perhaps the most commonly used agents in the treatment of aggressive behavior, even though it is believed that this effect is nonspecific (Miczek 1987). Both chlorpromazine (Campbell et al. 1982) and haloperidol (Campbell et al. 1984) were found to reduce both statistically and clinically significantly aggressive and explosive behavior in hospitalized children with conduct disorder. The powerful effects of these agents were shown under double-blind conditions with random assignment to treatment conditions, and in the study by Campbell et al. (1984) haloperidol was compared to lithium, and placebo served as control. Chlorpromazine was more sedative than haloperidol (Campbell et al. 1982), though the usefulness of haloperidol was also somewhat limited by its sedative effects (Campbell et al. 1982, 1984). The clinical usefulness of neuroleptics is limited not only by their sedative effect, but also by their long-term untoward effects: tardive or withdrawal dyskinesias (Campbell et al. 1988, 1997; Richardson et al. 1991). Development of dyskinetic movements was reported as early as after 4 weeks of treatment with molindone in an aggressive child with conduct disorder (Greenhill et al. 1985). An overview of the representative literature is presented in Table 16–2.

Lithium

Lithium has been used in children and adolescents with an aggressive profile in the past 25 years. As in all drugs used in the treatment of aggressiveness, the question is the behavioral specificity of the psychoactive agent to be employed (Miczek 1987): Are the doses of lithium at which aggressive behavior is reduced lower than the doses that reduce nonaggressive behavior? It appears that lithium does have specific

TABLE 16–2.
Neuroleptics: overview of representative studies

Author(s)	Psychoactive agents	Dose range in mg/d (mean)	Subjects[a]		Design	Results
			Age range in years (mean)	N		
Campbell et al. 1982	Chlorpromazine (vs. haloperidol and lithium)	100–200 (150)	6–11.9 (8.68)	5 (Total N = 15)	Double-blind randomized parallel groups	Positive; all three drugs equally effective
Campbell et. al. 1984	Haloperidol (vs. lithium)	1.0–6.0 (2.95)	5.2–12.9 (8.97)	20 (Total N = 61)	Double-blind, placebo-controlled, randomized parallel groups	Positive; haloperidol as effective as lithium; both superior to placebo
Greenhill et al. 1981	Molindone	18–155 (40.5)	6–11 (9.8)	6	Open pilot	Positive
Greenhill et al. 1985	Molindone (vs. thioridazine)	26.8	6–11	15 (Total N = 31)	Double-blind randomized parallel groups	Positive

[a]*Conduct disorder, aggressive type, in all samples with the exception of Campbell et al. (1982), which includes hyperkinetic reaction of childhood (6) and schizophrenia (3).*

antiaggressive properties (Eichelman 1987). In a well-designed study involving 66 subjects ages 16 to 24 years (mean = 19), lithium was shown to have strong antiaggressive effects (Sheard et al. 1976). All subjects were inmates convicted for serious aggressive crimes with a history of chronic aggressive behavior and/or impulsive antisocial behavior. Lithium was as effective as haloperidol in reducing aggressiveness and explosiveness in hospitalized children diagnosed as conduct disorder with a profile of aggressive and explosive behavior (Campbell et al. 1984). However, lithium had fewer side effects than haloperidol as rated by clinical staff and as experienced subjectively by the children (Campbell et al. 1984); furthermore, lithium had fewer adverse effects on performance in the laboratory (Platt et al. 1984). The most common side effect associated with haloperidol was excessive sedation (in 16 of 20 children during dose regulation, and in 4 at optimal doses); no child was sedated on optimal doses of lithium and only 4 were so during dose titration (Campbell et al. 1984). The side effects of lithium in these children are detailed elsewhere (Campbell et al. 1972, 1984, 1991; Silva et al. 1992). Though both lithium and haloperidol were clinically and statistically highly superior to placebo in reducing aggressiveness and explosiveness, as well as hyperactivity at doses shown in Table 16–3, lithium was rated superior to haloperidol by clinical and research staff on Global Clinical Judgments Scale, a consensus measure (Campbell et al. 1984). The therapeutic profiles of these two drugs were well stated by the head nurse of the ward: Haloperidol made the children more "manageable," whereas in the children receiving lithium the pathological aggressiveness was channeled in a more socially acceptable way. A few children who were constantly fighting and breaking the furniture became leaders of the ward.

In a subsequent study involving 50 hospitalized children randomly assigned to lithium or placebo under double-blind conditions, the superiority of lithium over placebo was again demonstrated (Campbell et al. 1995). However, the effects of lithium were not as powerful as in the previous study (Campbell et al. 1984) even though the same inclusion and exclusion criteria were employed for patients and the same assessment instruments and raters were used. The clinical effectiveness of lithium in this population of children was not related to comorbidity with depression or underlying affective disorder; these dis-

TABLE 16–3.

Lithium carbonate: overview of representative studies

Author(s)	Dose range in mg/d (mean)	Serum levels in mEq/l (mean)	Subjects[a] Age range in years (mean)	N	Design	Results
Campbell et al. 1982	1,250–2,000 (1,800)	0.76–1.24 (0.993)	6–11.9	5 (Total N = 15)	Double-blind (lithium vs. chlorpromazine vs. haloperidol)	Positive; all three drugs equally effective
Campbell et al. 1984	500–2,000 (1,166)	0.32–1.51 (0.993)	5.2–12.9 (8.97)	21 (Total N = 61)	Double-blind, placebo-controlled, randomized parallel groups (lithium vs. haloperidol)	Positive; lithium as effective as haloperidol; both superior to placebo
Campbell et al. 1995	600–1,800 (1,248)	0.53–1.79 (1.12)	5.1–12 (9.4)	21 (Total N = 50)	Double-blind, placebo controlled, randomized parallel groups	Positive
DeLong and Aldershof 1987	Not given	Not given	6.8–16 (12.3)	9 (Total N = 190)	Open	Positive (5 of 9 improved)
Siassi 1982	900–2,100 (1,475)	1.0–1.5 (1.21)	7–13 (9.8)	14 (Total N = 28)	Open	Positive

[a] *Conduct disorder, aggressive type, in all samples with the exception of Campbell et al. (1982), which includes hyperkinetic reaction of childhood (6) and schizophrenia (3). DeLong and Aldershof (1987) and Siassi (1982) contain a heterogeneous diagnostic sample with or without aggression.*

orders were among exclusion criteria in both clinical trials (Campbell et al. 1984, 1995). Furthermore, these children were not rated depressed on the 9 depression items of the Children's Psychiatric Rating Scale (CPRS; Psychopharmacology Bulletin 1985).

Carbamazepine

Not all children and adolescents with conduct disorder and target symptoms of aggressiveness and explosiveness respond to lithium, as indicated by double-blind and placebo-controlled studies (Campbell et al. 1984, 1995; Klein 1991; Rifkin et al. 1989; Sanchez et al. 1994) as well as clinical reports (DeLong and Aldershof 1987). Because of this, other psychoactive agents are sought and carbamazepine, another drug with reported antiaggressive properties, has been of interest. Carbamazepine has a similar clinical profile to that of lithium, although some of their side effects are divergent (Post 1987).

Although approximately a total of 800 children and adolescents with a profile of aggression have participated in studies of carbamazepine, there are only seven placebo-controlled studies in this population and they have methodological flaws (for review see Remschmidt 1976). Most knowledge regarding the effectiveness of carbamazepine in psychiatric patients is based on reports involving adults (for review see Post 1987); the information on safety in children is mainly derived from those treated with carbamazepine for seizure disorders (Gamstorp 1976; Sillanpaa 1981). Post (1987) suggested that different subgroups of patients with manic-depression respond to carbamazepine than to lithium, which is supported by some evidence. In a pilot study of carbamazepine involving 10 hospitalized children with conduct disorder and target symptoms of aggression and explosiveness, 5 children failed to respond to lithium prior to their treatment with carbamazepine (Kafantaris et al. 1992). Of the 5 who did not respond to lithium, 3 showed marked and 1 moderate improvement on carbamazepine, and the fifth child failed to respond to either drug. Those children who did not respond to lithium responded the best to carbamazepine; of the 4 children in the sample of 10 who responded markedly to carbamazepine, 3 did not respond to lithium. However, administration of carbamazepine (4.8–7.6 μg/ml) was associated with side effects including diplopia, dysarthria, and blurred vision, as well as transient slight decrease of white blood count (in 4 children). In a double-blind and placebo-controlled study carbamazepine was commonly associated with untoward effects and was not superior to placebo (Cueva et al. 1997). An overview of the representative studies is shown in Table 16–4.

Beta-Blockers

This class of drugs was explored in a variety of psychiatric patients and persons with mental retardation, characterized by treatment resistant aggression (for review see Campbell et al. 1992). The reported findings, sometimes dramatic reduction in aggression and rages, are mainly based on case reports, and some of the patients continued to receive other psychoactive agents when placed on propranolol. Two studies with propranolol are summarized in Table 16–5.

Psychosocial Influences and Response to Treatment

As the subtyping of aggression (into affective and "predatory") may have implications for treatment or type of treatment (Vitiello et al. 1990), the child's psychosocial environment, including adverse influences, may also affect response to treatment and predict response to treatment. Parental criminal behavior, alcoholism or substance abuse and dependence, violence, broken homes, marital discord, and socioeconomic status are among the adversities that contribute to risk of conduct disorder (Szatmari et al. 1989; for review see Kazdin 1987a). The effect of these contributing factors on treatment response has not been systematically examined in clinical drug trials involving children with conduct disorder. The observation has been made that a substantial number of children with conduct disorder who are hospitalized because of repetitive and severe aggressiveness and explosiveness show a

TABLE 16–4.

Carbamazepine: overview of representative studies

| Author(s) | Dose range in mg/d (mean) | Plasma level in µg/ml (mean) | Subjects[a] | | | Design | Results |
			Age range in years (mean)	N			
Groh 1976	Not given	Not given	8–14	20		Double-blind, placebo-controlled crossover	Ten children improved markedly on carbamazepine and only one on placebo
Puente 1976	200–300	Not given	5–13 (8.7)	27		Double-blind, placebo-controlled crossover; not randomized	More children improved on carbamazepine than on placebo
Kafantaris et al. 1992	600–800 (630)	4.8–10.4 (6.2)	5.25–10.92 (8.27)	10		Open pilot	Significant decrease of fighting, bullying, and temper outbursts from baseline to the end of treatment ($P < .005$)
Cueva et al. 1996	400–800 (683)	4.98–9.1 (6.81)	5.33–11.7 (8.97)	22		Double-blind, placebo-controlled, parallel groups, randomized	Negative

[a]*Conduct disorder, aggressive type, in Kafantaris et al. (1992) and in Cueva et al. (1996). In Groh (1976) and Puente (1976) subjects have no specific psychiatric diagnosis, but all have behavior problems including aggression.*

TABLE 16-5.

Beta blockers: overview of representative studies

Author(s)	Psychoactive agents	Dose range in mg/d (mean)	Subjects[a] Age range in years (mean)	N	Design	Results
Williams et al. 1982	Propranolol	50–960 Median = 160	7–35 (11 children; 15 adolescents; 4 adults)	30	Open	75% of sample had reduction in aggression
Kuperman and Stewart 1987	Propranolol	80–280 (164 ± 55)	4–24 (13.4) (8 children; 4 adolescents; 4 adults)	16	Open	63% of sample had reduction in aggression

[a]In both reports subjects were diagnostically heterogeneous but all were characterized by aggressiveness. In Williams et al. (1982), 25 subjects had conduct disorder and 13 were mentally retarded. In Kuperman and Stewart (1987), eight subjects were mildly to severely mentally retarded.

445

decline in these target symptoms during the pretreatment placebo baseline period while in the highly structured therapeutic environment of the hospital ward (Campbell et al. 1984). Sanchez et al. (1994) wished to differentiate those who responded to placebo from those who did not over the six-week treatment period in a double-blind study of lithium employing parallel groups design. The following adverse psychosocial environmental factors were rated: home violence, criminality in parents, parental substance abuse, and unstable home. The sample consisted of 25 children, 24 males and 1 female, ages 6.25 to 11.95 years who were assigned to placebo treatment following a two-week placebo baseline period (Campbell et al. 1995). Among the reasons for the placebo baseline period was the objective to eliminate some children who responded to placebo. In an earlier report, 16 children were dropped from the study because their aggressiveness and explosiveness ceased by the end of the two-week pretreatment placebo period, a number that represented almost one-quarter of the study sample (Campbell et al. 1984). Other investigators have had similar findings (Malone et al. 1997). In the report by Sanchez et al. (1994) those who responded to placebo ($n = 10$) did not differ significantly from those who failed to respond to placebo ($n = 15$) in regard to age, full-scale IQ, and baseline severity of symptoms as measured by the CPRS and Clinical Global Impressions (CGI; Psychopharmacology Bulletin 1995) scores with one exception. The hyperactivity factor of the CPRS was lower in those who responded to placebo than those who did not ($P = .055$).

Though adverse psychosocial factors were rated in most children, those who responded to placebo had significantly more adversities than those who did not respond, particularly violence in home and criminally charged parents ($P < .05$). Furthermore, even low level of hyperactivity contributed to failure to respond to placebo. These findings were based on a small sample of patients and require replication in a large sample. If these types of findings can be confirmed, they could serve as a guide for therapeutic intervention. Thus if a child comes from an undesirable home environment and is not hyperactive, focus should be on psychosocial interventions, including parental involvement, if feasible, and pharmacotherapy should not be considered at first. We plan to study in a more systematic fashion the effect of these factors on drug response.

Future Research

Reanalysis of some of the data of two clinical trials of lithium (Campbell et al. 1984, 1995) was conducted because of the discrepancies found in the effectiveness of lithium. As discussed earlier, the ability of lithium to reduce aggressiveness in the earlier trial (Campbell et al. 1984) was more powerful than in the subsequent study. At the present time, we can only speculate what may account or contribute to the differences in results between the two studies, even though the same design, methodology, assessment instruments, and the same raters were employed in both. The study published in 1984 was conducted in the old Bellevue Psychiatric Hospital, on a large ward where the patient census was high. The more recent study was conducted in a newer building, in a highly structured environment, with a smaller number of patients but the same number of staff. These changes in the child's hospital environment may have influenced the results of our studies. For example, whereas 16 children (19.5% of the sample) showed a considerable reduction in aggressiveness during the two-week pretreatment placebo period in the earlier study (Campbell et al. 1984), in the subsequent study, 23 children did so (29%) and therefore were not enrolled in the treatment phase (Campbell et al. 1995). The prevalence of conduct disorder is reported to be higher now (Loeber 1990; Thornberry et al. 1995) than in the late 1970s and early 1980s, when the study published in 1984 was conducted. Due to changes in society in recent years, adverse psychosocial environmental factors are more severe and numerous in the lives of this population of children. These changes may have contributed to our patients' aggressiveness, which in turn may have increased their response to placebo (see Sanchez et al. 1994) thus reducing the differences between placebo and lithium treatment conditions. Finally, the current sample is only mildly hyperactive, whereas the previous sample was markedly so; in the current sample, hyperactivity is inversely related to age, whereas in the previous sample it was present across all ages. In the study of Sanchez et al. (1994) even mild hyperactivity contributed to the failure to respond to placebo. It is conceivable that the presence of moderately severe hyperactivity as rated on the CPRS contributed to the favorable and strong response to lithium (Campbell et al. 1984), whereas in the more recent study the very low level of hyperactivity on the CPRS contributed to greater response to placebo (Campbell et al. 1995).

Future research is needed to advance understanding of aggressive behavior, with the objective to improve treatment and to predict responders to specific treatment modalities, including treatment with psychoactive agents. It is imperative to study both neurobio-chemical mechanisms of aggression as well as psychosocial-environmental influences. Preliminary data suggest that for a subgroup of children with conduct disorder, intensive psychosocial interventions are indicated, whereas for others, an appropriate psychoactive agent should be part of a comprehensive treatment program. Pharmacotherapy should be compared to psychosocial intervention(s) and the combination of both should be critically assessed. Such research should have high priority, because the outcome for children afflicted by this condition is at best guarded.

References

Achenbach TM, Edelbrock C: Manual for the Child Behavior Checklist and Revised Child Behavior Profile. Burlington, VT, Department of Psychiatry, University of Vermont, 1983

Arnold LE, Kirilcuk V, Corson SA, Corson EO: Levoamphetamine and dextroamphetamine: differential effect on aggression and hyperkinesis in children and dogs. Am J Psychiatry 130:165–170, 1973

Baron M, Gruen R, Asnis L: Age-of-onset in schizophrenia and schizotypal disorders. Neuropsychobiology 10:199–204, 1983

Barrnett RJ, Docherty JP, Frommelt GM: Special article: a review of child psychotherapy research since 1963. J Am Acad Child Adolesc Psychiatry 30(1):1–14, 1991

Bradley C: The behavior of children receiving benzedrine. Am J Psychiatry 94:577–585, 1937

Brent DA, Zelenak JP, Bukstein O, Brown RV: Reliability and validity of the structured interview for personality disorder. J Am Acad Child Adolesc Psychiatry 29:349–354, 1990

Campbell M, Palij M: Behavioral and cognitive measures used in psychopharmacological studies of infantile autism. Psychopharmacol Bull 21(3):1047–1053, 1985

Campbell M, Fish B, Korein J, et al: Lithium and chlorpromazine: a controlled crossover study of hyperactive severely disturbed young children. J Aut Child Schizophr 2:234–263, 1972

Campbell M, Cohen IL, Small AM: Drugs in aggressive behavior. J Am Acad Child Psychiatry 21:107, 1982

Campbell M, Small AM, Green WH, et al: Behavioral efficacy of haloperidol and lithium carbonate: a comparison in hospitalized aggressive children with conduct disorder. Arch Gen Psychiatry 41:650–656, 1984

Campbell M, Adams P, Perry R, et al: Tardive and withdrawal dyskinesia in autistic children: a prospective study. Psychopharmacol Bull 24:251–255, 1988

Campbell M, Silva RR, Kafantaris V, et al: Predictors of side effects associated with lithium administration in children. Psychopharmacol Bull 27:373–380, 1991

Campbell M, Gonzalez NM, Silva RR: The pharmacologic treatment of conduct disorders and rage outbursts. Psychiatr Clin North Am 15:69–85, 1992

Campbell M, Adams PB, Small AM, et al: Lithium in hospitalized aggressive children with conduct disorder: a double-blind and placebo controlled study J Am Acad Child Adolesc Psychiatry 34:445–453, 1995

Campbell M, Armenteros JL, Malone RP, et al: Neuroleptic-related dyskinesias in autistic children: a prospective, longitudinal study. J Am Acad Child Adolesc Psychiatry 36:835–843, 1997

Conners CK: A teacher rating scale for use in drug studies with children. Am J Psychiatry 126:884–888, 1969

Conners CK, Kramer R, Rothschild GH, et al: Treatment of young delinquent boys with diphenylhydantoin sodium and methylphenidate. Arch Gen Psychiatry 24:156–160, 1971

Cueva JE, Overall JE, Small AM, et al: Carbamazepine in aggressive children with conduct disorder: a double-blind and placebo-controlled study. J Am Acad Child Adolesc Psychiatry 35:480–490, 1996

DeLong GR, Aldershof AL: Long-term experience with lithium treatment in childhood: correlation with clinical diagnosis. J Am Acad Child Adolesc Psychiatry 26:389–394, 1987

Dodge KA, Coie JD: Social-information-processing factors in reactive and proactive aggression in children's peer groups. J Pers Soc Psychol 53: 1146–1158, 1987

Dostal T: Antiaggressive effect of lithium salts in mentally retarded adolescents, in Depressive States in Childhood and Adolescence. Edited by Annell AL. Stockholm, Almquist & Wiksell, 1972, pp 491–498

Eichelman B: Neurochemical and psychopharmacologic aspects of aggressive behavior, in Psychopharmacology: Third Generation of Progress. Edited by Meltzer HY. New York, Raven, 1987, pp 697–704

Eichelman B: Aggressive behavior: from laboratory to clinic: quo vadit? Arch Gen Psychiatry 49:488–492, 1992

Gadow KD, Nolan EE, Sverd J, et al: Methylphenidate in aggressive-hyperactive boys: I. Effects on peer aggression in public school settings. J Am Acad Child Adolesc Psychiatry 29:710–718, 1990

Gamstorp I: Carbamazepine in the treatment of epileptic disorders in infancy and childhood, in Epileptic Seizures-Behaviour-Pain. Edited by Birkmayer W. Baltimore, MD, University Park Press, 1976, pp 98–103

Goldstein M, Deutch AY, Shimizu Y, et al: Anatomical correlates of dopamine agonist-induced self-mutilative biting behavior in the primate. Soc Neurosci Abstr No 26814, p 972, 1986a

Goldstein M, Kusano N, Meller E, et al: Dopamine agonist induced self-mutilative biting behavior in monkeys with unilateral ventromedial tegmental lesions of the brain-stem: possible pharmacological model for Lesch-Nyhan syndrome. Brain Res 367:114–120, 1986b

Greenhill LL, Barmack JE, Spalten D, et al: Molindone hydrochloride in the treatment of aggressive, hospitalized children. Psychopharmacol Bull 17:125–126, 1981

Greenhill LL, Solomon M, Pleak R, et al: Molindone hydrochloride treatment of hospitalized children with conduct disorder. J Clin Psychiatry 46(8, Sec. 2):20–25, 1985

Groh C: The psychotropic effect of Tegretol in non-epileptic children, with particular reference to the drug's indications, in Epileptic Seizures-Behaviour-Pain. Edited by Birkmayer W. Baltimore, MD, University Park Press, 1976, pp 259–263

Hinshaw SP: Stimulant medication and the treatment of aggression in children with attentional deficits. J Clin Child Psychol 20:301–312, 1991

Hinshaw SP, Henker B, Whalen CK: Self-control in hyperactive boys in anger-inducing situations: effects of cognitive-behavioral training and of methylphenidate. J Abnorm Child Psychol 12:55–77, 1984

Hinshaw SP, Henker B, Whalen CK, et al: Aggressive, prosocial, and nonsocial behavior in hyperactive boys: dose effects of methylphenidate in naturalistic settings. J Consult Clin Psychol 57:636–643, 1989

Kafantaris V, Lee D, Magee H, et al: The Overt Aggression Scale in a child psychiatry inpatient unit: a pilot study. Paper presented at the annual meeting of the American Academy of Child and Adolescent Psychiatry, San Francisco, October 1991

Kafantaris V, Campbell M, Padron-Gayol MV, et al: Carbamazepine in aggressive children: a pilot study. Psychopharmacol Bull 28:193–199, 1992

Kaplan SL, Busner J, Kupietz S, et al: Effects of methylphenidate on adolescents with aggressive conduct disorder and ADDH: a preliminary report. J Am Acad Child Adolesc Psychiatry 29:719–723, 1990

Kazdin AE: Conduct Disorders in Childhood and Adolescence. London, Sage, 1987a

Kazdin AE: Treatment of antisocial behavior in children: current status and future directions. Psychol Bull 102:187–203, 1987b

Keller MB, Lavori PW, Beardslee WR, et al: The disruptive behavioral disorder on children and adolescents: comorbidity and clinical course. J Am Acad Child Adolesc Psychiatry 31:204–209, 1992

Klein R: Preliminary results: lithium effects in conduct disorders. CME Syllabus and Proceedings Summary, the 144th Annual Meeting of the American Psychiatric Association, New Orleans, LA, 1991, pp 119–120

Klein RG, Mannuzza S: The long-term outcome of the ADD/hyperkinetic syndrome, in Attention Deficit Disorder: Clinical and Basic Research. Edited by Sagvolden T, Archer T. Hillsdale, NJ, Lawrence Erlbaum Associates, 1989, pp 71–91

Kruesi MJP, Hibbs ED, Zahn TP, et al: A 2-year prospective follow-up study of children and adolescents with disruptive behavior disorders. Prediction by cerebrospinal fluid 5-hydroxyindoleacetic acid, homovanillic acid, and autonomic measures. Arch Gen Psychiatry 49:429–435, 1992

Kuperman S, Stewart MA: Use of propranolol to decrease aggressive outbursts in younger patients. Psychosomatics 28:315–319, 1987

Kutscher SP, Marton P, Korenblum M: Adolescent bipolar illness and personality disorder. J Am Acad Child Adolesc Psychiatry 29:355–358, 1990

Lefkowitz MM, Eron LD, Walder LO, et al: Growing Up to Be Violent: A Longitudinal Study of the Development of Aggression. New York, Pergamon, 1977

Loeber R: Development and risk factors of juvenile antisocial behavior and delinquency. Clin Psychol Rev 10:1–41, 1990

Loeber R, Schmaling KB: The utility of differentiating between mixed and pure forms of antisocial child behavior. J Abnorm Child Psychol 13:315–336, 1985a

Loeber R, Schmaling KB: Empirical evidence for overt and covert patterns of antisocial conduct problems: a metaanalysis. J Abnorm Child Psychol 13:337–352, 1985b

Malone RP, Luebbert J, Pena-Ariet M, et al: The Overt Aggression Scale in a study of lithium in aggressive conduct disorder. Psychopharmacol Bull 30:215–218, 1994

Malone RP, Luebbert JF, Delaney MA, et al: Nonpharmacological response in hospitalized children with conduct disorder. J Am Acad Child Adolesc Psychiatry 36:242–247, 1997

Malone RP, Bennett DS, Luebbert JF, et al: Aggression classification and treatment response. Psychopharmacol Bull 34:41–45, 1998

McDougle CJ, Price LH, Volkmar FR, et al: Clomipramine in autism: preliminary evidence of efficacy. J Am Acad Child Adolesc Psychiatry 31:746–750, 1992

McNair DM, Lorr M, Droppelman LF: Profile of Mood States: Manual. San Diego, CA, Educational and Industrial Testing Service, 1971

Miczek KA: The psychopharmacology of aggression, in Handbook of Psychopharmacology: New Directions in Behavioral Pharmacology. Edited by Iversen LL, Iversen SD, Snyder SH. New York, Plenum, 1987, pp 183–328

Murphy DA, Pelham WE, Lang AR: Aggression in boys with attention deficit-hyperactivity disorder: methylphenidate effects on naturalistically observed aggression, response to provocation, and social information processing. J Abnorm Child Psychol 2:451–466, 1992

O'Leary KD, Johnson SB: Psychological assessment, in Psychopathological Disorders of Childhood, 2nd Edition. Edited by Quay HC, Werry JS. New York, Wiley, 1979, pp 210–246

Pallmeyer TP, Petti TA: Effects of imipramine on aggression and dejection in depressed children. Am J Psychiatry 136:1472–1473, 1979

Patterson GR: Coercive Family Process. Eugene, OR, Castalaia, 1982

Pelham WE, Hoza J: Behavioral assessment of psychostimulant effects on ADD children in a summer day treatment program, in Advances in Behavioral Assessment of Children and Families, Vol 3. Edited by Prinz R. Greenwich, CT, JAI Press, 1987, pp 3–33

Platt J, Campbell M, Green WH, et al: Cognitive effects of lithium carbonate and haloperidol in treatment-resistant aggressive children. Arch Gen Psychiatry 41:657–662, 1984

Post RM: Mechanisms of action of carbamazepine and related anticonvulsants in affective illness, in Psychopharmacology: The Third Generation of Progress. Edited by Meltzer HY. New York, Raven, 1987, pp 567–576

Price JM, Dodge KA: Reactive and proactive aggression in childhood: relations to peer status and social context dimensions. J Abnorm Child Psychol 17:455–471, 1989

Psychopharmacology Bulletin: Special Feature: rating scales and assessment instruments for use in pediatric psychopharmacology research, 21(4), 1985

Puente RM: The use of carbamazepine in the treatment of behavioural disorders in children, in Epileptic Seizures-Behaviour-Pain. Edited by Birkmayer W. Baltimore, MD, University Park Press, 1976, pp 243–247

Quay HC: Measuring dimensions of deviant behavior. The behavior problem checklist. J Abnorm Child Psychol 5:277–287, 1977

Quay HC: Conduct disorders, in Psychopathological Disorders of Childhood. Edited by Quay HC, Werry JS. New York, Wiley, 1986, pp 35–72

Rapoport JL, Quinn PO, Bradbard G, et al: Imipramine and methylphenidate treatments of hyperactive boys. Arch Gen Psychiatry 30:789–793, 1974

Reis D: Brain monoamines in aggression and sleep. Clin Neurosurg 18:471–502, 1971

Reis D: Central neurotransmitters in aggression. Res Publ Assoc Res Nerv Ment Dis 52:119–148, 1974

Remschmidt H: The psychotropic effect of carbamazepine in non-epileptic patients, with particular reference to problems posed by clinical studies in children with behavioural disorders, in Epileptic Seizures-Behaviour-Pain. Edited by Birkmayer W. Baltimore, MD, University Park Press, 1976, pp 253–258

Richardson MA, Haugland G, Craig TJ: Neuroleptic use, parkinsonian symptoms, tardive dyskinesia, and associated factors in child and adolescent psychiatric patients. Am J Psychiatry 148:1322–1328, 1991

Rifkin A, Doddi S, Dicker R, et al: Lithium in adolescence with conduct disorder. Paper presented at the Annual New Clinical Drug Evaluation Unit Meeting, Key Biscayne, FL, May 1989

Robins LN: Sturdy childhood predictors of adult antisocial behavior: replications from longitudinal studies. Psychol Med 8:611–622, 1978

Robins LN: Epidemiological approaches to natural history research: antisocial disorders in children. J Am Acad Child Psychiatry 20:566–680, 1981

Rogeness GA, Hernandez JM, Macedo CA, et al: Biochemical differences in children with conduct disorder socialized and undersocialized. Am J Psychiatry 139:307–311, 1982

Rogeness GA, Javors MA, Maas JW, et al: Plasma dopamine-B-hydroxylase, HVA, MHPG, and conduct disorders in emotionally disturbed boys. Biol Psychiatry 22:1155–1158, 1987

Romanczyk RG, Kent RN, Diament C, et al: Measuring the reliability of observational data: a reactive process. J Appl Behav Analysis 6:175–184, 1973

Sanchez LE, Armenteros JL, Small AM, et al: Placebo response in aggressive children with conduct disorder. Psychopharmacol Bull 30:126, 1994

Sheard MH, Marini JL, Bridges CL, et al: The effect of lithium on impulsive aggressive behavior in man. Am J Psychiatry 133:1409–1413, 1976

Siassi I: Lithium treatment of impulsive behavior in children. J Clin Psychiatry 43:482–484, 1982

Sillanpaa M: Carbamazepine. Pharmacology and clinical uses. Acta Neurol Scand 64(suppl 88):145–161, 1981

Silva RR, Campbell M, Golden RR, et al: Side effects associated with lithium and placebo administration in aggressive children. Psychopharmacol Bull 28:319–326, 1992

Sokol MS, Campbell M, Goldstein M, et al: Attention deficit disorder with hyperactivity and the dopamine hypothesis: a case presentation with theoretical background. J Am Acad Child Psychiatry 26:428–433, 1987

Stoff DM, Friedman E, Pollack L, et al: Elevated platelet MAO is related to impulsivity in disruptive behavior disorders. J Am Acad Child Adolesc Psychiatry 28:754–760, 1989

Szatmari P, Boyle M, Offord, DR: ADDH and conduct disorder: degree of diagnostic overlap and difference among correlates. J Am Acad Child Adolesc Psychiatry 28:865–872, 1989

Thornberry TP, Huizinga D, Loeber R: Prevention of serious delinquency and violence, in Sourcebook on Serious, Violent, and Chronic Juvenile Offenders. Edited by Howell JC, Krisberg B, Hawkins JD, et al. Thousand Oaks, CA, Sage Publications, 1995, pp 213–227

Vitiello B, Behar D, Hunt J, et al: Subtyping aggression in children and adolescents. J Neuropsychiatry Clin Neurosci 2:189–192, 1990

Waizer J, Hoffman SP, Polizos P, Englehardt DM: Outpatient treatment of hyperactive school children with imipramine. Am J Psychiatry 131:587–591, 1974

Walker M: The psychomotor stimulants, in Drugs and Mental Retardation. Edited by Breuning SE, Poling AD. Springfield, IL, Charles C Thomas, 1982, pp 309–352

Werry JS, Wollersheim JP: Special article: behavior therapy with children and adolescents: a twenty-year overview. J Am Acad Child Adolesc Psychiatry 28(1):1–18, 1989

Williams DT, Mehl R, Yudofsky S, et al: The effect of propranolol on un-controlled rage outbursts in children and adolescents with organic brain dysfunction. J Am Acad Child Psychiatry 21:129–135, 1982

Winsberg BG, Bialer I, Kupietz S, et al: Effects of imipramine and dextro-amphetamine on behavior of neuropsychiatrically impaired children. Am J Psychiatry 128:1425–1431, 1972

Yepes LE, Balka EB, Winsberg BG, et al: Amitriptyline and methylphenidate treatment of behaviorally disordered children. J Child Psychol Psychiatry 18:39–52, 1977

Yudofsky SC, Silver JM, Jackson W, et al: The overt aggression scale for the objective rating of verbal and physical aggression. Am J Psychiatry 143:35–39, 1986

CHAPTER 17

Temperament and the Pharmacotherapy of Depression

Peter R. Joyce, M.D.

Roger T. Mulder, M.D.

C. Robert Cloninger, M.D.

The introduction of DSM-III (American Psychiatric Association 1980) in 1980, with a separate axis (II) for personality disorders, has been a major stimulus to research on personality and its disorders over the past two decades. However, while there has seldom been debate about the importance of personality to an understanding of psychopathology, there has never been a consensus on how to conceptualize, understand, and assess personality. Even the issue of categorical and/or dimensional approaches to personality has remained controversial.

In the validation of Axis I disorders, the approach exemplified by Robins and Guze (1970) has been fruitful. In this process, there are five phases in validation: clinical description, laboratory studies, delimitation from other disorders, follow-up studies, and family studies. Although this approach has been of major importance, it has led to a proliferation of sets of diagnostic criteria and may have limitations if the disorders of interest are essentially dimensional rather than truly discrete entities (Cloninger 1989). Of the current Axis II personality disorders, probably only antisocial personality disorder has been sufficiently validated.

With the growing interest and diversity of approaches to personality, there will be no real progress or consensus on which approaches to use, until steps toward validation by the traditional Robins and Guze phases are employed. In personality research, there has been ever growing use of family and genetic approaches (Plomin 1990). Interest has also been increasing in linking biologic and laboratory measures to personality (Mulder 1992), and as Zuckerman (1991) has elegantly argued, progress in personality research must be linked to understanding the biologic substrate of personality.

Another challenge for research into personality is to seek validation of personality measures by follow-up studies. These may take the design of following up individuals who were considered to have certain personality traits or disorders. The classic work in this area is by Lee Robins (1966), who showed the links between childhood conduct disorder and adult antisocial personality disorder. An alternative follow-up strategy is to determine how personality measures influence the outcome of other mental or physical disorders, such as major depression.

Personality and the Outcome of Depression

The expanding interest in personality has led to renewed interest in the possibility that certain personality traits or the presence of a comorbid personality disorder adversely affects the treatment outcome for patients with major depression. Many studies have reported that traits such as high neuroticism predict a worse outcome in patients with depression (Andrews et al. 1990; Duggan et al. 1990; Kerr et al. 1970; Weissman et al. 1978). Similarly, many studies find that patients with depression and a comorbid personality disorder have a poorer treatment outcome (Peselow et al. 1992a; Pfohl et al. 1984, 1987; Shea et al. 1990). However, not all studies have found that the presence of a comorbid personality disorder is associated with a worse treatment outcome (Downs et al. 1992; Joffe and Regan 1989).

Shea and colleagues (1993), in reviewing the studies looking at the treatment implications for patients with depression and comorbid personality disorders, stressed the need for a dimensional approach to the assessment of personality traits. Joyce and Paykel (1989), when reviewing the prediction of drug response in depression, suggested that the Cloninger Tridimensional Model of Personality (Cloninger 1986, 1987) provided an interesting new framework for investigating the relationships between personality, biological markers, and antidepressant response.

The Christchurch Prediction of Antidepressant Response Study

The objectives of this study were to examine predictors of outcome in a six-week double-blind trial of clomipramine versus desipramine in patients suffering from a current major depressive episode. In addition to examining for clinical predictors of antidepressant response, a major focus was on whether personality traits or disorders predicted the short-term antidepressant response.

Methods

This study included 104 patients suffering from a current major depressive episode and judged by their treating psychiatrist to need treatment with an antidepressant drug. All patients were aged 18 to 60, physically healthy, drug free (except occasional benzodiazepine or oral contraceptive), and had a score of 14 or greater on the 17-item Hamilton Rating Scale for Depression (HRSD; Hamilton 1960). Patients were referred to the study from a wide variety of sources, and most had not had prior treatment for their current major depressive episode. Patients with comorbid mental disorders or personality disorders, except for those with schizophrenia and current alcohol or drug dependence, were allowed into the study. Indeed, as personality traits and disorders were being examined as predictors of antidepressant response, we explicitly encouraged referral sources to send patients with personality disorders and major depression.

Before antidepressant treatment and after giving informed consent, all patients underwent a detailed clinical and biologic assessment. This included an interview with the treating psychiatrist for Axis I and II disorders using the Structured Clinical Interview for DSM-III-R (SCID-P and SCID-II; Spitzer et al. 1992), and for assessment of depression severity (Hamilton 1960). Patients completed a number of self-report questionnaires including the SCL-90 (Derogatis et al. 1973), the social adjustment scale (Cooper et al. 1982; Weissman and Bothwell 1976), the Tridimensional Personality Questionnaire (TPQ; Cloninger et al. 1991), Eysenck personality questionnaire (EPQ; Eysenck and Eysenck 1975), the Parental Bonding and Intimate Bonds Measure (PBI, IBM; Parker et al. 1979; Wilhelm and Parker 1988). The biologic assessment included a fenfluramine challenge test, thyrotropin releasing hormone test, tryptophan to large neutral amino acid ratio, mean afternoon cortisol level, urinary catecholamines, and tyramine sulphate excretion test.

After completion of the assessment, patients were treated for six weeks with either clomipramine or desipramine in a randomized double-blind antidepressant trial. Treating psychiatrists were able to adjust dosages of the tricyclics at their discretion and used regular drug levels as aids to optimal dosages. At six weeks, the mean daily dosages were 144 mg (range 75–250 mg) for clomipramine and 199 mg (range 100–350 mg) for desipramine. During the treatment trial, patients were rated on the HRSD after two, four, and six weeks.

Results

Of the 104 patients with depression who were randomized to treatment, 84 completed the six-week antidepressant trial and 20 failed to complete. Of the 20 who did not complete, 15 had been randomized to clomipramine and only 5 to desipramine ($\chi^2 = 6.19$, df $= 1$, $P <$ .02). During the first two weeks of treatment, 12 withdrew and 11 had been randomized to clomipramine. Table 17–1 compares the clinical characteristics of the 84 patients with depression who completed and

TABLE 17–1.

Clinical characteristics of the depressed patients who completed or did not complete the 6-week antidepressant trial

	Completers		Noncompleters	
	Mean	(SD)	Mean	(SD)
Male/female	39/45		11/9	
Age	31.3	(10.1)	32.2	(11.2)
Age at onset of depression	25.0	(15.1)	23.0	(8.9)
HRSD (baseline)	21.8	(4.6)	22.6	(4.3)
HRSD (six weeks)	8.4	(6.2)	—	—
HARS	17.7	(5.6)	16.9	(4.5)
Melancholic symptoms	3.8	(1.8)	3.6	(2.2)
Melancholic/nonmelancholic	34/50		8/12	
Single episode/recurrent	35/49		5/15	
Percentage time depressed in past 5 years:				
<6 months	15		3	
6–24 months	29		7	
25–36 months	17		1	
>36 months	23		9	
Desipramine/clomipramine[a]	47/37		5/15	
Temperament (TPQ)				
Novelty seeking (NS)	16.5	(5.7)	16.4	(4.7)
Harm avoidance (HA)	23.2	(6.7)	22.8	(6.4)
Reward dependence (RD)	17.0	(4.9)	16.7	(3.8)
Lifetime comorbidity				
Panic disorder (%)	16	(19%)	4	(20%)
Social phobia (%)	12	(14%)	5	(25%)
Simple phobia (%)	8	(10%)	1	(5%)
Alcohol abuse/depend (%)	24	(29%)	9	(45%)
Cannabis abuse/depend (%)	14	(17%)	6	(30%)

[a]$\chi^2 = 6.19$, P < .02.
Source. *Reprinted from Joyce et al. 1994b, p. 37, with permission from Elsevier Science Publishers.*

the 20 patients with depression who did not complete the six-week antidepressant trial.

Table 17–2 shows the treatment outcome for the patients with depression by gender and by drug. Although women randomized to desipramine tend to have a less favorable outcome, this did not reach

TABLE 17-2.
Treatment outcome for depressed patients by gender and drug (desipramine or clomipramine)

| | | Number of patients | | HRSD | | | | | |
| | | | | Week 0 | | Week 6 | | % Improved | |
Gender	Drug	Entered	Completed	Mean	SD	Mean	SD	Mean	SD
M	Clomipramine	25	16	20.7	(2.9)	7.6	(6.2)	62.8	(30.4)
M	Desipramine	25	23	21.8	(3.7)	8.0	(6.6)	62.9	(29.9)
F	Clomipramine	27	21	22.0	(5.1)	7.0	(4.8)	66.5	(22.4)
F	Desipramine	27	24	23.1	(5.7)	10.6	(6.7)	53.6	(28.4)
M + F	C + D	104	84	22.0	(4.6)	8.4	(6.2)	61.1	(27.8)

statistical significance. Table 17–3 compares the outcome for the patients with depression in the Christchurch Prediction of Antidepressant Response Study with the outcome for the patients with depression in the NIMH Treatment of Depression Collaborative Study (Elkin et al. 1989). Both studies used comparable entry criteria, notably an initial HRSD score of 14 or more, although in the Christchurch study a small minority were inpatients, three had histories of mania, and outcome was at 6 rather than 16 weeks.

Clinical Predictors of Treatment Outcome

A wide range of possible clinical variables were examined as predictors of percentage improvement over six weeks of antidepressant treatment. These clinical variables included age, gender, marital status, depression severity, depression onset, depression duration, melancholia, individual melancholic symptoms, recurrence, anxiety, and social functioning. Subsequent clinical variables examined included lifetime comorbid anxiety disorders or substance abuse or dependence. The only variable that predicted outcome was the presence of a lifetime simple phobia, which marginally predicted a better treatment response ($b = 0.22$, $F = 4.30$, $P = .04$). However, given the number of variables examined, it is possible that this finding as regards simple phobia is a false positive.

The Prevalence and Treatment Implications of Personality Disorders

In this sample of patients with depression, 50% met criteria on clinician interview for one or more personality disorders and, of those with any personality disorder(s), about two-thirds had more than one. In rank order, the most common personality disorders were avoidant, borderline, paranoid, self-defeating, dependent, obsessive-compulsive, and antisocial. Only one met criteria for schizoid personality disorder (Mulder et al. 1994).

TABLE 17–3.

Comparison of treatment outcome in this study (at 6 weeks) and the NIMH Treatment of depression Collaborative Program (at 16 weeks)

		Collaborative program	
	This study	Imipramine	Placebo
Number	104	57	62
Number completing	84	37	34
Baseline HRSD	22.0	19.2	19.1
Final HRSD	8.4	7.0	8.8
Completer patients			
Initial HRSD < 20 ($n = 31$)			
% with final HRSD ≤ 6	51%	55%	38%
% with final HRSD ≤ 7	58%		
% > 60% improved	55%		
Initial HRSD ≥ 20 ($n = 53$)			
% with final HRSD ≤ 6	47%	60%	15%
% with final HRSD ≤ 7	53%		
% ≥ 60% improved	60%		
Intention to treat			
Initial HRSD < 20 ($n = 35$)			
% with final HRSD ≤ 6	46%	44%	30%
% ≥ 60% improved	49%		
Initial HRSD > 20 ($n = 69$)			
% with final HRSD ≤ 6	37%	41%	7%
% ≥ 60% improved	46%		

The mean percentage improvement for those patients with depression who also had a personality disorder was the same as for those without a personality disorder. Although there was not even a trend for those with any personality disorder to have a poorer treatment response, when individual personality disorders were examined, there was a trend ($P = .09$) for those with borderline personality disorder to have a worse treatment response.

In this sample of patients with depression neuroticism did not predict a poorer treatment outcome.

Temperament as a Predictor of Outcome

Two of the important issues emphasized in the Biosocial Theory of Personality (Cloninger 1986, 1987) are its biologic substrate and that it is the combination of traits, rather than any one in isolation, that determines temperament. In the initial paper, Cloninger (1986) speculated that hypercortisolemia in patients with depression would be related to temperament and, especially, reward dependence. In this sample of patients with depression, temperament was related to the hypercortisolemia, with the strongest relation being between morning cortisol levels and reward dependence (Joyce et al. 1994a).

As Cloninger (1987) postulated, the existence of eight temperament types based on the combinations of the three temperament dimensions of novelty seeking (NS), harm avoidance (HA), and reward dependence (RD), each of these three measures was dichotomized as high or low, based on the means for this depressed sample (NS 16/17, HA 22/23, RD 16/17). Table 17–4 shows that when the patients with depression are divided into these eight temperament types, temperament type is a strong predictor of treatment outcome, regardless of which drug is used, explaining 25% of the variance (Joyce et al. 1994b).

Within the sample of 84 patients who completed treatment, 53 had an initial HRSD score of 20 or more. In these patients who were more severely depressed, response is more likely to be due to the antidepressant drug than to nonspecific treatment effects. When the analysis shown in Table 17–4 was repeated on the 53 patients who were more severely depressed, the classification of patients with depression by temperament type explained 40% of the variance in treatment outcome ($F = 4.36$, df = 7, 45, $P < .001$).

As the dichotomizing of continuous scales at the mean is, to some large degree, arbitrary, we checked to ensure that the results could not be explained by idiosyncratic cut points on the temperament scales. However, there was no evidence that the results could be explained in this way.

Although temperament type had already emerged as a strong predictor of antidepressant response over six weeks, we ran a series of stepwise multiple regression analyses adding gender and drug to the temperament scales. Table 17–5 shows the results from a stepwise mul-

TABLE 17–4.

Treatment outcome by Cloninger temperament type

| Temperament type | Entered | Number of patients | | Mean % improvement | | |
		Completed	Responded	Males	Females	Total
Schizoid (nhr)	9	7	7	88	88	88
Pass-aggress (NHR)	14	12	9	70	75	73
Pass-depend (nHR)	17	14	9	79	68	71
Histrionic (NhR)	14	11	6	62	56	59
Obsessional (nHr)	18	15	7	55	57	56
Explosive (NHr)	17	13	6	60	47	54
Antisocial (Nhr)	5	4	1	27	49	38
Cyclothymic (nhR)	10	8	3	38	36	37

Note. *The combination of temperament traits is indicated in parentheses: high or low novelty seeking (N or n), harm avoidance (H or h), and reward dependence (R or r).*

Analysis of variance on treatment outcome by temperament type:
F = 3.59 (df 7, 76), P = .002.

In multiple regression:
Multiple R = 0.50, R2 = 0.25, (i.e., temperament type explains 25% of the treatment outcome).

Source. *Reprinted from Joyce et al. 1994, p. 40, with permission from Elsevier Science Publishers.*

TABLE 17–5.

Results of a stepwise multiple regression on outcome

Source	df	F	P
RD × HA	1	5.02	.028
RD × drug × gender	1	11.75	.001
HA × drug × gender	1	8.63	.004

Note. *N = 84, Multiple R = 0.42, R2 = 0.18.*

tiple regression that entered the five variables (three temperaments, gender, and drug) plus two- and three-way interactions.

The results of this multiple regression can be interpreted as showing that those with high HA and high RD had a favorable outcome regardless of drug. This is consistent with the data in Table 17–4, which showed that those with high HA and RD had an above average treatment response. For women, a good response to clomipramine was predicted by high RD, whereas a favorable response to desipramine was predicted by high HA. Table 17–6 shows the correlations of each TPQ scale and subscale with outcome in the depressed women prescribed clomipramine or desipramine.

Temperament and the Pharmacotherapy of Depression: Summary and Discussion

In this study on predicting drug response in patients with major depression, temperament type predicted drug response regardless of

TABLE 17–6.

Regression coefficients of the TPQ scales and subscales on treatment outcome in depressed women who received either desipramine or clomipramine

	Clomipramine	Desipramine
Novelty seeking total	0.30	−0.23
NS1 (exploratory excitability)	0.27	−0.44*
NS2 (impulsiveness)	0.11	−0.03
NS3 (extravagance)	0.10	0.03
NS4 (disorderliness)	0.25	−0.19
Harm avoidance total	−0.23	0.48*
HA1 (anticipatory worry)	−0.16	0.37
HA2 (fear of uncertainty)	−0.28	0.44*
HA3 (shyness with strangers)	−0.22	0.20
HA4 (fatigability)	−0.08	0.44*
Reward dependence total	0.58**	−0.20
RD1 (sentimentality)	0.52*	−0.26
RD2 (persistence)	0.23	−0.08
RD3 (attachment)	0.48*	−0.25
RD4 (dependence)	0.34	0.17

Note. *Subjects completing study:* N = 21 *(clomipramine);* N = 24 *(desipramine).*
*P < .05. **P < .01.
Source. *Reprinted from Joyce et al. 1994b, p. 42, with permission with Elsevier Science Publishers.*

which antidepressant was used, and in depressed women there was an interaction between temperament and response to the noradrenergic or serotonergic antidepressant drug. These findings, that temperament predicted antidepressant response, stand in contrast to the general lack of clinical predictors of response. When the temperament and two possible clinical predictors of response were included in multiple regression analyses, both clinical variables (simple phobia and borderline personality disorder) ceased to be significant predictors, but both temperament factors remained as shown in Table 17–7. The multiple regression that was initially run using the whole sample ($n = 84$) was repeated on those with an initial HRSD of greater than or equal to 20 ($n = 53$). With the sample as a whole, temperament explained 38% of the variance in treatment outcome but, in the more severely depressed, temperament explained 49% of the variance in treatment outcome.

In the literature on antidepressant response, no clear finding comparable to our results suggests that temperament type is a major predictor of antidepressant response, regardless of which antidepressant is used. Perhaps the most comparable finding is the study by Peselow et al. (1992b) that reported that the personality traits of sociotropy and

TABLE 17–7.

Results from stepwise multiple regression analyses of TPQ variables on treatment outcome

Source	df	F	P
Total sample[a]			
Temperament type	7	3.49	.003
RD × drug × gender	1	10.54	.002
HA × drug × gender	1	7.72	.007
Severe sample[b]			
Temperament type	7	4.48	.001
RD × drug × gender	1	6.42	.015
HA × drug × gender	1	4.18	.047

[a]$N = 84$, *Multiple R* $= 0.59$, R2 $= 0.38$.
[b]$N = 53$, *Multiple R* $= 0.70$, R2 $= 0.49$.
Source. *Reproduced from Joyce et al. 1994b, p. 42, with permission from Elsevier Science Publishers.*

autonomy, but not the endogenous–nonendogenous dichotomy, predicted antidepressant drug response. Both of these studies therefore raise the possibility that personality and not Axis I symptoms or diagnoses will be the major determinant of antidepressant response. While the trait of autonomy does not easily relate to any of the temperament variables, it could well be that sociotropy is related to the temperament trait of RD.

The finding that in women RD predicts clomipramine response may be compatible with the growing literature on atypical depression where phenelzine is superior to imipramine, which is superior to placebo (Liebowitz et al. 1988; Quitkin et al. 1988, 1989). Perhaps clomipramine and selective serotonin reuptake blockers would also be superior to imipramine in atypical depression, and that the temperament trait of RD underlies the personality traits of sensitivity to interpersonal rejection.

It also appears possible that the dysfunctional attitudes, often displayed by patients with depression, in which they judge their own worth by how others see them, could also be related to RD. It is of interest that, in the NIMH Treatment of Depression Collaborative Research Program, high scores on dysfunctional attitudes predicted a better response to interpersonal psychotherapy and a poorer response to imipramine (Sotsky et al. 1991). If the speculative hypothesis that dysfunctional attitudes is related to RD is correct, then patients with depression and high dysfunctional attitudes may well do better with clomipramine or phenelzine than with imipramine.

If the findings from these study can be replicated and temperament shown to be a major predictor of antidepressant response, then an important step in the validation of a system for understanding personality will have occurred. At the very least, these findings suggest the need for an increased interest in personality traits for the understanding of response to psychopharmacologic drugs.

Joffe et al. (1993), in a study of 40 depressed outpatients treated with desipramine or imipramine, reported that a better response to these tricyclic antidepressants occurred in those with low HA. Tome et al. (1997) in a study of 54 patients with depression randomized to paroxetine or paroxetine and pindolol found that paroxetine responsiveness at six weeks was associated with high RD and low HA, whereas for patients on paroxetine and pindolol high NS and low HA predicted a better outcome at six weeks and six months. Furthermore, Tome et al. (1997) found that the character dimension of self-directedness predicted a better outcome, a finding replicated in a new antidepressant study with random allocation to fluoxetine and nortriptyline.

A number of studies have examined whether temperament measures change with improvement in depression and there is agreement that while NS and RD are largely independent of mood, HA decreases with successful treatment of depression (Joffe et al. 1993; Mulder and Joyce 1994). Given that HA is negatively correlated with self-directedness, it would be anticipated that self-directedness would improve upon recovery from depression, which has now been reported (Black and Sheline 1997).

References

American Psychiatric Association: Diagnostic and Statistical Manual of Mental Disorders, 3rd Edition. Washington, DC, American Psychiatric Association, 1980

Andrews G, Neilson M, Hunt C, et al: Diagnosis, personality and the long-term outcome of depression. Br J Psychiatry 157:13–18, 1990

Black KJ, Sheline YI: Personality disorder scores improve with effective pharmacotherapy of depression. J Affective Disord 43:11–18; 1997

Cloninger CR: A systematic method for clinical description and classification of personality variants. Arch Gen Psychiatry 44:573–588, 1987

Cloninger CR: A unified biosocial theory of personality and its role in the development of anxiety states. Psychiatr Dev 3:167–226, 1986

Cloninger CR: Establishment of diagnostic validity in psychiatric illness: Robins and Guze's method revisited, in The Validity of Psychiatric Diagnosis. Edited by Robins LN, Barrett JE. New York, Raven, 1989, pp 9–18

Cloninger CR, Przybeck TR, Svrakic DM: The Tridimensional Personality Questionnaire: U.S. normative data. Psychol Rep 69:1047–1057, 1991

Cooper P, Osborn M, Gath D, et al: Evaluation of a modified self-report measure of social adjustment. Br J Psychiatry 141:68–75, 1982

Derogatis LR, Lopman RS, Covi L: SCL-90: an outpatient psychiatric rating scale—preliminary report. Psychopharmacol Bull 9:13–28, 1973

Downs NS, Swerdlow NR, Zisook S: The relationship of affective illness and personality disorders in psychiatric outpatients. Ann Clin Psychiatry 4:87–94, 1992

Duggan CF, Lee AS, Murray RM: Does personality predict long-term outcome in depression? Br J Psychiatry 175:19–24, 1990

Elkin I, Shea MT, Watkins JT, et al: National Institute of Mental Health Treatment of Depression Collaborative Research Program: general effectiveness of treatments. Arch Gen Psychiatry 46:971–982, 1989

Eysenck HJ, Eysenck SBJ: Manual of the Eysenck Personality Questionnaire. Kent, Hodder & Stoughton, 1975

Hamilton M: A rating scale for depression. J Neurol Neurosurg Psychiatry 23:56–62, 1960

Joffe RT, Regan JJ: Personality and response to tricyclic antidepressants in depressed patients. J Nerv Ment Dis 177:745–749, 1989

Joffe RT, Bagby RM, Levitt AJ, et al: The Tridimensional Personality Questionnaire in major depression. Am J Psychiatry 150:959–960, 1993

Joyce PR, Paykel ES: Predictors of drug response in depression. Arch Gen Psychiatry 46:89–99, 1989

Joyce PR, Mulder RT, Cloninger CR: Temperament and hypercortisolemia in depression. Am J Psychiatry 151:195–198, 1994a

Joyce PR, Mulder RT, Cloninger CR: Temperament predicts clomipramine and desipramine response in major depression. J Affective Disord 30:35–46, 1994b

Kerr TA, Schapira K, Roth M, et al: The relationship between the Maudsley Personality Inventory and the course of affective illness. Br J Psychiatry 116:11–19, 1970

Liebowitz MR, Quitkin FM, Stewart JW, et al: Antidepressant specificity in atypical depression. Arch Gen Psychiatry 45:129–139, 1988

Mulder RT: The biology of personality. Aust N Z J Psychiatry 26:364–375, 1992

Mulder RT, Joyce PR: The relationships of the Tridimensional Personality Questionnaire to mood and personality measures in depressed patients. Psychol Rep 75:1315–1325, 1994

Mulder RT, Joyce PR, Cloninger CR: Temperament and early environment influence comorbidity and personality disorders in major depression. Compr Psychiatry 35:225–233, 1994

Parker G, Tupling H, Brown LB: A parental bonding instrument. Br J Med Psychol 52:1–10, 1979

Peselow ED, Fieve RR, DiFiglia C: Personality traits and response to desipramine. J Affective Disord 24:209–216, 1992a

Peselow ED, Robins CJ, Sanfilipo MP: Sociotropy and autonomy: relationship to antidepressant drug treatment response and endogenous — nonendogenous dichotomy. J Abnorm Psychol 101:479–486, 1992b

Pfohl B, Stangl D, Zimmerman M: The implications of DSM-III personality disorders for patient with major depression. J Affective Disord 7:309–318, 1984

Pfohl B, Coryell W, Zimmerman M, et al: Prognostic validity of self-report and interview measures of personality disorder in depressed inpatients. J Clin Psychiatry 48:472–486, 1987

Plomin R: The role of inheritance in behaviour. Science 248:183–188, 1990

Quitkin FM, McGrath PJ, Stewart JW, et al: Phenelzine and imipramine in mood reactive depressives. Further delineation of the syndrome of atypical depression. Arch Gen Psychiatry 46:787–793, 1989

Quitkin FM, Stewart JW, McGrath PJ, et al: Phenelzine vs imipramine in probable atypical depression: defining syndrome boundaries of selective MAOI responders. Am J Psychiatry 145:306–312, 1988

Robins LN: Deviant Children Grown Up. Baltimore, Williams & Wilkins, 1966

Robins E, Guze SB: Establishment of diagnostic validity in psychiatric illness: its application to schizophrenia. Am J Psychiatry 126:107–111, 1970

Shea MT, Pilkonis PA, Beckham E, et al: Personality disorders and treatment outcome in the NIMH Treatment Of Depression Collaborative Research Program. Am J Psychiatry 147:711–718, 1990

Shea MT, Widiger TA, Klein MH: Comorbidity of personality disorders and depression: implications for treatment. J Consult Clin Psychol 60:857–868, 1993

Sotsky SM, Glass DR, Shea MT, et al: Patient predictors of response to psychotherapy and pharmacotherapy: findings in the NIMH Treatment Of Depression Collaborative Research Program. Am J Psychiatry 148:997–1008, 1991

Spitzer RL, Williams JBW, Gibbon M, et al: The structured clinical interview for DSM-III-R. I. History, rationale and description. Arch Gen Psychiatry 49:624–629, 1992

Tome MB, Cloninger CR, Watson JP, et al: Serotonergic autoreceptor blockade in the reduction of antidepressant latency: personality variables and response to paroxetine and pindolol. J Affective Disord 44:101–110, 1997

Weissman MM, Bothwell S: Assessment of social adjustment by patient self-report. Arch Gen Psychiatry 33:1111–1115, 1976

Weissman MM, Prusoff BA, Klearman GL: Personality and the prediction of long-term outcome of depression. Am J Psychiatry 35:797–800, 1978

Wilhelm K, Parker G: The development of a measure of intimate bonds. Psychol Med 18:225–234, 1988

Zuckerman M: Psychobiology of Personality. Cambridge, England, Cambridge University Press, 1991

Treatment of Borderline Personality Disorder With Rational Emotive Behavior Therapy

Albert Ellis, Ph.D.

I have worked with thousands of people with personality disorders for the last 50 years, first as a psychoanalyst and later as a practitioner of rational emotive behavior therapy (REBT), and I have naturally given much thought to how these disorders originate and what are some of the best methods to help people alleviate or cope with this serious problem. After much thought and experimentation, I have come up with some hypotheses that seem original to me but that may merely be restatements of other clinicians' ideas. In any event, I shall try to state them clearly in the hope that they may be clinically and experimentally tested.

How Do Personality Disorders Originate?

My first hypothesis is hardly startling but follows REBT theory: All "emotional" disturbances tend to have strong cognitive, emotive, and behavioral elements, and that this is particularly true of the personality disorders and of the so-called borderline personality states. Individuals with these conditions usually show severe dysfunction in their thinking, feeling, and behaving; so-called neurotics show less dysfunction and so-called psychotics often show more severe dysfunction in these three areas. (American Psychiatric Association 1987; Beck et al. 1990; Benjamin 1993; Ellis 1988; Kernberg 1984, 1985; Klein 1984, Kohut 1971, 1991; Linehan 1993; Masterson 1981; Young 1990).

People with personality disorders almost always have cognitive, emotive, and behavioral organic deficits for various reasons, including hereditary predispositions. They (and most properly diagnosed psychotics) have anomalies of their brain and central nervous system (as well as, often, other physiological defects), that significantly contribute, along with other environmental factors, to their personality disorders (Adler 1992; Brown 1991; Ellis 1985, 1988; Gazzinga 1993; Gottesman 1991; Huessy 1992; Larson and Agresti 1992; Pies 1992).

As I pointed out in my first paper on REBT (Ellis 1958), thinking, feeling, and behavior are not separate processes but

> thinking . . . is, and to some extent has to be, sensory, motor, and emotional behavior . . . Emotion, like thinking and the sensory-motor processes, we may define as an exceptionally complex state of human reaction which is integrally related to all the other perception and response processes. It is not one thing, but a combination and holistic integration of several seemingly diverse, yet actually closely related phenomena . . . Thinking and emoting are so closely interrelated that they usually accompany each other, act in a circular cause and effect relationship, and in certain (though hardly all) respects are essentially the same thing, so that one's thinking becomes one's emotion and emotion becomes one's thought. (pp. 35–36)

As I have also pointed out (Ellis 1991) and as Hayes and Hayes (1992) and other contextualists have indicated, thought, feeling, and action always take place in environmental contexts and backgrounds, so that people and their situations interactively influence and affect each other. Humans have goals and purposes; in various environments, and especially in their social relationships, they construct thoughts, feelings, and behaviors that actualize or defeat themselves, thereby creating conditions of "mental health" and "emotional disturbance."

Virtually all humans are born with strong, constructive self-changing and self-actualizing tendencies, and even when they are clearly not in a disordered personality or a psychotic state they also have strong self-defeating irrational tendencies. To a varying degree they are almost always neurotic or needlessly self-destructive; and although they tend to learn, acquire, or become conditioned to disturbed thoughts, feelings, and actions, they also have innate tendencies to construct or create these neurotic conditions. Few, if any, of them are consistently self-helping and socially appropriate (Brown 1991; Ellis 1962, 1965, 1976, 1985, 1988; Ellis and Dryden 1990; Gilovich 1992).

What we call neurosis includes and largely (though not completely) stems from people's dysfunctional, irrational, and self-defeating thinking or basic philosophy. As I, Beck, Meichenbaum, and other rational emotive behavior and cognitive-behavior theorists and therapists have pointed out since 1955 (Beck 1976, 1991; Ellis 1957, 1956, 1962, 1985, 1988, 1992; Meichenbaum 1977), anxious, depressed, and enraged people have many dysfunctional ideas or irrational beliefs by which they largely create their neurotic disturbances; and as the theory of REBT holds, these beliefs almost always seem to consist of or be derived from unrealistically, illogically, and rigidly raising their nondisturbing wishes and preferences into godlike absolutist musts, shoulds, demands, and commands. Thus, they tend to create neurotic ego problems, and consequent anxiety and depression, when they strongly insist, "I absolutely must perform well and be approved by significant others or else I am an inadequate, unlovable person!" They tend to create interpersonal and social problems, and especially feelings of rage, when they powerfully demand, "Other people must completely treat me well and fairly or else they are no damned good!" And they tend to create problems with the world, low frustration tolerance (LFT), and feelings of depression, when they command, "Things and conditions absolutely must be the way I want them to be or else it's *awful*, I *can't stand* it, and my life is no good!" (Ellis 1957, 1962, 1985, 1988; Ellis and Becker 1982; Ellis and Harper 1997).

People's functional and appropriate cognitions, feelings, and behaviors are rarely, if ever, pure and separate, but instead importantly interact with and influence each other. Thus, their thoughts tend to create their feelings and behaviors, their emotions and acts lead to thought and acts, and their actions lead to ideas and feelings (Ellis 1962, 1985, 1991). REBT, along with most of the other cognitive behavioral therapies, theorizes that when people experience activating events or activating experiences (A), their beliefs (B) about these As largely create their emotional and behavioral consequences (C). But REBT also theorizes that A, B, and C often powerfully interact so that As influence Bs and Cs. Bs influence As and Cs; and Cs influence As and Bs. Thus, people's serious failures and loss of approval (A) often lead to negative beliefs (B) and to withdrawal (C). Negative beliefs (B) often encourage failures and lack of approval (A) as well as withdrawal (C). And withdrawal (C) often encourages serious failures and loss of approval (A) and negative beliefs (B). It seems to be the nature of virtually all humans to be importantly affected by both their environment and their own (partly inherited) biology and to have their thoughts, feelings, and behaviors significantly interact with and to cause and affect each other.

Thus, following Skinner (1938, 1987, 1989), the radical behaviorists and contextualists are probably correct in holding that humans (and other animals) do not function outside of the environment and are inevitably and crucially affected by environmental changes (Biglan 1993; Hayes and Hayes 1992). But the cognitive-behaviorists are also correct in holding that humans have interacting thoughts, feelings, and behaviors, all of which significantly affect each other, and that their thinking prominently influences and changes their feelings and their actions. Significant changes in human functioning can therefore be effected by environmental changes—most of which they have to plan and execute themselves—but can also be effected by their choosing to work at their thoughts, emotions, and behaviors. Why are both of these change processes crucial to human functions? Because so-called human nature has strong hereditary components, which are also subject to evolutionary environmental influences (Davidson and Cacioppo 1992; Ellis 1992; Eysenck 1967; Gazzinga 1993; Ruth 1992; Wilson 1975).

All humans seem to be both self-actualizing and self-defeating (or what I shall call neurotic). The three main neurotic processes may be seen as 1) self-downing (damning oneself for poor performances and rejection); 2) hostility and rage (damning others for poor performances and unkind reactions); and 3) LFT (damning things and the world for poor, dislikable conditions). These three main "emotional" disturbances tend to be experienced individually and/or collectively at times by almost all humans, and when two or more coexist (which they frequently do) they tend to interact with other and exacerbate one another. They particularly add to and exacerbate personality disorders, as I shall show in detail later (Ellis 1991; Ellis and Dryden 1997, 1990, 1991; Ellis and Harper 1997).

There are many personality disorders, such as narcissism, borderline personality disorder (BPD), obsessive-compulsive disorder (OCD), schizoid personality, histrionic personality disorder, narcissistic personality disorder, avoidant personality disorder and dependent personality disorder. They vary in intensity, often accompany each other, and often go along with other severe neurotic disorders, such as neurotic depression, panic states, and self-hatred (Ellis 1965, 1988; Kernberg 1985; Masterson 1981).

Because they are so varied and complex, I shall mainly limit myself in this chapter to discussing the borderline personality, a quite complex and varied entity that is often (or usually) accompanied by serious neurotic disturbances and sometimes includes psychotic episodes. The main characteristics of the borderline personality includes a pattern of unstable relationships, self-damaging impulsiveness, affective instability, intense inappropriate anger, recurrent suicidal threats, marked and persistent identity disturbance, chronic feelings of emptiness or boredom, and frantic efforts to avoid real or imagined abandonment (American Psychiatric Association 1987).

How Do People With BPD Get That Way?

We can start almost anywhere to examine the main causes of the problems of BPD, but let me arbitrarily start with organic deficits, which I hypothesize clients with BPD largely inherit. They seem to be born with several innate tendencies that interact with their experiences to produce several deficits. Thus, cognitively they often exhibit (probably from childhood onward) attention deficit disorders, rigid ways of thinking, inability to organize well, impulsive thinking, forgetfulness, inconsistent images of others, inability to maintain a sense of time as an ongoing process, learning disability, perceptual disability, proneness to be doublebound, a tendency to exaggerate the significance of things, rigidity, demandingness, severe self-downing, purposelessness, impairment in recalling and recognition and deficient semantic encoding. Neurotic individuals may have all these cognitive organic deficiencies too, but they usually demonstrate them much less intensively, adjust to and cope with them better, and exhibit them largely under stressful environmental conditions, whereas individuals with BPD tend to have them more endogenously and more severely (Barkley 1990; Benjamin 1993; Cohen and Gara 1992; Cohen and Sherwood 1991; Gold et al. 1992; Kazdin 1992; Lenzenweger et al. 1991; Linehan 1993; Rhodes and Wood 1992; Rosenbaum et al. 1988; Rourke and Fuerst 1991; Swanson and Keogh 1990; Yee et al. 1992).

Individuals with emotionally borderline personalities, I again hypothesize, have innate emotional difficulties and deficits. Thus they are frequently dysthymic, depressive, easily enraged, overexcitable, high-strung, easily panicked, and histrionic (Adler and Buie 1979; Andreason 1979; Barinaga 1992; Berenbaum and Poltmanns 1992; Bowlby 1969; Davis 1992; Hauser 1992; Pediaditakis 1991; Plutchik 1990; Plutchik and Kellerman 1990; Sperling and Sharp 1991).

Behaviorally, individuals with BPD, again, are often born with distinct tendencies to be hyperactive, hypervigilant, impulsive, obstreperous, interruptive, excessively restless, temper ridden, and antisocial, or they often are alienated, addictive, overdependent, inattentive, and purposeless (Cole 1991; Iocono 1989).

Again, neurotic individuals may at times and to some degree have the same emotional and behavioral traits, but persons with BPD tend to have them more intensely, severely, frequently, consistently, and endogenously (American Psychiatric Association 1987; Benjamin 1993; Ellis 1988; Kernberg 1985; Linehan 1993; Masterson 1981).

Let us assume, for the moment, that people with BPD have some serious cognitive deficits. How will they neurotically react to them? First of all, they will on some levels, according to REBT theory, tend to observe or sense these deficits and put themselves down for having them. They will often note that they have poor intellectual functioning, demand that they *must* not act inadequately, berate themselves for having them, and more easily feel like *inadequate* people—which people with BPD often tend to feel anyway, and which will now be significantly exacerbated.

If, as I theorize, individuals with BPD have *real* cognitive deficiencies, they will often tend to be jealous and hostile toward less dysfunctional people, will insist that these individuals *must* not have greater advantages than they themselves have, and will often show, as DSM-III-R notes, "intense anger or lack of control of anger, e.g., frequent displays of temper, constant anger, recurrent physical fights" (American Psychiatric Association 1987, p. 347).

If individuals with BPD, as I again theorize, often have innate behavioral problems, such as hyperactivity and temper tantrums, they will tend to create or exacerbate their natural LFT by demanding, "I *must* not be as handicapped by and looked down upon for these handicaps, as I indubitably am!" So they will easily have and aggravate, as DSM-III-R observes, "marked and persistent identity disturbance" and "frantic efforts to avoid real or imagined abandonment" (p. 347).

If I am right about this, and if people with cognitive, emotional, and behavioral handicaps very often tend to severely down themselves, hate other people, and hate the world, why should people with BPD, who may well have all three of these handicaps, not come up with similar—or worse—hatred of themselves and of others? Biologically, they may be *more* prone to hating themselves, others, and the world than are the rest of us, the neurotic population. But even if they are not directly so, their other specific cognitive, emotive, and behavioral handicaps would, interacting with their general neurotic tendencies, tend to produce these grim results.

To make matters still worse, if individuals with BPD are, first, innately handicapped in important ways; if they are naturally neurotic or whining about these handicaps; and if they then directly and indirectly produce their borderline conditions, these conditions themselves are quite cognitively, emotionally, and behaviorally handicapping, which, unless they are exceptionally stupid or defensive, they could hardly fail to observe. If and when they do observe their borderline characteristics and the real handicaps they bear in our society, they will then *once again* tend to neurotically demand, 1) "I must do better than I am actually doing!" 2) "Other people *absolutely must not* treat me unfairly for my handicaps!" and 3) "The conditions under which I live must not be so handicapping! It's *awful* and *I can't stand it* when they are!" If they neurotically think in these ways, individuals with BPD will make themselves more disturbed—and more borderline! (Leaf et al. 1991a, 1991b; Priester and Clum 1993).

Moreover, they will usually then tend to take their hatred of themselves, of others, and of their handicaps into their therapy, upset themselves about it and about their therapists, and again make their condition and their potential for improvement much worse. As Benjamin (1993), Linehan (1993), and other authorities indicate, their extreme social difficulties will often include interpersonal problems with their often quite devoted therapists.

I am proposing, then, that individuals with BPD (as well as most other individuals with serious personality disorders) have several levels of disturbances all of which interact with and affect each other, and which had better be considered together if we are to understand the main causes and effects of BPD. Let me make a summary list of these levels.

Level 1:   Individuals with BPD usually have cognitive, emotional, and behavioral deficits, some of which they are innately (and probably genetically) predisposed to have. Some of their borderline behavior may directly stem from these deficits and some of their individual and social inadequacies almost certainly do.

Level 2:   Individuals with BPD (like neurotic individuals) also have innate and acquired tendencies to *demand* that they must succeed in work, love, and play and to denigrate themselves when they fail; and they have innate and acquired tendencies to insist that they *must* not be very frustrated or handicapped and to have LFT, anger, and self-pity when they are seriously balked. They therefore tend to be at least as

and probably more neurotic and self-defeating then are individuals without personality disorders.

Level 3:   Because of their innate cognitive, emotive, and behavioral
impairments, and because of self-downing and LFT about
these impairments, individuals with BPD became even more
psychobiologically impaired and dysfunctional; their neurotic self-deprecation and discomfort about their impairment
then tends to make them still more impaired, still more disturbed about their dysfunctions, and still more impaired. A
vicious cycle ensues, in the course of which impairment encourage neurosis, neurosis promotes more impairment, and
greater impairment encourages more neurosis.

This vicious circle can be partially alleviated if individuals with
BPD are helped to minimize their self-denigration and their LFT. But
their original cognitive, emotional, and behavioral deficits—which often present them with tendencies to hold on to *must*urbatory, rigid
demands that lead to self-downing and intolerance of frustration—
block them from alleviating their neurosis and often seriously exacerbate it. They may also be biologically prone to bringing on secondary
neurotic symptoms by demanding that they *absolutely must not* be
anxious and depressed about 1) their original cognitive, emotional, and
behavioral deficits; 2) their neurotic nonacceptance of these deficits;
3) their severe symptoms; and 4) their unusual difficulty in achieving
self-improvement, either within or outside of therapy.

The vicious cycle already mentioned can also be partly or largely
alleviated if it is possible to make up for the original biosocial deficits
of persons with BPD. But these deficits are usually so varied and profound that our present medications and remedial teachings are often
helpful but only partially effective. Nothing indicates that they will be
truly curative in the near future.

So I think we had better face the reality that patients with BPD
are not hopelessly and totally incurable but are still so biologically,
psychologically, and socially handicapped that we can rarely help them
achieve what may be called a "real" cure. Sometimes we can help
them minimize their neurosis about their borderline condition but
even that may be limited, because they often rigidly cling to self-

deprecation and an abysmal LFT, and therefore have to work harder than normal neurotics to give them up. The catch-22 is that they rarely work hard at anything consistently because of their basic cognitive, emotional, and behavioral deficits (e.g., attentional deficit disorder and focusing deficits) and because their abysmal LFT and short-range hedonism interferes with sustained discipline.

Guidelines for Treating Clients With BPD

What, therapeutically, shall we do? Shall we expect very limited gains? Work mainly on the neurosis about their borderline condition? Train them to partially overcome or compensate for their basic cognitive, emotional, and behavioral deficits? Probably all of the above, depending on our own skills and patience as therapists and on the individual's inclination to get better, to do very hard and persistent therapeutic work, and to relate to anyone, including their therapist. What follows are some suggested guidelines for therapists who have the guts to work persistently with them.

Try for real improvement but expect limited gains with most of them. Even normal neurotic patients rarely improve as much as we would like them to do, and patients with BPD are much more disturbed and usually much more resistant to changing. Fully accept this reality and don't discourage yourself when you meet with it. Have abundant patience and fortitude!

Work on yourself to acquire unconditional acceptance for your clients with BPD. This is what Rogers (1961) called unconditional positive regard. Deplore and even hate their annoying, often hostile and antisocial traits, but accept *them* with their poor behavior. Often confront them with their obnoxious and self-defeating thoughts, feelings, and actions, but do so supportively, protectively, and utterly nondamningly. Forgive the sinner but not necessarily the sin.

Teach your clients specifically how to unconditionally accept themselves. My encouragement of you to teach diverges from Carl Rogers' writings. REBT presents clients with a less elegant and more elegant solution to this important human problem.

Less elegantly, you can teach your clients the existential, humanistic philosophy that they can accept themselves unconditionally *whether or not* they perform or relate well—just because they are human, just because they are alive, just because they *choose* to do so. All self-acceptance is really a choice and is definitional. When we have what is usually called self-esteem—probably the greatest emotional sickness of men and women—we wrongly *decide* to accept ourselves as "good" or "deserving" individuals on condition that we perform well and are lovable. This won't really work: Even when we meet these conditions today, we may well not meet them tomorrow, so we are always anxious and overconcerned about our performances.

When we decide to accept ourselves *unconditionally* with all our wants and failings, our sense of self or identity is still chosen and still definitional. But this time our defining ourselves as "good" or "worthy" is more practical and useful. For we will safely accept ourselves—as long as we are alive, and presumably will only have to worry about our identity when we are dead!

This solution to the problem of self-worth is somewhat inelegant, however, because it is not falsifiable. Thus, you can firmly say, "I fully accept myself as a worthwhile person because I am alive and human" and I (and other people) can object, "But I think that, because you are alive and human, you are no good and worthless. In fact, all humans are worthless and only deserve to die!"

Which of us, then, is right—you or I? I say that neither of us can substantiate or falsify our view of human worth—because both our views are definitional and tautological. Yours will probably *work* better than mine if your goal is to keep yourself and the human race alive, healthy, and happy. But it is still quite definitional.

REBT has, therefore, proposed for more than two decades a more elegant solution to the problem of human worth that you can teach to your borderline (and other) clients. They can choose to *only* rate or evaluate their thoughts, feelings, and behaviors and *not* fall into the dangerous error of rating or measuring their self, their essence, their being, or their totality. Thus, they can say, "Because I choose to stay alive and be healthy and reasonably happy, many of my *acts and traits* are 'bad,' 'harmful,' or 'against my purpose,' but I am too complex, *too much of an ongoing process,* to give any rating, good or bad, to my *self or being."*

This more elegant solution to self-acceptance is, I have found, difficult for most neurotic clients and clients with BPD to achieve. Why? I hypothesize that self-rating has, through the course of human evolution, some distinct advantages, is biologically predisposed, and is hard to surrender. But even clients with BPD can minimize it, if they are unconditionally accepted by their therapists and actively taught to accept themselves.

Show clients how LFT is self-defeating and how to ameliorate it. Clients with BPD, for reasons already mentioned, usually have both innate and acquired abysmal LFT, and LFT includes the irrational, dysfunctional beliefs that "Conditions *absolutely must not* be as hard as they are! It's *awful* and I *can't stand* it!" But these beliefs can be clearly revealed and forcefully disputed. As noted previously, LFT itself will stop clients from thinking and working hard to overcome their LFT! But you, as a therapist, can persist in teaching that LFT is self-defeating and amenable to improvement. Don't give up and give into our own LFT in this respect!

Many of the dysfunctional cognitions accompanying BPD can often be successfully reduced with the usual methods of REBT and cognitive-behavioral therapy. Complete cure in this regard is unlikely, but significant improvement can often be achieved (Beck et al. 1991; Benjamin 1993; Cahill 1993; Ellis 1985, 1988; Friedberg 1993; Leaf and DiGiuseppe 1992; Leaf et al. 1991b; Linehan 1993; Stone 1990; Yank et al. 1993; Young 1990).

The original and partially biological thinking, feeling, and behavioral deficits of BPD mentioned earlier in this chapter are not easy to improve, but can often be ameliorated. You, as a therapist, can try to help your clients with BPD in this respect, or you can refer them to other suitable professionals: neuropsychologists, rehabilitation counselors, teachers. As both Benjamin (1993) and Linehan (1993) indicate skill training, which may partially compensate for their deficits, is almost mandatory with many clients with BPD.

At times it pays to be clever at unraveling, revealing, and disputing some of the thinking of the client with BPD. Such clients often think in what may be called "perverse" or "intentionally self-defeating ways," underneath which may be found a method to their madness. At one and the same time they may attempt suicide to control others and have them surrender to their overweening need for attention and support. But they may also try to kill themselves, as one of my own clients attempted, because she wanted to convince me how really sick she was and that I was wrong in trying to show her that she could live and have a happy existence.

Several techniques may work to make disputing clients effective at therapy: the dialectical or oppositional persuasive techniques of Linehan (1993), the use of the client as a consultant methods of Benjamin (1993), or the paradoxical and metaphorical methods that Hayes (Hayes et al. 1991) uses with agoraphobic patients (but that can also sometimes be used with BPD). Because these clients are often fiendishly clever in holding on to their disturbances the therapist who is equally clever disputing sometimes wins out.

Although clever and well-calculated therapist ripostes sometimes win the game, sticking to the strategy of regular cognitive-behavior therapy is probably more effective in the long run.

Because clients with BPD are often so unpredictable and unique, cognitive-behavior therapy seems to be the best general choice. REBT, like Lazarus's (1990) multimodal therapy, includes a large number of cognitive, emotive, and behavioral methods, so that when the usual ones do not seem to be working, I try some of the less usual ones and sometimes find that they work well. Thus, although I teach my clients that rage is almost always self-destructive, I induced one of my clients to give up all thoughts of killing herself because her arch-rival for her lover's affection would certainly live and be deliriously happy. So I encouraged my client, at least temporarily, to keep and to vent her rage against her rival and thereby motivate herself to live and work for her own happiness.

Psychopharmacological treatment sometimes works well but often does not. I frequently recommend that my clients experimentally try antidepressants or other medications, and if they don't work and/or find taking them too obnoxious, they can always return to psychotherapy alone. My helping them increase their frustration tolerance and decrease their medication phobias frequently serves to get them to try

proper medication and to put up with the side effects of some medications. Conversely, being on an antidepressant and/or a tranquilizer
sometimes helps them think better and benefit more from REBT. But,
being tricky, they also may use pharmacological treatment as an excuse
not to work hard to change their thinking, feeling, and acting.

*Experience has brought me to abandon psychoanalysis for BPD,
except for some of its relationship aspects, and heavily use cognitive-
behavior therapy instead.* Other cognitive-behavior therapists, and I
think therapists in general, have found cognitive-behavioral methods
quite useful with clients with BPD (Beck et al. 1991; Benjamin 1993;
Ellis 1962, 1985, 1988; Linehan 1993). As for psychoanalysis, I now
feel that it is exceptionally wasteful for most neurotic individuals and
fairly iatrogenic for most clients with BPD. Kohut's (1971) methods
are basically Rogerian and probably less harmful than other psychoanalytic techniques. Kernberg (1984, 1985) and Masterson (1981) are
more confrontative but too sidetrackingly psychoanalytic for my prejudiced tastes!

Case Presentation

Rona was a woman of 25 when I began treating her for what she called
severe depression. She worked as a bookkeeper in a small office because she was afraid of human contacts. She considered herself "hor-
ribly ugly," although she was quite attractive. She strongly felt that she
was a basket case; she was on one side of the human race and every
other person was on the other side—the good side. She had no social
relationships and was sure that she couldn't make any because of her
extreme shyness, need for love, and self-rejection. She had made suicide attempts at the ages of 16 and 21 but was saved by her parents
each time and rushed to the hospital. She was briefly hospitalized each
time, refused to take medication after leaving the hospital, and went
back to living with her critical parents. Rona hated them but couldn't
set herself free. She felt they abandoned her and was determined to
never risk abandonment again. She also felt continually bored and
empty and spent her leisure hours sleeping or looking at television,

although she was quite intelligent and had achieved an MBA degree with honors. Typically, Rona made no friends in college and none at work. Her one relationship, just before she came to see me, was a brief one with John, who was quite attracted to her, who pushed her for dates, but who was soon turned off by her intermittent hostility and dire need to be constantly assured that he really, really loved her and would never abandon her.

Rona came to see me when she was severely depressed after John had broken off with her. I could see quickly, from her history, her unstable emotionality, her complete focus on herself, and her phobic and panicked reactions, that she was hardly a nice neurotic and that she would most probably be a "DC" (or difficult customer).

I was right. She alternatively was very seductive and very hostile to me. She knew about REBT but was very skeptical of it because of her nine years of previous psychoanalytic therapy, which she considered "deep" but "highly ineffective." She threatened to stop seeing me from the first session onward and, during the three years I saw her, she quit twice for a month at a time. She at first identified me with her hated supercritical father, but later became overattached to and overdependent on me. She was very resentful when I went out of town for a few days for talks, workshops, and conferences and would insist on phone sessions at the hotels where I was staying.

Following REBT principles, I fully accepted Rona with her difficultness and tried to teach her, over and over again, how to unconditionally accept herself, accept her critical parents, and accept her borderline, quite handicapped condition. I honestly and firmly kept showing her that she was probably innately disturbed—as were both her parents—and that she often behaved hostilely and had better—not *must*—change her hostility for her own sake.

Although Rona strongly objected to the REBT philosophy of fully accepting herself and others, I persistently showed her that the results she was getting from her self-hatred, withdrawal, and hostility weren't worth it and that only something like unconditional self-acceptance would bring better results. My efforts finally prevailed and within six months of therapy she started to "get it" and to become a devotee of undamning acceptance. She joined one of my regular therapy groups and consistently came to my regular Friday night workshop, where I demonstrate REBT with volunteers who have sessions of public ther-apy. She also attended a record number of four-hour-long public work-shops that are given every other week at the Albert Ellis Institute in New York City. At the group and workshop sessions she vigorously kept convincing other participants of the value of unconditionally accepting themselves and others.

I had greater difficulty helping Rona reduce her abysmal LFT, but I was finally able to convince her that demanding immediate gratifi-cation at the expense of later pain wasn't worth it. No matter how uncomfortable she felt, she began to go through difficult dates, make and keep friendships with somewhat unreliable people, work in a larger office, force herself to overcome her public speaking phobia, accept my absences from her therapy sessions when I was out of town, stop smoking, and do many other uncomfortable things for her later satis-faction.

I, her therapy group, and her workshop groups helped Rona ac-quire several skills in which she was deficient. In the course of this skill training she became quite assertive, began to listen more atten-tively to others, learned how to actively break the ice and meet new people, became adept at job interviewing, and took courses that led to her becoming a CPA. At the same time, her innate and acquired ten-dencies to be unfocused, to think impulsively, to exaggerate the sig-nificance of things, to be emotionally labile, and to be purposeless definitely improved or interfered less with her social and work behavior.

I still see Rona for occasional therapy sessions and as a visitor at some of my Friday night workshops; and I hear about her from several of her friends and relatives whom she keeps sending to me for therapy. By all visible standards she is now only moderately neurotic—like most of the human race. But as a trained clinician, I can still see some of the remnants of her BPD showing through her outward demeanor. She now makes herself angry and depressed on relatively few occasions, but when she does, she becomes quite discombobulated, stutters and stammers, and for several days is disorganized and distraught. She has good social relationships but never becomes too deeply involved with anyone. She displays little overt hostility, but underneath she is very jealous of successful people and somewhat paranoid about being exploited by her friends. She is a successful CPA but sometimes feels that her life is meaningless and purposeless and that she is not truly integrated into the human race.

Rona, although vastly improved, is not quite whole. I have said for many years that REBT can help people overcome their neurosis about their psychosis and about BPD; and by working very hard to fully accept herself and to acquire higher frustration tolerance, Rona has used it to become much less neurotic. But I don't fool myself into believing that she or any of the other individuals with psychosis and BPD I have helped with REBT for the last 43 years have been truly cured. Nor have I seen any other therapists' clients with borderline and psychotic disorders who, even after many years of treatment, are now truly healthy. Some are significantly and even magnificently improved, but all still have underlying psychotic or borderline disorders.

Being something of an optimist as well as a realist, I think that both the arts of psychotherapy and of psychopharmacology are in their infancy stages and that someday they will combine to help individuals with BPD do more than they do today, perhaps even cure them of their borderline states, and leave them, like the rest of the human race, only neurotic. Meanwhile, working with clients with BPD is damned difficult, but it can also be quite challenging and rewarding, for clients as well as for therapists.

References

Note: Some of Dr. Ellis's published articles have been reprinted and are available from the Albert Ellis Institute, 45 East 65th Street, New York, NY 10021.

Adler D, Buie DH: Aloneness and borderline pathology and psychopathology. Int J Psychoanal 60:83–96, 1979

Adler T: Personality, like plaster, is pretty stable over time. APA Monitor 23(10):19, 1992

American Psychiatric Association: Diagnostic and Statistical Manual of Mental Disorders, 3rd Edition, Revised. Washington, DC, American Psychiatric Association, 1987

Andreason NC: Affective flattening and the criteria for schizophrenia. Am J Psychiatry 135:944–947, 1979

Barinaga M: How scary things get that way. Science 258:887–888, 1992

Barkley BA: Attention Deficit Hyperactivity Disorder. New York, Guilford, 1990

Beck AT: Cognitive Therapy and the Emotional Disorders. New York, International Universities Press, 1976

Beck AT: Cognitive therapy: a 30-year retrospective. Am Psychol 46:382–389, 1991

Beck AT, Freeman AT, et al: Cognitive Therapy of Personality Disorders. New York, Guilford, 1990

Benjamin LS: Interpersonal Diagnosis and Treatment of Personality Disorders. New York, Guilford, 1993

Berenbaum HJ, Poltmanns TE: Emotional experience and expression in schizophrenia and depression. J Abnorm Psychol 101:37–44, 1992

Biglan A: Capturing Skinner's legacy to behavior therapy. Behavior Therapist 16:3–5, 1993

Bowlby J: Attachment and Loss. New York, Basic Books, 1969

Brown DE: Human Universals. Philadelphia, PA, Temple University Press, 1991

Cahill K: Cognitive therapy frontiers extend to addictions phobias. Psychiatric Times 10(1):1–2, 1993

Cohen BD, Gara MA: Self-structure in borderline personality disorder. Am J Orthopsychiatry 62:618–625, 1992

Cohen CP, Sherwood VR: Becoming a Constant Object in Psychotherapy With the Borderline Patient. Northvale, NJ, Aronson, 1991

Cole CA: Preliminary support for the competency-based model of depression in children. J Abnorm Psychol 100:181–190, 1991

Davidson G, Cacioppo J: New developments in the scientific study of emotion. Psychol Sci 3:21–22, 1992

Davis M: The role of the amygdala in fear and anxiety. Annu Rev Neurosci 15:353–365, 1992

Ellis A: How to Live With a Neurotic: At Home and at Work, Revised Edition. Hollywood, CA, Wilshire Books, 1975.

Ellis A: Rational psychotherapy. J Gen Psychol 59:35–49, 1958.

Ellis A: Reason and Emotion in Psychotherapy. Secaucus, NJ, Citadel, 1962

Ellis A: The Treatment of Borderline and Psychotic Individuals, Revised Edition. New York, Albert Ellis Institute, 1988.

Ellis A: Workshop in rational-emotive therapy. New York, Institute for Rational-Emotive Therapy, September 8, 1965

Ellis A: The biological basis of human irrationality. J Individual Psychol 32:145–168, 1976.

Ellis A: Overcoming Resistance: Rational-Emotive Therapy With Difficult Clients. New York, Springer, 1985

Ellis A: How to Stubbornly Refuse to Make Yourself Miserable About Anything—Yes Anything! Secaucus, NJ, Lyle Stuart, 1988

Ellis A: The revised ABCs of rational-emotive therapy (RET). J Rational-Emotive Cognitive-Behav Ther 9:139–172, 1991

Ellis A: Rational-emotive therapy and evolutionary psychology. Paper presented at a conference on evolutionary psychology, McLean Hospital, Boston, MA, April 1992

Ellis A, Becker IL: A Guide to Personal Happiness. North Hollywood, CA, Wilshire Books, 1982

Ellis A, Dryden W: The Practice of Rational-Emotive Therapy. New York, Springer, 1997

Ellis A, Dryden W: The Essential Albert Ellis. New York, Springer, 1990

Ellis A, Dryden W: A Dialogue With Albert Ellis: Against Dogma. Philadelphia, PA, Open University Press, 1991

Ellis A, Harper RA: A Guide to Rational Living. North Hollywood, CA, Wilshire Books, 1997

Eysenck HJ: The Biological Basis of Personality. Springfield, IL, Charles C Thomas, 1967

Friedberg RD: Inpatient cognitive games cognitive therapists play. Behavior Therapist 16:41–42, 1993

Gazzinga MS: Nature's Mind. New York, Basic Books, 1993

Gilovich T: How We Know What Isn't So: The Fallibility of Human Reason on Everyday Living. New York, Free Press, 1992

Gold JM, Randolph C, Carpenter CJ, et al: Forms of memory failure in schizophrenia. J Abnorm Psychol 191:487–494, 1992

Gottesman IJ: Schizophrenia Genesis: The Origins of Madness. San Francisco, Freeman, 1991

Hauser P (ed): Brain Imaging and the Pathology of Affective Disorders. Washington, DC, American Psychiatric Press, 1992

Hayes SC, Hayes LJ: Some clinical implications of contextualist behaviorism: the example of cognition. Behavior Therapy 23:225–250, 1992

Hayes SC, McMurry SM, Afari N, et al: Acceptance and Commitment Therapy (ACT). Reno, NV, Context Press, 1991

Huessy HR: The varied adult psychopathologies of children's behavior disorders. J Psychiatry Neurosci 17:147–157, 1992

Iocono WS: Eye movement abnormalities in schizophrenia and affective disorders, in Neuropsychology of Eye Movement. Edited by Johnston CW, Pirozzolo FJ. Hillsdale, NJ, Lawrence Erlbaum Associates, 1989, pp 115–145

Kazdin AE: Child and adolescent dysfunction and paths toward maladjustment: targets for intervention. Clin Psychol Rev 12:793–817,1992

Kernberg O: Object Relations and Clinical Psychoanalysis. Northvale, NJ, Jason Aronson,1984

Kernberg O: Borderline Conditions and Pathological Narcissism. Northvale, NJ, Jason Aronson, 1985

Klein M: Envy and Gratitude and Other Works. New York, Free Press, 1984

Kohut H: The Analysis of the Self. New York, International Universities Press, 1971

Kohut H: The Search for the Self: Selected Writings of Heinz Kohut. Madison, CT, International Universities Press, 1991

Larson PC, Agresti AA: Counseling psychology and neuropsychology: an overview. Counseling Psychologist 20:549–553, 1992

Lazarus AA: The Practice of Multimodal Therapy. Baltimore, MD, Johns Hopkins University Press, 1990

Leaf RC, DiGiuseppe R: Review of A. T. Beck et al: Cognitive Therapy of Personality Disorders. J Rational-Emotive Cognitive-Behav Ther 10:105–106, 1992

Leaf RC, Ellis A, DiGiuseppe R, et al: Rationality, self-regard and the "healthfulness" of personality disorder. J Rational-Emotive Cognitive-Behav Ther 9:3–36, 1991a

Leaf RC, Allington DE, Mass R, et al: Personality disorders, life events, and clinical syndromes. J Personal Disord 5:264–2800, 1991b

Leaf RC, Allington DE, Ellis A, et al: Personality disorders, underlying traits, social problems, and clinical syndromes. J Personal Disord 6:130–142, 1992

Lenzenweger MF, Cornblatt BA, Putnick M: Schizotype and sustained attention. J Abnorm Psychol 100:84–89, 1991

Linehan M: Cognitive Behavioral Treatment of Personality Disorders. New York, Guilford, 1993

Masterson JF: The Narcissistic Borderline Disorders. New York, Brunner/Mazel, 1981

Meichenbaum D: Cognitive-Behavior Modification. New York, Plenum, 1977

Pediaditakis N: Boredom: the unexplored and rarely mentioned phenomenon. Psychiatr Times, p 49, November 1991

Pies RW: Splitting the discipline of psychiatry: modern Manichaen. Psychiatr Times, pp 13–14, April 1992

Plutchik R: Emotions and psychotherapy: a psychoevolutionary perspective in Emotion: Theory, Research, Research and Practice, Vol 5. Edited by Plutchik R, Kellerman H. San Diego, CA, Academic Press, 1990, pp 3–20

Plutchik R, Kellerman H: Emotion, Psychopathology, and Psychotherapy. San Diego, CA, Academic Press, 1990

Priester MJ, Clum GA: Perceiving solving ability as a predictor of depression, hopelessness, and suicide ideation in a college population. J Counseling Psychol 40:79–85, 1993

Rhodes NB, Wood W: Self-esteem, intelligence and affect influence-ability: the mediating role of message reception. Psychol Bull 111:156–171, 1992

Rogers CR: On Becoming a Person. Boston, MA, Houghton Mifflin, 1961

Rosenbaum G, Shapiro DL, Chapin K: Attention deficit in schizophrenia and schizotypy. J Abnorm Psychol 97:41–47, 1988

Rourke BF, Fuerst DB: Learning Disabilities and Psychosocial Dysfunctioning. New York, Guilford, 1991

Ruth WJ: Irrational thinking in human: An evolutionary proposal for Ellis' genetic postulate. J Rational-Emotive Cognitive-Behav Ther 10:3–20, 1992

Skinner BF: The Behavior of Organisms. New York, Appleton-Century, 1938

Skinner BF: On Further Reflection. Englewood Cliffs, NJ, Prentice-Hall, 1987

Skinner BF: Recent Issues in the Analysis of Behavior. Columbus, OH, Merrill, 1989

Sperling MB, Sharp JL: On the nature of attachment in a borderline population: a preliminary investigation. Psychol Rep 68:543–546, 1991

Stone MH: The Fate of Borderline Patients. Successful Outcome and Psychiatric Practice. New York, Guilford, 1990

Swanson HL, Keogh B (eds): Learning Disabilities: Theoretical and Research Issues. Hillsdale, NJ, Lawrence Erlbaum Associates, 1990

Wilson EO: Sociobiology: The New Synthesis. Cambridge, MA, Harvard University Press, 1975

Yank GR, Bentley KJ, Hargrove DS: The vulnerability-stress model of schizophrenia: advances in psychosocial treatment. Am J Orthopsychiatry 63:55–69, 1993

Yee CM, Deleon PJ, Miller GA: Early stimulus processing in dysthymia and anhedonia. J Abnorm Psychol 101:230–233, 1992

Young J: Cognitive Therapy for Personality Disorders. Sarasota, FL, Professional Resources Exchange, 1990

Index